D1710781

CLINICS IN DEVELOPMENTAL MEDICINE NO. 122
CURRENT CONCEPTS IN SPINA BIFIDA AND HYDROCEPHALUS

Clinics in Developmental Medicine No. 122

CURRENT CONCEPTS IN SPINA BIFIDA AND HYDROCEPHALUS

Edited by
CARYS M. BANNISTER
BRIAN TEW

1991
Mac Keith Press

Distributed by:
OXFORD: Blackwell Scientific Publications Ltd
NEW YORK: Cambridge University Press

©1991 Mac Keith Press
5a Netherhall Gardens, London NW3 5RN

First published 1991

British Library Cataloguing in Publication Data

Current concepts in spina bifida and hydrocephalus.—
  (Clinics in developmental medicine; 122)
  I. Bannister, Carys M.   II. Tew, Brian
  III. Series
  618.9273043

ISBN (UK) 0 901260 91 6
     (USA) 0 521 41279 X

Printed in Great Britain at The Lavenham Press Ltd, Lavenham, Suffolk
Mac Keith Press is supported by **The Spastics Society, London, England**

CONTENTS

v

CONTRIBUTORS

CARYS M. BANNISTER   Consultant Neurological Surgeon, Department of Neurosurgery, Booth Hall Children's Hospital, Blackley, Manchester.

JOHN BANTA   Associate Professor of Surgery, University of Connecticut School of Medicine, Department of Orthopaedics; and Director, Myelomeningocele Program, Newington Children's Hospital, Connecticut, USA.

STANFORD BOURNE   Consultant Psychotherapist and Psycho-Analyst, Perinatal Bereavement Unit, Tavistock Clinic, Belsize Lane, London NW3.

R. BRAUNER   Pediatric Endocrinology Unit, Hôpital des Enfants Malades, 149 Rue de Sèvres, 75015 Paris, France.

JANET CARR   Regional Tutor in the Psychology of Mental and Multiple Handicap, Department of Psychology, St George's Hospital Medical School, London SW17.

PAT EDSER   Counselling Coordinator, Association for Spina Bifida and Hydrocephalus, Park Road, Peterborough.

M. FONTOURA   Pediatric Endocrinology Unit, Hôpital des Enfants Malades, 149 Rue de Sèvres, 75015 Paris, France.

J. M. HAWNAUR   Senior Lecturer in Diagnostic Radiology, University Department of Diagnostic Radiology, Manchester; and Honorary Consultant Radiologist, University Hospital of South Manchester.

EMANUEL LEWIS   Consultant Psychotherapist, Tavistock Clinic, Belsize Lane, London NW3.

ANTONIO V. LORENZO   Director of Neurosurgical Laboratory, Children's Hospital Medical Center, 300 Longwood Avenue, Boston, Massachusetts 02115, USA.

M. J. A. MARESH

Consultant Obstetrician/Gynaecologist, Department of Obstetrics, St Mary's Hospital, Whitnorth Park, Manchester.

R. RAPOPORT

Pediatric Endocrinology Unit, Hôpital des Enfants Malades, 149 Rue de Sèvres, 75015 Paris, France.

GORDON ROSE

Late Director of the Orthotic Research and Locomotor Assessment Unit (ORLAU); and Honorary Consultant Orthopaedic Surgeon, Robert Jones and Agnes Hunt Orthopaedic Hospital, Oswestry.

DAVID I. ROWLEY

Head, Department of Orthopaedic and Trauma Surgery, University of Dundee.

DICK SMITHELLS

Emeritus Professor, University of Leeds.

CAROLE SOBKOWIAK

Superintendent Physiotherapist, Memorial Hospital, Hollyhurst Road, Darlington, Co. Durham.

BRIAN TEW

Lecturer in Educational Psychology, University of Wales College of Cardiff.

GILLIAN WARD

Principal Clinical Psychologist, Booth Hall, Children's Hospital, Blackley, Manchester.

KEASLEY WELCH

Emeritus Professor of Neurosurgery, Harvard Medical School, Boston, Massachusetts 02115, USA.

FOREWORD

Hydrocephalus is an almost constant accompaniment of open spina bifida. It is therefore convenient to discuss the two together, and also to include hydrocephalus arising from other causes, both congenital and acquired.

There have been enormous changes in the conception, management and outcome of spina bifida and hydrocephalus in the past four decades. Up to the late 1950s few infants born with these defects were treated actively and there was a wish, usually realised, that they would die. Attempts at drainage of hydrocephalus usually failed after a short time and there was no prospect of lifelong control.

With the introduction of the ventriculo-atrial shunt, there was an immediate improvement in the prognosis of hydrocephalus, and a growing perception that early surgery for the spinal lesion of spina bifida would give the best chance of preserving neuromuscular function. This led to an enormous effort throughout the 1960s to start active treatment in the neonatal period of virtually all infants with spina bifida. The result was a huge increase in survival, not so much because of the surgery, but because of the greatly improved general care the infants received and the expectation that they would live.

Before the end of the 1960s it was becoming clear that the survivors were not always improved mentally or physically and that large numbers were doomed to suffer long years of severe disability.

The 1970s were characterised by retrenchment, with selection for active treatment of the most favourable cases and the expectation that those not selected for treatment would soon die. At the same time, methods of prenatal diagnosis were developed, allowing the parents to be offered termination of the abnormal fetus. Thus the numbers of livebirths fell dramatically, helped by some ill understood epidemiological changes.

The 1980s have been notable for greatly increased understanding of the prognosis of spina bifida when actively treated from birth. This has been made possible by close study of the development of the huge cohort of children born in the 1960s, enabling many improvements in management to be made. At the same time, there has been rapid improvement in imaging techniques, both for *in utero* diagnosis of spina bifida and for later management of hydrocephalus. By far the most exciting prospect is the possibility of true prevention by the use of vitamin supplementation during the crucial periconception period. This has at last culminated in clear recognition of the anti-teratogenic role of folic acid with the possibility of cheap, universal prophylaxis.

Not only has there been an increase in the ability to treat the physical and mental defects, but there has been a greatly improved understanding of the need for support of the family with a disabled child, and also those grieving for the loss of a fetus or a child.

Though the number of infants born with spina bifida has greatly declined, hydrocephalus alone is still seen; indeed, the improved survival of very low-birthweight babies has led to an increase in hydrocephalus resulting from intraventricular haemorrhage.

Among the prospects for the 1990s must be counted the application of fetal surgery to modify the fetal course of hydrocephalus. This is not yet a realistic option but is likely to become so in the near future. More remote is the possibility of closing the spinal lesion in the fetus with spina bifida.

For the effective management of both spina bifida and hydrocephalus there is a need for a multidisciplinary approach. It is the aim of this book to give guidance to all those who try to help children and adults with these conditions.

DUNCAN FORREST FRCS
October 1991

1
PREVENTION OF SPINA BIFIDA AND HYDROCEPHALUS

Dick Smithells

Developmental abnormalities of the central nervous system (CNS) are among the most prevalent and widely studied of all birth defects. Spina bifida and anencephaly are neural tube defects (NTDS). They arise from failure of neurulation or canalisation of the primitive neural tube, and share many epidemiological and aetiological features. Isolated hydrocephalus and encephalocele have more diverse origins, and their epidemiology is less well documented.

The possibility of preventing spina bifida and hydrocephalus implies that we can count cases: that there is some mechanism for ascertaining and recording these defects, and for deciding whether any reduction in numbers results from any particular preventive measure. This is not as simple as appears at first sight.

First we must agree on definitions. For spina bifida, whatever terms are used (myelocele, meningomyelocele, meningocele), the lesions encountered in clinical practice present the least problem of definition. At the extremes of severity, some arbitrary decisions may be necessary. Spina bifida occulta (the least severe) is commonly excluded because precise definition is difficult, ascertainment may be incomplete and clinical importance is very variable. At the other extreme—complete rachischisis—it is easy to recognise an open neural tube, but when anencephaly and spina bifida coexist, the usual convention is to classify the infant or fetus as anencephalic so that one case is not counted as two. Similarly, when spina bifida and hydrocephalus coexist, the infant is usually recorded only under the head of spina bifida.

The definition of hydrocephalus is more difficult because we are dealing with continuous variables: head size, ventricular size and their rate of increase. It is not hard to decide when hydrocephalus requires clinical intervention, but lesser degrees (including some examples of 'arrested hydrocephalus') are sometimes diagnosed on a somewhat arbitrary basis.

Until recently birth defects were not ascertained in spontaneously aborted fetuses, largely because of the enormous practical difficulties. As this was universal practice, it did not significantly affect comparisons. Now that prenatal diagnosis with termination of NTD-affected pregnancies is widespread, comparisons between regional or national NTD rates are often meaningless. Within the European registries of birth defects contributing to EUROCAT (European Study of Congenital Abnormalities and Twins), ascertainment begins anywhere from 20 to 28 weeks of gestation. In the United Kingdom, where ascertainment for the national birth defects register begins at 28 weeks, the apparent fall in NTD rate since the mid-1970s has been far more dramatic than the real fall.

If ascertainment includes defects diagnosed by ultrasound scanning, further caution is needed. The possibility of overlooking spina bifida is not significant in this context, but whenever a pregnancy is terminated for prenatally diagnosed hydrocephalus, skilled post-mortem examination is mandatory because ventricles sometimes turn out to be less enlarged than they appeared.

Despite these difficulties, birth prevalence data for spina bifida and hydrocephalus are available from many centres and covering many decades. They reveal a very wide variation in prevalence in different parts of the world, in different ethnic and social groups within individual countries, and from one decade to another in a given population. This variability in all three dimensions of epidemiology (time, place and person) is in marked contrast to data for congenital heart disease (CHD). Although data are not so numerous for CHD as for NTD, the overall prevalence is remarkably constant at 7 to 8 per 1000 births. Before prenatal diagnosis created the problems already described, NTD prevalence worldwide ranged from over 10 to less than 0.1 per 1000 births (Elwood and Elwood 1980).

One particular epidemiological feature of NTD underlies the current nutritional approach to the primary prevention of spina bifida: that is the social class difference in birth prevalence. This phenomenon, whereby NTDs are least common among more prosperous, better educated, professional families and most common in the families of unskilled manual workers, has been reported from many parts of the world. It has also been noted to diminish or vanish when and where NTD birth prevalence is low.

This social class gradient should offer a clue to the causation of NTD. In view of the rapidity with which prevalence can change, the underlying factors cannot be purely, or even predominantly, genetic. A nutritional factor is only one of many possibilities related to the lifestyle of different social classes: and if nutrition was shown to affect NTD causation, it would not rule out other factors.

Within the broad field of nutrition there are several reasons for concentrating on vitamins (and possibly also trace metals), especially folic acid, rather than on energy sources—carbohydrate, fat and protein.

1. Animal experiments over more than half a century have shown that malformations, including those of the CNS, can be induced in many animal species by feeding the pregnant mothers with diets which either are deficient in one vitamin or another, or contain a vitamin excess. Harmful effects from excess have been largely confined to vitamin A: effects of deficiency have been shown mainly with vitamin A, riboflavin and folic acid (Kalter 1968).

2. Ireland has an exceptionally high birth prevalence of NTD, though the country has not experienced malnutrition since the potato famines of the 19th century. The birth prevalence of NTD is very low in the poor countries of Africa, where protein-energy malnutrition is rife but access to water-soluble vitamins in fruit and vegetables may remain sufficient.

2

3. The teratogenic action of aminopterin, a folic acid antagonist drug, was recognised in 1952 (Thiersch 1952).

4. Folic acid deficiency in pregnancy, first recognised by Lucy Wills in India (Wills and Mehta 1930), is the only common vitamin-deficiency disorder in well nourished populations.

Most of the clinical management of spina bifida (and most of this book) is about tertiary prevention, which seeks to prevent deterioration, to preserve and improve function in conditions which are already irreversibly established.

Secondary prevention seeks to avoid the undesirable consequences of an irreversible disorder. For some disorders (*e.g.* congenital hypothyroidism), early diagnosis and treatment are so effective that secondary prevention looks remarkably like cure, until the patient stops taking the tablets. For spina bifida, unless and until some major advance in early intrauterine surgery comes along, the only option for secondary prevention rests in prenatal diagnosis and the termination of affected pregnancies.

Prenatal diagnosis of spina bifida rests partly on ultrasound scanning of the spine and skull (see Chapter 5) and partly on the determination of levels of alpha-fetoprotein (AFP) and acetyl-cholinesterase in amniotic fluid. Estimation of AFP in maternal serum may be used as a screening test but is not diagnostic. Amniotic fluid AFP may be raised in conditions other than NTD, hence the need to measure acetyl-cholinesterase which is an enzyme specific to neural tissue.

AFP concentration in both amniotic fluid and serum is a continuous variable, and the distinction between 'normal' and 'raised' is an arbitrary one: the cut-off point is determined by the laboratory to minimise the numbers of 'false positives' and 'false negatives'. (They are not truly false, in that they can only indicate the probability of a fetus being affected.) As ultrasound equipment and ultrason-ographers become increasingly discriminating, scanning contributes increasingly to the prenatal diagnosis of spina bifida. As the consequences of misdiagnosis either way are profound, it is wise to use all available tools.

This is not the place to debate the difficult moral and human issues relating to the abortion of malformed fetuses, nor to discuss the cost/benefit and risk/benefit ratios of various clinical policies and procedures. However, it is generally agreed that an effective method of primary prevention, ensuring that a baby who would otherwise have had NTD is born unaffected, is a highly desirable objective.

Observational studies
Diet in pregnancy in relation to social class and NTD
Before reviewing the results of studies in Yorkshire, South Wales and Western Australia, it is important to underline the difficulties and limitations of dietary studies. First, diet is only one aspect of nutrition, albeit a crucial one. If the diet is inadequate, nutrition cannot be good. The reverse, however, is not necessarily true. Following ingestion, the processes of digestion, absorption, transport and metabolism must also be in good order to establish good nutrition. In the present

TABLE 1.I

Mean daily intakes of selected nutrients of 179 women in the first trimester of pregnancy, by social class

Nutrient	Social class		Statistical
	$I+II$ $N\ 40$	$III+IV+V$ $N\ 139$	significance of difference P
Energy (kcal)	2183	1892	<0.001
Protein (g)	76.4	65.2	<0.001
Iron (mg)	12.6	10.4	<0.001
Riboflavin (mg)	1.89	1.33	<0.001
Ascorbic acid (mg)	83.4	58.6	<0.001
Cholecalciferol (IU)	95.8	64.0	<0.005
Total folate (μg)	176.8	139.6	<0.001
Free folate (μg)	82.2	62.3	<0.001

Social-class differences were of the same order of significance for all other nutrients.

context there is an added complication, in that our 'subject' is the developing embryo and fetus which is nourished by proxy. We know little of the transport of nutrients to the early human conceptus, and even less of embryonic metabolism. In considering the closure and canalisation of the neural tube we are concentrating on the first four to five weeks of embryonic life, or the first six to seven weeks of 'pregnancy' as usually calculated.

It is also remarkably difficult to record dietary intakes with any degree of accuracy, as only those who have attempted it fully realise. The fact that your eating habits are being recorded creates a strong incentive to change them, especially if you are under the supervision of a dietitian who, you suspect, might not think very highly of them. As diet often varies from day to day, especially at weekends, the record of a single day (24-hour recall) gives limited information. A seven-day record is more comprehensive, but is more difficult and more tedious for the subject, so accuracy and compliance may suffer. A broad idea of diet may be obtained from a checklist of foods, asking the subject how often they eat the principle sources of major nutrients. But every method is open to criticism, and the methods which are best from a scientific point of view may defeat the very people in whose diets we are most interested.

If information is required about individual nutrients (*e.g.* folic acid) as distinct from a broad nutritional picture, the dietary record must be converted into its nutrient components. This in turn requires that the dietary record be not only accurate but also specific (*e.g.* detailing brand names).

The Yorkshire study, based in Leeds, used the seven-day weighed record of food intake of 200 mothers in the first trimester of pregnancy (Smithells *et al.* 1977, Rogozinski *et al.* 1983). None gave birth to an infant with NTD, and the data were analysed with reference to social class and recommended daily allowances (RDAS).

4

There was a highly significant social-class difference in mean daily intakes of all nutrients when social classes I and II were compared with classes III, IV and V (Table 1.I).

Recommended daily allowances, which differ from country to country and are periodically revised, provide a good margin of safety. They indicate that a person consuming the RDA of a particular nutrient is eating enough of it. They do not mean that a person eating less is necessarily deficient. In the Yorkshire study, the only nutrient for which mean daily intakes (all social classes) were widely different from the RDA was vitamin D. Most women were taking less than the RDA for non-pregnant women: none was taking the RDA for pregnant women. The probable explanation is that the RDA is over-generous.

Two dietary studies based in Cardiff were carried out between 1969 and 1979 (Laurence *et al.* 1980, 1983). Both took as their index subjects women who had previously given birth to a child with NTD, recorded their diets during the first trimester of the next pregnancy, and observed the rate of recurrence of NTD. The first study used a simple checklist of important foods: the second used a rather more detailed method. In both studies the diets were classified as good, fair or poor: in the second study 'poor' diets were subdivided into those that were adequate but with an excess of refined carbohydrates and fat, and those that were generally inadequate. All NTD recurrences in both studies (13 cases from 362 pregnancies), and all eight miscarriages in the first study, were to women judged to be on poor diets.

The most recent study in this group comes from Western Australia, based in Nedlands, Perth (Bower and Stanley 1989). It combined a checklist of foods with 24-hour recall to assess the dietary intakes of 77 mothers of infants with isolated NTD, 77 mothers of infants with non-NTD malformations and 154 mothers of healthy babies. The most significant finding was that the risk of NTD decreased as the intake of folate increased. This applied particularly to free folate. Adjustment for confounding variables slightly strengthened the association. Similar trends were shown with vitamin C, riboflavin, carotene, calcium and dietary fibre. The intakes of individual nutrients are closely correlated with one another: free folate and possibly vitamin C showed the strongest negative association with NTD.*

Blood vitamin levels in relation to social class and NTD
The concentrations of vitamins in blood are likely to provide more significant information than dietary intakes. For one thing, they reflect digestion and absorption as well as ingestion. For another, they overcome the problem that arises from the variation in human size. It may well be appropriate for a small person to

---

*Dietary folate is partly in the form of small molecules (mono-, di- and tri-glutamates, usually referred to as free folate) which are readily absorbed from the gut, and partly in the form of polyglutamates which must be broken down by intestinal folate conjugase enzymes before they can be absorbed. Folic acid in tablets is all in the monoglutamate form. This is potentially relevant when considering the possible protective mechanism of folic acid.

eat less than a large person with similar energy expenditure. Adult height correlates quite closely with social class so that, other things being equal, it is appropriate that a woman from social class V should eat less than one from class I. As blood volume is closely correlated with bodyweight, blood levels should tell us the same thing about women of widely varying height and weight.

Nevertheless it is not easy to interpret blood vitamin levels, whether measured in plasma/serum, red cells or white cells. The vitamin content of red cells is relatively stable, and as the average life of a red cell is about three months, red cell values measured today are likely to tell us something of what was going on a few weeks ago. White blood cells have a much shorter lifespan on the whole, and their contents reflect much more recent history. Plasma levels are the most contemporary of all, but also the most ephemeral and variable. A single estimation of a plasma level is very hard to interpret. Quite a small oral dose of folic acid, for example, will cause an impressive rise in plasma folate in less than an hour, which may return to the base level within four hours. Vitamins (or any other chemicals) in plasma are for the most part in transit between the site of absorption and the sites of utilisation or storage. Their levels indicate their availability at the moment the blood sample is taken: they may not indicate much else. But it is likely that the plasma is the only source of nutrients available to the feto-placental (or embryo-trophoblastic) unit.

When vitamins are measured in relation to pregnancy, we have to remember that mean levels may vary according to the stage of gestation, and that levels in pregnancy may be very different from those in the same women when not pregnant. Pregnant women with overt folic acid deficiency, manifest as macrocytic anaemia, may regain normal folate levels within a week of delivery without therapeutic intervention, only to become deficient again in the early stages of their next pregnancy (Hibbard and Hibbard 1966).

Vitamins may be measured directly (although the congener which is measured is not necessarily the biologically important one), or indirectly by measuring a vitamin-dependent process. If we consider folic acid, for example, whether in food or in biological fluids, it is a cocktail of folate congeners (vitamers) of which the most important biologically is 5-methyltetrahydrofolic acid. The most widely used methods of folate assay (bioassay using *Lactobacillus casei* and radiometric binding assays) do not distinguish between vitamers. An older, but still valid, method of assessing folate status is the FIGLU test. After an oral loading dose of histidine, urinary excretion of formiminoglutamic acid is measured. The conversion of histidine to FIGLU is folate dependent: poor conversion reflects poor folate status.

The FIGLU test was used by Hibbard and Smithells (1965) to compare the folate status of 35 mothers of NTD infants with 35 controls, the tests being done in late pregnancy or within three days of delivery. The results were considered to indicate folate deficiency in 69 per cent of NTD mothers and 17 per cent of controls.

In the South Wales studies of Laurence *et al.* (1980, 1983) referred to earlier, serum and red cell folate were measured on 411 non-pregnant women who had previously given birth to a NTD infant. Mean values of both were highest in mothers judged to be taking a good diet, lowest in those on a poor diet. The relationship between folate levels and NTD recurrence in subsequent pregnancies will be discussed later.

Smithells *et al.* (1977) studied approximately 1000 mothers, unselected except that they had agreed to give a blood sample, in the first trimester of pregnancy. Folic acid was measured in serum and red cells, vitamin C in white cells, riboflavin in red cells and vitamin A in serum. The findings were analysed in relation to the social class of the mothers and the occurrence of NTD. As regards social class, those in classes I and II had significantly higher mean values of all vitamins measured except serum folate. The mothers of six infants or fetuses with NTD had significantly lower mean levels of red cell folate and white cell vitamin C: serum folate and red cell riboflavin tended in the same direction.

Yates *et al.* (1987) measured serum and red cell folate (and other vitamins) in non-pregnant women with a history of NTD and in controls. They found significantly lower levels of red cell folate (but not of other vitamins measured) in the NTD mothers, and a tendency for levels to be lowest in mothers who had had the greatest number of previous NTDS.

Bower and Stanley (1989) measured serum and red cell folate postpartum in mothers of NTD infants or fetuses and controls, and were unable to demonstrate any significant difference. However, many mothers were taking vitamin supplements at the time of blood sampling, which made interpretation difficult.

Self-administered vitamins in relation to NTD
Three case-control studies have been reported from the United States (where the consumption of over-the-counter vitamin preparations is widespread), comparing the vitamin consumption of mothers of NTD infants in the period around conception with that of controls. A comparable study has also been carried out in Western Australia, looking at vitamin supplements whether self-administered or prescribed.

This kind of study inevitably depends on maternal recollections, without any documentation from which memories might be confirmed. It is important for such a study to know exactly when medication was started and ended in relation to the relevant conception, and the name or nature of the vitamin preparation taken. The longer the interval between the medication and the enquiry, the less confidence one feels in the accuracy of the replies. Nevertheless, if there is no recall bias as between subjects and controls, the degree of accuracy is likely to be similar in the two groups. In fact, in only one of these four studies was the enquiry made before the mother knew whether or not her infant/fetus was affected, and there is a real possibility of recall bias in the other three.

It is often suggested that, if enquiries are made after the end of pregnancy about medication early in that pregnancy, the mothers of malformed infants will report a higher rate of drug use than will controls. It is argued that they have a greater incentive to search their memories to find a reason for the malformation. If

7

such a bias exists, it would lead to an over-reporting of vitamin intake by the mothers of affected infants, unless they were aware of the suggested protective effect of vitamins. There is, in fact, evidence that although post-delivery recall of drug use in pregnancy is inaccurate, particularly with regard to the stage of pregnancy at which drugs were taken, the recall bias of mothers of malformed infants does not differ from that of mothers of healthy babies (Klemetti and Saxen 1967).

Mulinare *et al.* (1988) conducted telephone interviews with 347 mothers of NTD infants and 2829 controls, including questions about vitamin supplements taken before and after the relevant conception. The interviewers were blind as to pregnancy outcome. The index births, both cases and controls, had been up to 16 years previously. Mothers who claimed to have taken vitamin supplements continuously from three months before until three months after conception were compared with mothers who had taken none during those six months. Vitamin consumption was significantly less common among the mothers of NTD infants than among the mothers of both malformed (non-NTD) and normal controls.

Mills *et al.* (1989) carried out a similar study, but all mothers were interviewed within five months of the end of pregnancy. Mothers were classified as fully supplemented, partially supplemented or unsupplemented on a complex basis. Among the several criticisms of their classification, perhaps the most serious (although affecting a relatively small number of women) is that those starting supplements after conception were classified as unsupplemented, even if they started before the time of neural tube closure. No difference in vitamin supplementation history was found between index mothers and controls.

Milunsky *et al.* (1989) obtained information about diet and vitamin supplements from 22,776 women who had undergone amniocentesis, the interviews being carried out before the mothers knew the results of the test (with a few exceptions), thus avoiding recall bias. Their definition of 'supplemented' required only that mothers had taken vitamins at least once weekly. Forty-nine women had an infant/fetus with NTD. The most significant findings in this study were (i) that the NTD prevalence ratio in mothers taking vitamins in the first six weeks of pregnancy (0.32:95 per cent CI 0.15–0.66) was significantly lower than in those starting supplements after six weeks (0.91:95 per cent CI 0.45–1.80); and (ii) that the protective effect was seen with supplements containing folate rather than with other vitamins.

In the same study dietary folate was estimated for women not taking folate supplements. A protective effect was shown with daily intakes of 100μg or more.

The dietary study in Western Australia discussed earlier (Bower and Stanley 1989) showed a protective effect against NTD from folates, combining dietary folate and supplements. When the data were analysed in relation to folate supplements only, comparing 77 mothers of NTD infants with 77 mothers of malformed (non-NTD) infants and 154 mothers of normal infants, a small but non-significant protective effect was shown (Bower 1990). When all vitamin supplements were considered, no effect was seen. The rather small numbers of mothers reduce the power of this study.

Summary of observational studies
Three widely different approaches to the NTD/vitamin problem (diet, blood chemistry, vitamin supplements) carried out in three continents (Europe, North America, Australasia) over a period of 20 years are unlikely to reach precisely the same conclusions, particularly as the methodology of each study is unique to itself. It is not surprising to find significant differences in nutritional parameters between social classes, but it is surprising that so many of these observational studies point to a protective effect from folate taken before conception and/or in the first six weeks of pregnancy.

Intervention studies
The principle behind all the relevant intervention studies is simple—to find out whether the administration of vitamin supplements to the mother will prevent or reduce the risk of NTD (including spina bifida) in the offspring. The practice has proved to be rather more difficult. The three fundamental questions in designing such a study are:
1. What group of mothers will be offered supplements?
2. What supplement, in what dose, and over what time period, is to be given?
3. With what control group should study mothers be compared?

At the time of writing, three intervention studies have been published (the largest in a series of papers) and another three are known to be in progress. In each of the six studies the methodology differs in some respects from that of the other five.

1. *UK multicentre trial*
For admission to this study, mothers had to: (i) have had one or more previous NTD infants or fetuses, (ii) not be pregnant, and (iii) be considering a further pregnancy. They were recruited largely through genetic counselling clinics in Leeds (York-shire), Belfast (Northern Ireland), London (South-East England), Manchester and Chester (Cheshire). They were given Pregnavite Forte F*, one tablet three times a day, and advised to take it for at least 28 days before conceiving again and to continue until they had missed two menstrual periods. Mothers who conceived less than 28 days after starting tablets, or who missed taking tablets on more than one day of the minimum period specified, were classified as 'partially supplemented'.

The outcome of their pregnancies was compared with that of unsupplemented mothers with similar histories who delivered in the same areas over the same period

*Three tablets of Pregnavite Forte F (the normal daily dose) provides the following: vitamin A 4000 IU, vitamin D 400 IU, thiamine 1.5mg, riboflavin 1.5mg, pyridoxine 1mg, nicotinamide 15mg, ascorbic acid 40mg, folic acid 0.36mg, calcium phosphate 480mg, ferrous sulphate equivalent to 75.6mg Fe.

of time. No placebo was used and the mothers were not randomly allocated to 'vitamin' and 'no vitamin' groups. The most common reason for mothers not receiving vitamins was that they were already pregnant when first referred and therefore failed to meet the criteria for admission to the study.

The last report from the multicentre group (Smithells *et al.* 1983) showed three NTD recurrences among 454 fully supplemented mothers (0.7 per cent), no recurrences among 114 partially supplemented, and 24 recurrences among 519 unsupplemented mothers (4.7 per cent), a highly significant difference. Later comparison between the supplemented and the unsupplemented mothers in regard to a variety of clinical and demographic features of possible relevance showed no significant difference, suggesting that selection bias did not contribute substantially to the difference in recurrence rate (Wild *et al.* 1986).

Subsequently, later data from continuing studies in Yorkshire, Northern Ireland and South-East England have been published. The overall results from Yorkshire (Smithells *et al.* 1989) showed one NTD recurrence among 315 infants/fetuses born to 274 fully supplemented mothers (0.3 per cent) and none among 57 infants born to 58 partially supplemented. There were 18 recurrences among 320 infants/fetuses born to unsupplemented mothers (5.6 per cent). In Northern Ireland there had been four recurrences among 511 infants/fetuses born to supplemented mothers (0.8 per cent), compared to 17 of 353 unsupplemented (4.8 per cent). In South-East England there is no substantiated figure for unsupplemented mothers, but it is believed to be 4 per cent. There were eight NTD recurrences among 457 infants/fetuses born to supplemented mothers (1.8 per cent) (Nevin and Seller 1990).

2. *South Wales study* (Laurence *et al.* 1981)

Mothers who had previously had one or more NTD infants/fetuses were allocated randomly to receive folic acid, 2mg twice daily, or placebo. This study overlapped in time and place with the dietary intervention study reviewed earlier. Four mothers in the placebo group and two in the folic acid group had NTD recurrences, a non-significant difference. The 111 mothers in the study had given blood samples at six to nine weeks' gestation. When these samples were later analysed, it was decided that mothers with levels below 10μg/L could not have been taking their tablets. When these 'non-compliant' mothers were added to the placebo group, all recurrences were in that group, the difference between six and zero being significant.

3. *The Cuba study* (Vergel *et al.* 1990)

Folic acid 5mg daily was given to 81 women with a history of previous NTD birth, from not less than one menstrual period before conception until the 10th week of pregnancy. Pregnancy outcome was compared with that of 124 unsupplemented mothers who were already pregnant when referred. There were no NTD recurrences in 80 fully, and 19 partially, supplemented mothers (although one of the latter miscarried a fetus with hydrocephalus), compared to four NTD recurrences (3.5 per cent) in the unsupplemented group.

4. *The UK Medical Research Council study* (Wald and Polani 1984)
In this multinational study, which is still in progress, mothers with a previous history of NTD are randomly allocated to one of four groups. One receives folic acid 4mg daily; one receives a multivitamin comparable to Pregnavite Forte F but without folic acid; one receives both the foregoing; one receives the iron/calcium component of all three of the foregoing, without vitamins.

5. *The Dublin study* (Kirke 1983)
This is similar to the Medical Research Council study above but excludes the 'no vitamin' group. Mothers are randomly allocated to one of the three vitamin groups.

6. *The Budapest study* (Cziezel and Rode 1984)
This important study differs from all the others in that the mothers entering the study have not previously had a NTD infant/fetus. They are randomly allocated to receive a multivitamin preparation, including folic acid 0.8mg daily and broadly comparable to Pregnavite Forte F, or placebo. Interim results indicate a possible protective effect from vitamin supplements, but numbers are not yet large enough to permit a firm conclusion.

The particular significance of the Budapest study lies in the fact that it seeks to prevent first occurrence of NTD rather than recurrence. As recurrences account for no more than 5 per cent of all NTDs, the outcome will be of particular importance.

Summary of intervention studies
Although none of the published studies is in itself conclusive, the results are all consistent with a protective effect from vitamins, especially folic acid, and are therefore consistent with the findings of the majority of the observational studies reviewed above. While awaiting with interest the outcome of intervention studies still in progress (none of which will be conclusive on its own), it seems reasonable to accept such an effect as a working hypothesis. This being so, doctors involved with affected families (general practitioners, obstetricians, clinical geneticists) need to consider the practical implications (see below), and research effort needs to turn towards the mechanisms of the protective effect.

Possible mechanisms of protection by folic acid
Folic acid is a precursor of nucleic acid and therefore essential to all cell division. So far as is known, however, it is of no greater importance to the cells of the CNS than to any other cells and there is no evidence that vitamin/folate supplements prevent any other birth defects, with the possible exception of facial clefts. Furthermore, the studies already cited suggest that although dietary folate deficiency may be one aetiological factor, it is unlikely to explain the whole protective effect.

The embryology of the neural tube is remarkably complicated, involving not only neural tube closure, but canalisation of the lower part of the spinal cord, a rather abrupt change in embryonic attitude from extension to flexion, and a good deal of cell migration. It is possible that cell division must be exceptionally rapid at crucial stages in development, with correspondingly great demands for folate. However, the size of the human embryo at this stage is so small that the folate requirement cannot be substantial in absolute terms.

The metabolic pathways of many nutrients are inextricably intertwined, so that folate, vitamin B12, vitamin C and zinc, for example, all interact with one another. It may be an oversimplification to consider a single nutrient (in this case, folic acid) as responsible. Nevertheless, folate seems a good place to start.

An interesting recent observation (Steegers-Theunissen et al. 1991) is the high (31 per cent) incidence of abnormal methionine loading tests, possibly indicative of heterozygosity for the homocystinuria gene, among mothers of NTD infants. Folic acid, vitamin B12 and vitamin B6 are all involved in the metabolism of methionine and homocysteine.

The curly-tail mouse, which is genetically predisposed to NTD, has yielded much interesting information about vitamin A but little about folate. Vitamin A, paradoxically, can either increase or decrease the proportion of offspring with NTD depending upon the day of gestation on which it is administered (Seller et al. 1979). Rat embryos cultured in serum from folate-deficient rats grow poorly, have problems switching from the extended to the flexed position, abnormal kinking of the neural tube (though not NTD) and rather small brains (Miller et al. 1989).

In humans, it has been suggested that the mothers of NTD infants may metabolise folate differently from others. It has also been suggested that the metabolic problem may lie within the feto-placental unit. When human tropho-blasts are grown in culture in the presence of 14c-labelled methyltetrahydrofolic acid (MTHF), cells from NTD pregnancies tend to incorporate MTHF into DNA more slowly than controls (Habibzadeh et al. 1990). These last observations are preliminary, but suggest directions for future research into the aetiology of NTD and the protective effect of vitamins.

Prevention of hydrocephalus

It is customary, and appropriate, to consider hydrocephalus as distinct from anencephaly and spina bifida because it is known to be aetiologically hetero-geneous. It is arguable whether the surgical treatment of hydrocephalus should be regarded as tertiary or secondary prevention. The secondary prevention of isolated hydrocephalus by prenatal diagnosis and pregnancy termination requires skill and experience, especially in the less severe cases. Ventricular size as judged by fetal ultrasound scanning is sometimes at variance with the size of the same ventricles as seen at autopsy.

The opportunities for primary prevention of hydrocephalus can be summarised quite briefly.

1. As hydrocephalus is commonly associated with spina bifida, prevention of the latter by the use of vitamins may at the same time prevent hydrocephalus.

2. There is evidence (Lorber 1984) to suggest that some cases of isolated hydrocephalus may properly be regarded as part of the NTD spectrum. If a way can be found to identify these (other than by the preceding birth of a child with NTD), vitamin prophylaxis *might* be effective, but this is conjecture.

3. The family history may suggest x-linked inheritance in a few instances: genetic counselling can then be helpful. Hydrocephalus is also a feature of some other genetic syndromes.

4. The teratogenic effect of high-dose vitamin A, or more often of its analogues etretinate and isotretinoin, used in the treatment of severe acne, is often manifest as hydrocephalus. The use of these drugs in adolescent girls must always be accompanied by appropriate counselling.

Congenital toxoplasmosis is responsible for a few cases of hydrocephalus, but there is as yet no effective vaccine.

Practical implications

The evidence so far available, which has been reviewed in this chapter, is consistent with the hypothesis that vitamin supplements (particularly of folic acid) in very early pregnancy provide some degree of protection against recurrence of NTD. It is also consistent with a protective effect against the first occurrence of NTD, although this must be less certain until studies still in progress have been concluded. There is also evidence that 'physiological' doses of vitamins, approximating to RDA, cause no harm. It is reasonable, when counselling a couple who have had a baby or fetus with NTD, to suggest a suitable supplement (either folic acid alone or multivitamins including folic acid) to be taken in very early pregnancy. In practice this means advising that it should be started before the next conception.

Should further evidence support the idea that vitamin supplements can reduce the risk of first occurrence of NTD, the implications are far wider. First, if future work identifies a biochemical marker of maternal susceptibility to fetal NTD (preferably by means of a simple blood test) it could become possible to identify, before the first pregnancy, a subset of the population who needed additional vitamins. The problem could be viewed as a vitamin-dependency rather than a vitamin-deficiency disorder.

Second, it may be necessary to review the vitamin intake of adolescent and adult women, especially with regard to free folates, and to increase it. Although the prescription of appropriate supplements in pre-pregnancy (pre-conception) clinics might be the best in theory, in practice too many pregnancies are unplanned for this approach to be effective. The alternative is to reconsider RDA for folate (and other vitamins), and to achieve higher intakes by further fortification of staple dietary items. Fortified breakfast cereals are already the biggest single source of folic acid for large numbers of people. This principle could readily be extended. There is to date no evidence that folic acid intakes as much as 10 times current RDA are harmful to mother or fetus.

Finally, whatever the eventual outcome of this particular approach to the prevention of one major group of birth defects, it has perhaps encouraged a move away from the historically defeatist view that congenital malformations are inevitable, and towards a more positive and hopeful frame of mind.

Addendum

The United Kingdom Medical Research Council trial of vitamin supplementation for prevention of NTD recurrences has now been published (Lancet 1991, MRC Vitamin Study Research Group 1991). In an international, multi-centre study which yielded 1195 informative pregnancies, a clear preventive effect was found for folic acid 4mg daily. The observed NTD recurrences were 1.0 per cent in mothers receiving folic acid and 3.5 per cent in those not receiving folic acid (relative risk 0.28 : 95 percent CI 0.12–0.71). No effect was found for other vitamins. The authors suggested, very reasonably, that since folic acid can prevent recurrences it is likely to prevent first occurrences. They recommend that all high-risk mothers should receive folic acid supplements starting before conception, and that folic acid intake for all women of childbearing age should be increased, probably by fortification of staple foods (*e.g.* bread and cereals). It is undertood that the chief medical officer of the UK Department of Health is to set up an advisory group to make specific proposals.

REFERENCES

Bower, C. (1990) 'A case-control study of neural tube defects in Western Australia.' University of Western Australia: PhD thesis.
—— Stanley, F. (1989) 'Dietary folate as a risk factor for neural-tube defects: evidence from a case-control study in Western Australia.' *Medical Journal of Australia*, **150**, 613–619.
Cziezel, A., Rode, K. (1984) 'Trial to prevent first occurrence of neural tube defects by periconceptional multivitamin supplementation.' *Lancet*, **2**, 40.
Elwood, J.M., Elwood, J.H. (1980) *Epidemiology of Anencephalus and Spina Bifida*. Oxford: Oxford University Press.
Habibzadeh, N., Smithells, R.W., Schorah, C.J. (1990) 'Folic acid metabolism in placental cells associated with neural tube defects.' *In* Curtius, H.-Ch., Ghisla, S., Blau, N. (Eds) *Proceedings of the Ninth International Symposium on Pteridines and Folic Acid Derivatives; Chemical, Biological & Clinical Aspects*. Berlin: Walter de Gruyter.
Hibbard, B.M., Hibbard, E.D. (1966) 'Recurrence of defective folate metabolism in successive pregnancies.' *Journal of Obstetrics & Gynaecology of the British Commonwealth*, **73**, 428–430.
Hibbard, E.D., Smithells, R.W. (1965) 'Folic acid metabolism and human embryopathy.' *Lancet*, **1**, 1254.
Kalter, H. (1968) *Teratology of the Central Nervous System*. Chicago: University of Chicago Press.
Kirke, P.E. (1983) *In* Dobbing, J. (Ed.) *Prevention of Spina Bifida and Other Neural Tube Defects*. London: Academic Press. pp. 45, 117.
Klemetti, A., Saxen, L. (1967) 'Prospective vs retrospective approach in the search for environmental causes of malformations.' *American Journal of Public Health*, **57**, 2071–2075.
Lancet (1991) 'Folic acid and neural tube defects.' *Lancet*, **338**, 153–154. (Editorial.)
Laurence, K.M., James, N., Miller, M.H., Campbell, H. (1980) 'Increased risk of recurrence of

pregnancies complicated by fetal neural tube defects in mothers receiving poor diets, and possible benefits of dietary counselling.' *British Medical Journal*, **2**, 1592–1594.

—— —— —— Tennant, G.B., Campbell, H. (1981) 'Double-blind, randomised, controlled trial of folate treatment before conception to prevent recurrence of neural-tube defects.' *British Medical Journal*, **282**, 1509–1511.

—— Campbell, H., James, N.E. (1983) 'The role of improvement in the maternal diet and preconceptional folic acid supplementation in the prevention of neural tube defects.' *In* Dobbing, J. (Ed.) *Prevention of Spina Bifida and Other Neural Tube Defects.* London: Academic Press.

Lorber, J. (1984) 'The family history of uncomplicated congenital hydrocephalus: an epidemiological study based on 270 probands.' *British Medical Journal*, **289**, 281–284.

Miller, P.M., Pratten, M.K., Beck, F. (1989) 'Growth of 9.5-day rat embryos in folic-acid-deficient serum.' *Teratology*, **39**, 375–385.

Mills, J.L., Rhoads, G.G., Simpson, J.L., Cunningham, G.C., Conley, M.R., Lassman, M.R., Walden, M.E., Depp, O.R., Hoffman, H.J. (1989) 'The absence of a relation between the periconceptional use of vitamins and neural-tube defects.' *New England Journal of Medicine*, **321**, 430–435.

MRC Vitamin Study Research Group (1991) 'Prevention of neural tube defects: results of the Medical Research Council Vitamin Study.' *Lancet*, **338**, 131–137.

Milunsky, A., Jick, H., Jick, S.S., Bruell, C.L., MacLaughlin, D.S., Rothman, K.J., Willett, W. (1989) 'Multivitamin/folic acid supplementation in early pregnancy reduces the prevalence of neural tube defects.' *Journal of the American Medical Association*, **262**, 2847–2852.

Mulinare, J., Cordero, J.F., Erickson, J.D., Berry, R.J. (1988) 'Periconceptional use of multivitamins and the occurrence of neural tube defects.' *Journal of the American Medical Association*, **260**, 3141–3145.

Nevin, N.C., Seller, M.J. (1990) 'Prevention of neural-tube-defect recurrences.' *Lancet*, **335**, 178–179.

Rogozinski, H., Ankers, C., Lennon, D., Wild, J., Schorah, C.J., Sheppard, S., Smithells, R.W. (1983) 'Folate nutrition in early pregnancy.' *Human Nutrition: Applied Nutrition*, **37A**, 357–364.

Seller, M.J., Embury, S., Polani, P.E., Adinolfi, M. (1979) 'Neural tube defects in curly-tail mice. II. Effect of maternal administration of vitamin A.' *Proceedings of the Royal Society of London*, **206**, 95–107.

Smithells, R.W., Ankers, C., Carver, M.E., Lennon, D., Schorah, C.J., Sheppard, S. (1977) 'Maternal nutrition in early pregnancy.' *British Journal of Nutrition*, **38**, 497–506.

—— Nevin, N.C., Seller, M.J., Sheppard, S., Harris, R., Read, A.P., Fielding, D.W., Walker, S., Schorah, C.J., Wild, J. (1983) 'Further experience of vitamin supplementation for prevention of neural tube defect recurrences.' *Lancet*, **1**, 1027–1031.

—— Sheppard, S., Wild, J., Schorah, C.J. (1989) 'Prevention of neural tube defect recurrences: final report.' *Lancet*, **2**, 498–499.

Steegers-Theunissen, R.P.M., Boers, G.H.J., Trijbels, F.J.M., Eskes, T.K.A.B. (1991) 'Neural-tube defects and derangement of homocysteine metabolism.' *New England Journal of Medicine*, **324**, 199–200

Thiersch, J.B. (1952) 'Therapeutic abortions with a folic acid antagonist, 4-amino-pteroylglutamic acid (4 amino PGA) administered by the oral route.' *American Journal of Obstetrics and Gynecology*, **63**, 1298–1304.

Vergel, R.G., Sanchez, L.R., Heredero, B.L., Rodriguez, P.L., Martinez, A.J., (1990) 'Primary prevention of neural tube defects with folic acid supplementation: Cuban experience.' *Prenatal Diagnosis*, **10**, 149–152.

Wald, N.J., Polani, P.E. (1984) 'Neural-tube defects and vitamins: the need for a randomised clinical trial.' *British Journal of Obstetrics and Gynaecology*, **91**, 516–523.

Wild, J., Read, A.P., Sheppard, S., Seller, M.J., Smithells, R.W., Nevin, N.C., Schorah, C.J., Fielding, D.W., Walker, S., Harris, R. (1986) 'Recurrent neural tube defects, risk factors and vitamins.' *Archives of Disease in Childhood*, **61**, 440–444.

Wills, L., Mehta, M.M. (1930) 'Studies in "pernicious anaemia" of pregnancy. Part I. Preliminary report.' *Indian Journal of Medical Research*, **17**, 777–792.

Yates, J.R.W., Ferguson-Smith, M.A., Shenkin, A., Guzman-Rodriguez, R., White, M., Clark, B.J. (1987) 'Is disordered folate metabolism the basis for the genetic predisposition to neural tube defects?' *Clinical Genetics*, **31**, 279–287.

15

2

THE ROLE OF FETAL NEUROSURGERY IN THE MANAGEMENT OF CENTRAL NERVOUS SYSTEM ABNORMALITIES

Carys M. Bannister

A few years ago it would have been inconceivable to think of performing any kind of surgical procedure on a fetus. Today it is commonplace for umbilical vessels to be punctured repeatedly in order to obtain blood samples, administer drugs and give blood transfusions (De Crespigny *et al.* 1985, Nicolaides *et al.* 1986*a*, Berkowitz *et al.* 1987, Grannum *et al.* 1988, Lemery *et al.* 1988). Catheters are placed in distended bladders, fluid is withdrawn from the chests and peritoneal cavities of hydropic fetuses (Roberts *et al.* 1986), and shunts have been inserted to drain cerebrospinal fluid (CSF) from dilated lateral ventricles (Clewell *et al.* 1982, Frigoletto *et al.* 1982). A few fetuses have been temporarily delivered to allow complex surgical procedures to be carried out before being returned to the uterus to continue development (Harrison *et al.* 1982, Glick *et al.* 1985).

Yet only a short time ago the fetus was virtually ignored by most of the medical profession. This change in attitude has been brought about principally by the introduction of ultrasound scanning. Images of the fetus, although indistinct at first, raised the profession's awareness of the fetus as an individual, and the provision of clearer and more detailed pictures by subsequent advances in ultrasound technology have considerably reinforced this awareness. Practically every organ in the fetus's body can now be visualised, usually from an early stage of gestation, and real-time scanning has made it possible to analyse fetal limb and eye movements (Ianniruberto and Tejani 1981, Campbell *et al.* 1983, Awost and Levi 1984), the heart action (Truccone and Mariona 1986, Stewart and Wladimiroff 1987) and the emptying and filling of the bladder (Campbell *et al.* 1983).

While ultrasound scanning has been the predominant method of visualising the fetus, computed tomographic (CT) scans (Patterson *et al.* 1981, Kirkinen *et al.* 1982, Olund *et al.* 1983, Pretorius *et al.* 1985, Hanigan *et al.* 1986) and magnetic resonance imaging (MRI) (Vitzileos *et al.* 1983, Hanigan *et al.* 1986, Hill *et al.* 1988) have also been used in some centres. CT scanning has the disadvantage of exposing the fetus to a dose of radiation. The fetus has to be still during both CT and MR scanning, and this may require the injection of a paralysing agent. Because these two methods of investigation are not universally available, they will not be considered further here.

16

Inevitably, almost from its inception, ultrasound scanning revealed fetal abnormalities and in so doing identified a new category of patient. It became necessary to set up new departments, fetal therapy units, staffed by specialists with expertise and specific interests in the management of fetal disease. The constitution and role of fetal therapy units are discussed in Chapter 3.

While ultrasound scanning has brought many benefits, in the diagnosis and management of the sick fetus, it has also revealed new problems. In the CNS, and no doubt in other organs as well, the significance of some abnormalities that have been demonstrated remains unknown. We need much more information to correlate ultrasound appearances with the developmental outcome of affected fetuses. Without this information, it is an awesome responsibility to have to give advice about how these cases should be managed. Should the parents be reassured and encouraged to allow the pregnancy to continue to term? Should they be advised to seek a therapeutic abortion? Or should the fetus be subjected to an interventional procedure? As ultrasound techniques become more sophisticated, it is likely that more abnormalities will be identified and these challenging situations will have to be faced more frequently.

The identification of serious abnormalities will inevitably stimulate the medical profession to devise and test increasingly bold and innovative surgical procedures to deal with them, among the most challenging of which will be those affecting the CNS. We must ensure that intervention in these cases results in an individual with a worthwhile quality of life, and that we do not merely keep alive those who would otherwise perish either *in utero* or shortly after birth, and produce survivors whose quality of life is very poor.

All those who take on the responsibility of giving advice and information to the parents of an abnormal fetus must be sure that the fetus's life is not sacrificed unnecessarily. On the other hand, if the advice is to intervene, there must be no illusion about the fact that two lives (that of the mother and her fetus) will be put at risk. These risks can be justified only if there is no reasonable doubt about the benefits to be gained from performing the procedure, if there is a good chance the procedure will be successful, and furthermore if there is no safer way of achieving the same result. Everyone must consider all aspects of the problem, including clinical aspects and the relevant experimental data.

This chapter deals with conditions affecting the human brain, skull and spinal cord which can be diagnosed prenatally by ultrasound scanning and either deteriorate progressively or are thought likely to benefit from early surgical intervention because of observations made postnatally or because of evidence obtained in the laboratory from animal experimentation.

Conditions affecting the brain
Hydrocephalus and encephaloceles are the most common conditions affecting the fetal brain which are amenable or at least potentially amenable to intrauterine surgical intervention.

Hydrocephalus

CAUSES OF HYDROCEPHALUS

Surgically remedial hydrocephalus diagnosed *in utero* may be either congenital or acquired. It can occur in isolation or in association with other abnormalities of the CNS. The most common causes of isolated congenital hydrocephalus are (i) aqueduct stenosis, (ii) the Dandy-Walker complex, and (iii) failure of the subarachnoid spaces to develop normally. Less commonly it is caused by an aneurysm of the vein of Galen. Hydrocephalus associated with other congenital abnormalities is due to (i) the Arnold-Chiari malformation which generally accompanies spina bifida operta, and (ii) malformations of the fourth ventricle associated with posteriorly placed encephaloceles. Most cases of acquired hydrocephalus are due to infection of the fetal CNS by toxoplasmosis (Lorber and Bassi 1965), cytomegalovirus, mumps, rubella, varicella, Asian influenza, and other viruses (Bray 1972, Davis 1981, McCullough 1989), and to intraventricular haemorrhages following an intrauterine catastrophe. Acquired hydrocephalus is occasionally caused by cerebral tumours which may be malignant (Hill *et al.* 1988).

EFFECT OF HYDROCEPHALUS ON THE FETAL BRAIN

All the causes of hydrocephalus listed above result in a blockage of some part of the CSF pathways, leading to an accumulation of fluid proximal to the site of block. After birth, excessive build-up of fluid causes an increase in the intracranial pressure (ICP) which may not be particularly high (although it often is) and may not be raised all the time (although again it generally is). The evidence suggests that ICP is also raised in fetal hydrocephalus.

   CSF production plays a crucial role in the development of hydrocephalus. The fluid is actively secreted by the choroid plexuses, which continue production even when ICP is considerably raised. As the fluid accumulates and the ventricular system dilates, the brain is stretched and thinned. The raised ICP causes the cerebral perfusion pressure (CPP) to fall, and when this reaches a critical level the brain becomes ischaemic. It is not known in detail how this affects the growth and development of the fetal brain, but it is likely to be most damaging when ICP is raised early, reaches a high level and stays there a long time. Those areas of the brain undergoing the most active growth and development are likely to be the most affected.

   Repeated ultrasound examinations may show that hydrocephalus, which was progressing, has become stable. The reason for this, as in postnatal hydrocephalus, is that CSF can to some extent escape from the CSF pathways by diffusing across the ependymal lining of the ventricles. When the fluid reaches the brain parenchyma it is absorbed by capillaries in the periventricular region. Once the rate of fluid production is equal to the rate of escape, a balance is reached and the hydrocephalus becomes compensated. Compensation may occur for another reason if the Arnold-Chiari malformation is present with a myelomeningocele: because CSF can diffuse across the membranes of the spinal lesion and enter the

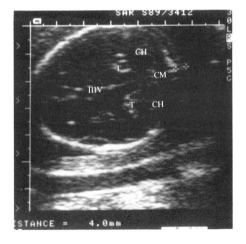

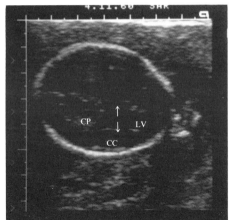

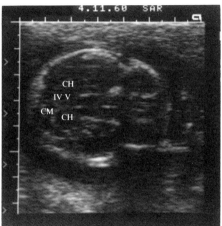

Fig. 2.1. Ultrasonographs of the brains of normal fetuses. *Above left:* third ventricle (III V), both thalami (T), cerebellar hemispheres (CH) and cisterna magna (CM) are clearly seen. White stars indicate the thickness of the nuchal tissues. *Above right:* medial and lateral walls of the lateral ventricle (LV) are indicated by the arrows. The choroid plexus (CP) and cortical mantle (CC) can be visualised. *Left:* fourth ventricle (IV V), cisterna magna (CM) and cerebellar hemispheres (CH) are seen in this view of the posterior fossa structures.

amniotic cavity. In addition the central spinal canal is often patent and CSF escapes from the fourth ventricle by flowing down it and emptying into the amniotic cavity via an opening on the surface of the neuroplaque which lies in the centre of the myelomeningocele.

In uncompensated hydrocephalus the ventricular system proximal to the site of the block dilates progressively, so that the head circumference may have reached grotesque proportions by the time the fetus reaches term. In the worst cases the wall of the lateral ventricles is reduced to a thin membrane, particularly in the occipital region, which is often the most affected area. By this stage, irreversible changes have already taken place. Raised ICP is generally accompanied by an increase in the head circumference, but this is not always the case. If the cortex fails to develop or existing brain substance is lost, the head may remain small even though the ventricular system is enlarged.

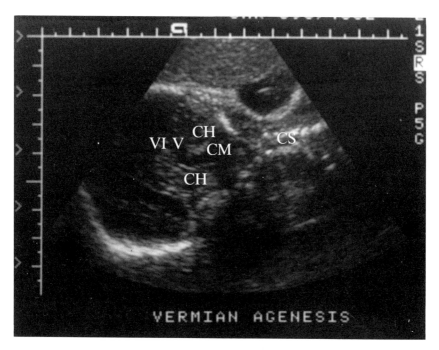

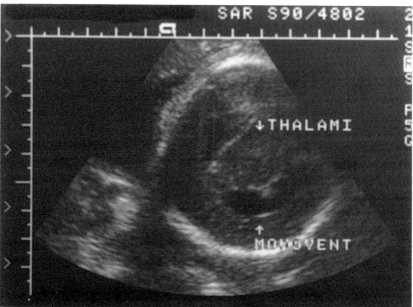

Fig. 2.2. Ultrasonograph of fetus with the Dandy-Walker complex. *Top:* fourth ventricle (IV V) lying between the two cerebellar hemispheres (CH) opens directly into the cisterna magna (CM). The vermis is absent. The cervical spine (CS) is seen. *Bottom:* visualisation of the supratentorial structures showed that the fetus had holoprosencephalus, the thalami were fused and there was only a single ventricle present.

As already stated, ultrasound scanning is currently the main method of investigation for fetal hydrocephalus.

Ultrasound scans rarely detect hydrocephalus before the 20th week of gestation. In the normal brain the lateral ventricles and choroid plexuses can be identified between the 10th and 12th week of gestation (Sanders and James 1985). By the 16th week much of the anatomy of the brain can be recognised, including the corpus callosum, thalami, cerebral peduncles, brainstem, cerebellar hemispheres, vermis and cisterna magna (Campbell *et al.* 1983, Pilu 1986, Hill *et al.* 1988). Up to the 20th week of gestation the comparatively large choroid plexuses completely fill the cavities of the lateral ventricles, and it is only in extremely severe hydrocephalus that CSF is seen separating the choroid plexuses from the walls of the ventricles at less than 20 weeks of gestation. After the 20th week, development of the brain leads to thickening of the cortical mantle and it is then much easier to appreciate that the lateral ventricles are dilated. It is very likely that hydrocephalus will be missed if ultrasound scans are only performed before the 20th week of gestation.

The third and fourth ventricles (Fig. 2.1) can also be seen on ultrasound scans from as early as the 14th week of gestation, making it possible to establish the cause of hydrocephalus in many cases. Cystic dilatation of the fourth ventricle occurs in the Dandy-Walker complex (Fig. 2.2). Some forms of the Dandy-Walker complex are associated with abnormalities in other parts of the CNS, and these include posterior encephaloceles, failure of development of the corpus callosum and haloprosencephaly. These abnormalities should always be looked for specifically during ultrasound examination when the Dandy-Walker complex is diagnosed because they adversely affect the prognosis. If the lateral ventricles are dilated and the posterior fossa structures are normal, the hydrocephalus is probably due to aqueduct stenosis (Fig. 2.3). In the Arnold-Chiari malformation the cerebellar hemispheres are small and the cerebellar tonsils, parts of the medulla oblongata and fourth ventricle are displaced downwards into the upper cervical spinal canal. This causes the posterior fossa to be reduced in size and the remaining cerebellum appears on ultrasound scanning to be banana-shaped (Fig. 2.4) (Nicolaides *et al.* 1986*b*). This, together with narrowing of the frontal region, causes the skull of a fetus with the Arnold-Chiari malformation in the middle trimester of pregnancy to have a characteristic lemon shape (Fig. 2.4) (Nicolaides *et al.* 1986*a*). Because of the high probability of an associated spina bifida operta, whenever the Arnold-Chiari malformation is identified, the whole length of the fetal spine must be examined to exclude a spinal defect (see below).

While infections of the CNS by toxoplasmosis, rubella, cytomegalovirus or herpes simplex can lead to obstructive hydrocephalus, they more commonly cause cerebral atrophy. The thinning of the cortical mantle leads to compensatory enlargement of the ventricular system. It can be difficult positively to differentiate severe hydrocephalus from cerebral atrophy accompanied by ventricular enlarge-

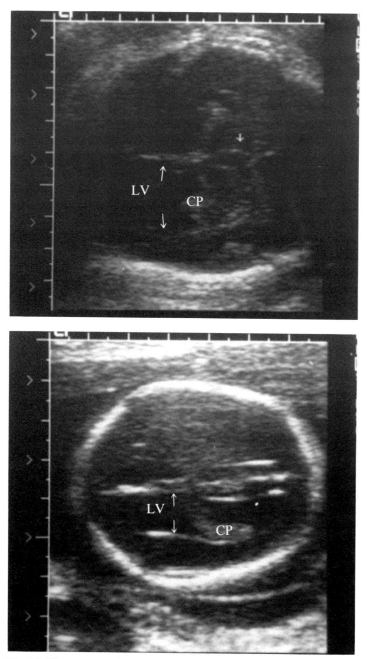

Fig. 2.3. Ultrasonographs of two fetuses with hydrocephalus. *Top:* mild dilatation of the lateral ventricle (LV) is indicated by arrows. The choroid plexus (CP) is dangling in the cavity of the ventricle. *Bottom:* grosser dilatation of the lateral ventricle (LV) is present, the medial and lateral walls of the ventricle are indicated by the large arrows. The third ventricle (TV) is also dilated (small arrow). The choroid plexus (CP) is present in the cavity of the lateral ventricle.

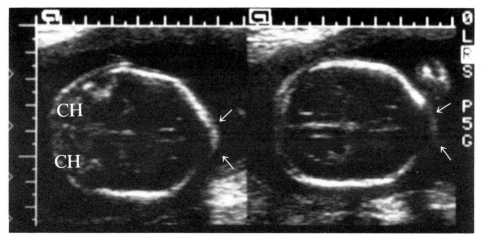

Fig. 2.4. Ultrasonographs of a fetus with the Arnold-Chiari malformation. The left scan shows the banana sign caused by the small cerebellar hemispheres (CM) effacing the cisterna magna. Bossing of the frontal region of the skull (arrows) is seen in both scans. This, together with the banana sign, causes the skull to be lemon-shaped.

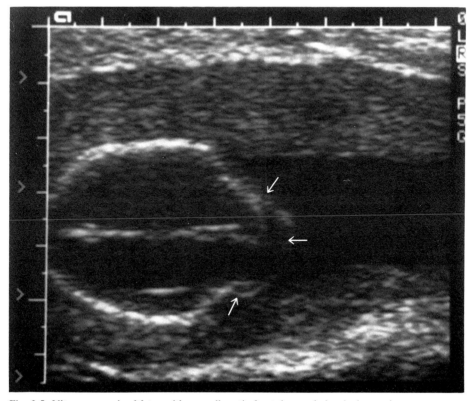

Fig. 2.5. Ultrasonograph of fetus with a small cystic frontal encephalocele (arrows).

ment or from hydranencephaly. A viral aetiology should be suspected if ultrasound examination shows intrauterine growth retardation, cerebral calcification and subtle changes in the texture of the brain (Clewell 1988). Porencephalic cysts lie within the cerebral substance and communicate with the ventricular system. They are frequently associated with hydrocephalus and are thought to be due either to an intracerebral haemorrhage, or to an intrauterine catastrophe causing occlusion of one of the major arteries supplying blood to the brain. An aneurysm of the vein of Galen causes hydrocephalus by obstructing the posterior end of the third ventricle. The aneurysm can be seen on ultrasound scans. If the bloodflow through the associated angioma is sufficiently large, it can cause heart failure and lead to hydrops fetalis (Hill *et al.* 1988). Cerebral tumours can obstruct the ventricular system and lead to hydrocephalus. They have been seen on fetal ultrasound scans (Lipman *et al.* 1985, Hill *et al.* 1988).

When enlarged ventricles are detected, ultrasound scans should be repeated at one- or two-weekly intervals to determine whether the hydrocephalus is arrested or progressing (Fig. 2.5). Measurements of head circumference and width of the lateral ventricles are taken for comparison with normal growth charts (Christie and Ivory 1984, Warsof and Griffin 1984). Simultaneous increase in ventricular size and head circumference suggests that ICP is raised. However, the pressure can also be raised when the head size is normal or even smaller than normal, as in cerebral atrophy and hydranencephaly when the ICP is not raised and the head circumference increases slowly or not at all.

Measurement of CPP would be of great benefit to diagnose, assess the outcome and decide how to treat fetal hydrocephalus. It would also be valuable if ICP could be recorded over a period of time. While at present it is not possible to measure CPP, single ICP measurements have been made by inserting a needle under ultrasound guidance into one of the fetus's lateral ventricles. However, because of the trauma and pain inflicted on the fetus by the puncture, and because the pressure probably varies with time, single measurements are of doubtful value and may not be an accurate representation of the true pressure. What is needed is a method of measuring ICP noninvasively.

Isolated hydrocephalus, but more particularly hydrocephalus coexisting with other congenital abnormalities of the CNS and other organs, may be associated with chromosomal abnormalities (Williamson *et al.* 1981). The karyotype is determined from culture of fetal cells obtained from the amniotic fluid, chorionic villus samples or blood collected from puncture of a vessel in the umbilical cord.

If a viral infection is suspected to be the cause of the hydrocephalus, a sample of amniotic fluid should be obtained for culture. However, viral culture techniques are highly specific and only common organisms such as the cytomegalovirus can usually be grown (Clewell 1988).

PHILOSOPHY OF TREATMENT OF HYDROCEPHALUS
For maximum benefit, measures to control fetal hydrocephalus should be carried

out as soon as possible. Since the ongoing damage in hydrocephalus is due to the raised ICP compressing the brain and reducing CPP, treatment is directed towards lowering ICP to within the normal range and keeping it there.

Hopes must not be set unrealistically high. There are many reasons in addition to raised ICP which can cause the hydrocephalic brain to develop abnormally. Infections and intracerebral haemorrhages may have a lasting and sometimes devastating effect on the ability of the brain to grow and develop, but other causes of hydrocephalus may have equally severe reasons for producing a poor outcome. Since these factors cannot be quantified, it is too optimistic to expect treatment in every case to achieve a good outcome; it is more realistic to hope that treatment will limit the amount of damage sustained.

Once hydrocephalus has been shown to be present, it must be determined whether it is arrested or progressing. If it is arrested, further scans are carried out at intervals to ensure that it has not started to progress again. If it is progressing, before a fetus is subjected to treatment it is imperative to ensure that the hydrocephalus is the only abnormality present, that the pregnancy is single, and that the fetus has a normal karyotype. The amniotic fluid is examined to exclude specific viral infections. A detailed ultrasound examination of the brain will usually be able to establish the cause of the hydrocephalus. Finally an estimate of the severity of the hydrocephalus is made by measuring the head circumference and determining the thickness of the cortical mantle. If the head circumference is very large for gestational age and the cortical mantle is only a few millimetres thick, treatment is unlikely to achieve a satisfactory outcome.

When all this information is available, the parents should be given a detailed explanation of the likely consequences of hydrocephalus on the growth and development of their child's brain, what outcome can be expected if treatment is not undertaken, and what treatment options are available. Armed with this knowledge the parents are in a position to make an informed decision about whether to continue the pregnancy or (if the gestational age allows) to terminate it.

TREATMENT OPTIONS

Non-intervention. The first option is to allow the pregnancy to proceed to term. If the head circumference is very large, the baby may have to be delivered by caesarean section. If a vaginal delivery is decided on, CSF may need to be aspirated from the fetal ventricular system at the time of delivery to reduce the size of the head sufficiently to allow it to pass through the birth canal. Shortly after birth a ventriculo-peritoneal shunt is inserted to control the hydrocephalus. The grave disadvantage of this treatment method is that if the hydrocephalus is diagnosed at about the 20th week of pregnancy, there will be a delay of about 20 weeks before treatment is carried out.

Early delivery. The second option is to intervene when the fetus has matured sufficiently to be able to live independently outside the uterus. At about the 32nd or 33rd week of pregnancy the lungs have generally developed sufficiently to allow the prematurely delivered infant to breathe without the aid of mechanical ventilation. The state of maturity of the fetal lungs is assessed by measuring the surfactant levels in the amniotic fluid. It may be necessary to perform an amniocentesis more than once before a satisfactory lecithin : sphingomyelin ratio is found. Administration of glucocorticoids to the mother may accelerate the maturation of the fetal lungs (Cosmi and DiRenzo 1989). The fetus is usually delivered by caesarean section and shortly afterwards a ventriculo-peritoneal shunt is inserted.

This method of treatment also imposes a considerable delay (12 to 13 weeks) between the diagnosis of the hydrocephalus and the institution of treatment. However, it is a relatively simple and safe form of treatment and does not require any special skills or equipment other than those available in most maternity units.

Intrauterine intervention. The third option is to insert a shunt to drain CSF from the fetal ventricular system into the amniotic cavity. Unfortunately, while the concept is simple, in practice it is fraught with difficulties.

In 1981 Birnholtz and Frigoletto performed the first intrauterine procedure on a human fetus with the specific object of treating hydrocephalus. Using ultrasound, they guided a needle through the mother's abdominal wall and uterus, and after entering one of the dilated lateral ventricles, they aspirated CSF. Because the fluid rapidly reaccumulated, the procedure had to be repeated to keep the hydrocephalus under control. This was impractical, and another solution was sought: inserting shunts to drain CSF from the ventricular system into the amniotic cavity (Clewell *et al.* 1982, Frigoletto *et al.* 1982).

Insertion of ventriculo-amniotic shunts. In this procedure a fine trocar and cannula is guided under ultrasound control through the mother's abdomen and the wall of the uterus and into one of the fetus's dilated lateral ventricles. A catheter, generally with a one-way flow system built into it, is threaded down the cannula. When the cannula is withdrawn, the proximal end of the catheter is left in the ventricle and the distal end lies free in the amniotic cavity.

In theory this procedure can be carried out on fetuses as young as 20 weeks, but in practice none younger than 25 weeks have been treated (Manning *et al.* 1986). If the shunt is functioning, ultrasound scans should show a decrease in the ventricular size and a thickening of the cortical mantle, and these changes have been observed in some treated fetuses (Clewell 1988). Ideally the shunt should remain in place and continue to function until the fetus reaches full term. After delivery the ventriculo-amniotic shunt is removed and replaced by a ventriculo-peritoneal shunt. In practice most of the treated fetuses have been delivered prematurely either because of shunt failure or because of spontaneous onset of preterm labour (Manning *et al.* 1986).

Complications of ventriculo-amniotic shunts. Inserting the shunt is by no means easy. One fetus is reported to have died during the procedure (Manning *et al.* 1986). A number of shunts have become dislodged after satisfactory placement and have had to be replaced. There is also a high risk of preterm labour. Chorio-amnionitis was reported in one case, with death of the fetus (Manning *et al.* 1986).

Results of insertion of ventriculo-amniotic shunts. Forty-four hydrocephalic fetuses in North America and Italy had ventriculo-amniotic shunts inserted. The details of these cases are recorded in the International Registry of Fetal Treatment (Manning *et al.* 1986). The gestational ages of the fetuses at the time of shunt insertion ranged from 25 to 33 weeks (Manning *et al.* 1986). Hydrocephalus was judged to be due to an aqueduct stenosis in 32 fetuses, due to communicating hydrocephalus in two, and to the Dandy-Walker complex in one. In nine fetuses the hydrocephalus was thought to be due to a variety of causes, but the diagnosis was not established for certain in any of them. Ten fetuses died during treatment or within three months of birth. Death was attributed to difficult shunt insertions, preterm delivery, chorioamnionitis or associated abnormalities of the CNS, heart, lungs or gastrointestinal tract. The survivors were followed up for two years: 12 of the 34 were reported to be normal, four had mild neurological abnormalities, and 18 had severe deficits, but in addition to hydrocephalus some had CNS malformations or abnormalities of other organs (Manning *et al.* 1986).

It is assumed that shunting CSF from the fetal ventricles into the amniotic cavity reduces ICP, but is this really so? Is the pressure differential between the fetal cranium and the amniotic cavity sufficient to allow this to happen? While indirect evidence from follow-up ultrasound scans of shunted fetuses (Clewell 1988), and from studies of shunted fetal monkeys and lambs with induced hydrocephalus (Edwards *et al.* 1984, Michejda *et al.* 1984), suggests that this is the case, definitive proof awaits the development of technology which will allow ICP to be measured noninvasively.

The obvious advantage of ventriculo-amniotic shunts, compared to the other two options, is that treatment can be instituted immediately after the diagnosis of hydrocephalus has been made. The procedure has now largely been suspended, because the shunts are difficult to insert and are easily dislodged, because of the danger of preterm delivery, unacceptably high fetal morbidity and mortality rates, and the uncertainty about whether shunts significantly improve outcome (Clewell 1988). The present moratorium means that ventriculo-amniotic shunts can no longer generally be considered as an option for the treatment of fetal hydrocephalus. Intrauterine intervention should currently be considered as an experimental procedure to be carried out only in specialised centres where the patients can be fully documented and the results analysed in detail.

If the results of insertion of ventriculo-amniotic shunts had proved satisfactory, there would be little argument about how fetal hydrocephalus should be managed. As it is, the question remains open. Deciding how to advise parents about the two remaining options is complicated by the fact that several key questions remain unanswered. It is still unknown in detail how hydrocephalus affects the growth and development of the fetal brain at different stages of gestation. It is crucial to know this, since neither the mother nor her fetus should be subjected to the risks of a procedure if it were shown, for instance, that treatment is of no value if carried out before or after certain gestational ages. Nor is it known for certain whether fetal hydrocephalus really does cause a rise in ICP, although the whole basis for treatment depends on the assumption that reducing ICP by removing CSF from the ventricular system allows the brain to develop to its maximum potential. Finally, it is important to know the outcome of patients treated in the various ways described above. Before proper conclusions can be drawn, there must be detailed follow-up studies of the survivors. As yet too few fetuses and babies have undergone treatment. Large series are needed if the numerous variables present are to be taken into account. The cause of hydrocephalus is one important variable. Different causes have different expected outcomes, which must be allowed for when the results of one treatment are compared with another. Patients must be followed up for a sufficient length of time. To make a comprehensive assessment of a child's mental and physical development, s/he must be at least five years old. But the reported assessments of most of the treated children were made at a much younger age (Manning *et al.* 1986), and are therefore of limited value in assessing outcome.

The foregoing may appear to present a rather gloomy picture of the current status of management of fetal hydrocephalus. It should not be viewed as such, but rather as a challenge to solve outstanding problems. There is experimental evidence that lesions made in the brains of postnatal animals and fetal rats and lambs during the second and third trimesters of pregnancy are very similar in many respects (Bannister and Chapman 1986, 1987; Chapman and Bannister 1989). The fetal brain, however, differs from the neonatal one in that widespread effects can also be detected in distant parts of the injured hemisphere (Bannister and Chapman 1987). This suggests that the deleterious effects of untreated hydrocephalus may be similar or perhaps even worse in fetuses than in neonates. This should strengthen the impetus to search for a safe, effective, and if possible simple way of treating fetal hydrocephalus as soon as it is diagnosed. It is not good enough to deliver the fetus when it is mature enough to live independently, and only then insert a ventriculo-peritoneal shunt to reduce ICP, or to wait for the baby to be delivered at full term. But until new ventriculo-amniotic shunts and better and safer methods of inserting them have been devised, and until ICP measurements can be made noninvasively so that the fetuses most likely to benefit from treatment can be identified and the results of shunt insertion monitored, it is the best we have to offer.

Further developments and experimentation will no doubt solve the outstanding problems. Only then is it likely that ventriculo-amniotic shunting will be generally resumed, unless it is found more satisfactory to insert a ventriculo-peritoneal shunt into the fetus as has already been done in experimental animals (Edwards *et al.* 1984).

Encephaloceles
Among the Western races the majority of encephaloceles arise either in the occipital region or in the posterior fossa. A smaller number occur in the frontal region, and the least common arise in the nose, base of skull and orbit.

Encephaloceles vary from about a centimetre in diameter, to lesions which can be several times larger than the circumference of the head. They may be covered by skin or membranes, and their contents are either cystic, solid, or more commonly a combination of the two. Cystic encephaloceles are generally connected to the intracranial contents by a narrow neck, while solid encephaloceles usually have broad necks containing neural tissue, which can have function. The remainder of the brain may be normal but often it is small and poorly developed. Hydrocephalus may accompany encephaloceles arising in any location, but it occurs most frequently with posterior lesions. Frontal encephaloceles are often associated with malformations of the upper part of the face, the most common of which are defects in the frontal bone, hypertelorism and malformations of the nose.

Encephaloceles develop early in gestation, probably during the embryonic period. They are often described as herniations of brain through defects in the skull. However, it has been suggested that they may arise at the point where the basement membranes of the developing neural tube and the surface ectoderm fail to separate from one another (Hoving 1990).

AIMS OF TREATMENT

The aims of surgical treatment are the removal of an unsightly and often cumbersome lesion and, if it is membranous, to get skin cover to eliminate the risk of infection. In frontal encephaloceles, reconstruction of the frontal and orbital bones is often necessary to correct the accompanying bony deformity.

PROGNOSIS

The outlook from the point of view of mental and physical development depends on the amount of neural tissue in the encephalocele, whether the rest of the brain has developed normally, and whether hydrocephalus is present. Very large lesions with small head size have a dismal prognosis; the child may be blind, grossly retarded mentally and physically, and prone to seizures. On the other hand, the outlook may be excellent with a good chance of normal mental and physical development if the lesion is cystic, the head size is normal and hydrocephalus is not present.

INVESTIGATIONS

Encephaloceles can usually be seen on ultrasound scans (Fig. 2.6) carried out during the first trimester of pregnancy. Because the prognosis depends on the size and site of the lesion, the nature of its contents and the presence or absence of hydrocephalus, these must be specifically looked for during ultrasound scanning and their implications discussed with the parents. The poor prognosis of large, solid encephaloceles means that many parents will opt for a termination of pregnancy if the fetus has such a lesion. Parents should be made aware of the more favourable prognosis of cystic encephaloceles, and those arising in the frontal region, before they come to a decision about what action to take. The accompanying

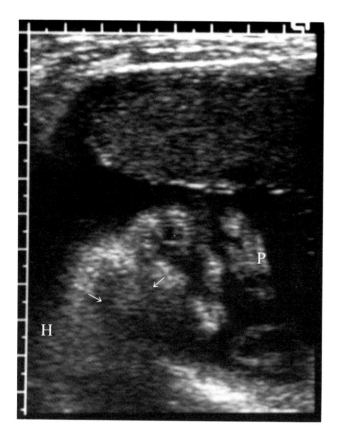

Fig. 2.6. Ultrasonograph of full-face view of fetus with bilateral facial clefts (arrows). The placenta (P) lies adjacent to left side of the face with one of the fetus's hands (H) close to the other side of the face.

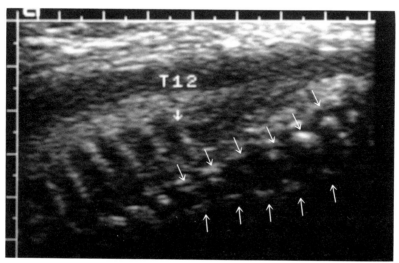

Fig. 2.7. Ultrasonograph of the spine of fetus with lumbar myelomeningocele. The divergence of the pedicles at the site of the lesion is indicated by the large arrows. The small arrow is at the level of the 12th rib.

hydrocephalus can be arrested or uncompensated; if the latter is the case, it may need to be managed if the pregnancy is allowed to continue.

EXPERIMENTAL STUDIES
In the laboratory, posterior encephaloceles have been induced in fetal monkeys by feeding teratogens to the mothers early in pregnancy (Michejda *et al.* 1984). Excision of the encephalocele and treatment of the associated hydrocephalus by draining CSF into the amniotic cavity has been reported to be followed by regeneration and reorganisation of the cytoarchitecture of the occipital lobes (Michejda *et al.* 1984). However, my colleagues and I did not find any evidence of regeneration following injury or excision of brain tissue in fetal rats and lambs (Bannister and Chapman 1986, Chapman and Bannister 1989).

The balance of evidence does not indicate that intrauterine treatment of encephaloceles should be considered at present. Further experimental work is needed to elucidate the effect of excising these lesions *in utero*.

CRANIOFACIAL MALFORMATIONS
Although bony craniofacial malformations frequently accompany frontal enceph-aloceles, the majority occur in isolation. They can be diagnosed by ultrasound scans during pregnancy (Fig. 2.7) (Strauss and Davis 1990). It has been suggested that because fetal skin wounds may heal without a scar, contracture or inflammation (Longaker *et al.* 1989, 1990; Siebert *et al.* 1990), intrauterine repair of hare-lips and cleft palates might produce better cosmetic results than surgery performed after birth. The same argument could be put forward for advocating surgery for fetuses with other craniofacial deformities. While there is experimental evidence that fetal skin wounds do heal with less scar formation than postnatal ones (Somasundaram and Prathap 1972; Krummel *et al.* 1982; Longaker *et al.* 1989, 1990; Siebert *et al.* 1989), we have shown recently that the healing processes of membranous bone can be altered by surgical manipulations carried out *in utero*; and bony defects in the calvarium, instead of ossifying, are permanently healed by membraneous tissue (Bannister *et al.* 1991). These findings, if confirmed, suggest that craniofacial deformities may not benefit from intrauterine surgery.

Conditions affecting the spinal cord and its covering membranes
Myelomeningoceles
Myelomeningoceles arise anywhere along the length of the spinal column but are most common in the mid-thoracic, thoracolumbar, lumbar and lumbosacral regions. The neuroplaque is that part of the neural groove which fails to separate from the ectoderm and remains exposed in the midline of the back. It may lie flush with the skin surface or on the dome of a CSF-filled cyst.

ULTRASOUND IMAGING OF THE FETUS WITH A MYELOMENINGOCELE
The accompanying defect in the vertebral column at the level of the meningomyelo-

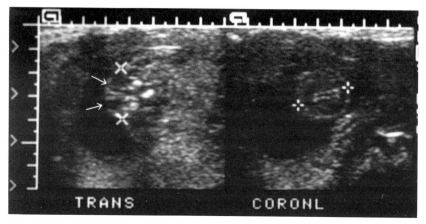

Fig. 2.8. Ultrasonographs of a fetus with a myelomeningocele. The left scan is a transverse view of one vertebra. The pedicles are marked X. Membranous sac protrudes between (*arrows*). The double white lines in the centre of the sac are abnormal neural tissue. The scan on the right is a coronal view of the same lesion. The periphery of the sac is indicated by the crosses.

cele is caused by failure of development of the spines and laminae of the associated vertebrae. Generally at least three and often more vertebrae are involved. The pedicles in the affected area are bent outwards to form a wide, shallow gutter which can be detected by ultrasound scanning from the 12th week of gestation. The pedicles in the normal section of the vertebral canal form parallel lines down the length of the spinal column, but at the level of the meningomyelocele they broaden out suddenly to form an oval-shaped defect (Fig. 2.8, *left*). If the fetus is scanned transversely, the open spinal canal can be imaged (Fig. 2.8, *right*). The sac can often be seen if the myelomeningocele is cystic. Myelomeningoceles at the thoracolumbar junction may be associated with maldevelopment of the bodies of the vertebrae, giving rise to a kypho-scoliosis (Barson 1970) which can also be seen on ultrasound examination.

Virtually every fetus with a myelomeningocele has the Arnold-Chiari malformation. As mentioned above (p. 21), in the Arnold-Chiari malformation cerebellar tissue together with the fourth ventricle lies into the upper cervical spinal canal. The remaining cerebellar tissue is different in shape from normal and the posterior fossa is small and shallow. These changes produce the banana-shaped deformity seen on ultrasound scans (Fig. 2.4) (Nicolaides *et al.* 1986*b*). The shallow posterior fossa and the forward bowing of the frontal bone gives the skull the lemon shape which is so characteristic of the Arnold-Chiari malformation (Fig. 2.4) (Nicolaides *et al.* 1986*b*). While progressive hydrocephalus may be present because the subarachnoid space at the level of the foramen magnum is blocked by neural tissue (p. 18), alternative pathways for escape of CSF exist in the Arnold-Chiari malformation. In many cases the hydrocephalus remains compensated throughout pregnancy, the ICP only rising after the escape routes are obliterated by surgical repair of the back lesion after birth.

Ultrasound examination of the fetus with a myelomeningocele should include an examination of the legs to see if orthopaedic deformities are present. It remains to be determined what is the significance of leg movements seen *in utero* (Warsof *et al.* 1988). It is tempting to believe that if movements are present, then paralysis is minimal or absent. But until these findings are correlated with neurological observations made after birth, great caution should be exercised in interpreting the significance of fetal leg movements, to avoid giving the parents an over-optimistic prognosis. In many affected fetuses the bladder is seen to fill and empty periodically. These findings do not mean that after birth the child will have normal bladder function (Warsof *et al.* 1988), and this should be explained to the parents.

Prognosis is affected by the spinal level of the myelomeningocele, the size of the lesion, whether or not it is cystic, the presence or absence of orthopaedic deformities and the degree of hydrocephalus present. It may be impossible to repair a large lesion lying flush with the skin surface, or if a kypho-scoliosis is present. In general the higher the lesion, the more severe the neurological deficits in the lower limbs and the more severe the accompanying hydrocephalus. Conversely, the lower the lesion, the fewer the neurological deficits and the less severe the hydrocephalus. However, almost all patients with a myelomeningocele have some degree of weakness and loss of sensation of the lower limbs, a neurogenic bladder and hydrocephalus. If the lesion is operable, shortly after birth most babies with a myelomeningocele will undergo operation to repair the back lesion. About seven to 10 days later the ICP has usually increased and a ventriculo-peritoneal shunt is inserted. These shunts frequently require revision especially within the first year of insertion (Sainte-Rose *et al.* 1989). The child will need long-term orthopaedic care which may include operations to correct orthopaedic deformities of the lower limbs and possibly also the kyphoscoliosis. The neurogenic bladder will require long-term management, probably by intermittent catheteris-ation, but many children also have operative procedures performed on the bladder and ureteric orifices.

The parents of a fetus with a myelomeningocele need to be given all these facts. They should also have the opportunity to discuss the implications of the ultrasound scan findings in their child with the appropriate specialists, so that they can make an informed decision about whether to terminate the pregnancy or allow it to continue to term.

EXPERIMENTAL STUDIES

In the laboratory no attempt has yet been made to carry out intrauterine repair of experimentally induced myelomeningoceles. However, fetal monkeys (Michejda *et al.* 1983) and sheep (Manning *et al.* 1984) have had their spinal cord exposed by lumbar laminectomy. Later some of the fetuses had the bony defect repaired with bone paste. In these animals rapid remodelling of the posterior vertebral arches took place and their spinal cords developed normally. The bone did not regenerate in the untreated fetuses, and the prolonged exposure of their spinal cords led to

33

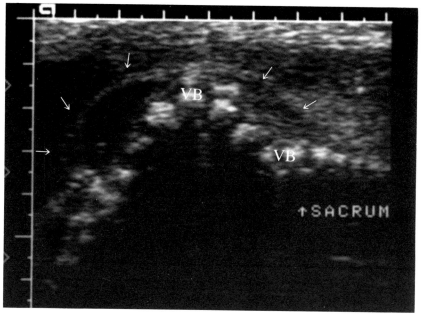

Fig. 2.9. Sagittal ultrasonograph of a fetus with myelomeningocele at the thoracolumbar junction. There is marked kyphosis at the level of the lesion. The dome of the cyst is indicated by the arrows. BV = the centres of ossification in the bodies of the vertebrae.

abnormalities which caused motor and sensory deficits in the lower limbs. It is difficult to assess the relevance of these findings to human fetuses with myelomeningoceles. The lesions in the laboratory animals were created at a relatively late stage of pregnancy, whereas myelomeningoceles develop in the embryological period. The response of the neuroplaque to closure of the bony canal is unlikely to be the same as that of the spinal cord. More laboratory investigations are needed to confirm and extend these observations before intrauterine intervention is considered for human fetuses with myelomeningoceles.

MANAGEMENT OF A FETUS WITH A MYELOMENINGOCELE

Shurtleff (1986) suggested that all fetuses with myelomeningoceles should be delivered by caesarean section because of the possibility that exposed neural tissue may be damaged during vaginal delivery. However, it has yet to be proved that neural tissue in the neuroplaque has significant function, and therefore it is difficult to justify subjecting the mother on these grounds to the risks of a caesarean section.

Currently, therefore, there are no positive indications for changing the present policy of management of fetuses with myelomeningoceles. If the condition is diagnosed early enough the parents have the option of terminating the pregnancy. If the diagnosis is made too late for this, the pregnancy is allowed to continue to term, and after delivery the baby is assessed for suitability for repair of the back lesion. A ventriculo-peritoneal shunt is inserted when the ICP rises.

Meningoceles

In a meningocele, membranes protrude through a defect in the posterior arch of the spinal column where the spines and laminae of one or two vertebrae have failed to develop. The open spinal gutter is shorter and narrower than that of most myelomeningoceles. Meningoceles occur anywhere along the length of the spine, but like myelomeningoceles they are commonest below the mid-thoracic level. Because of the absence of neural tissue in the lesion, patients with meningoceles do not generally have weakness or loss of sensation in the legs, and their bladder and bowel function is usually normal. Some patients have the Arnold-Chiari malformation and a few develop hydrocephalus requiring the insertion of a ventriculo-peritoneal shunt.

Meningoceles can be diagnosed during fetal life by ultrasound scans (Fig. 2.9). Because of their good prognosis, it is essential to distinguish them from myelomeningoceles. Even though the number of vertebrae involved in a meningocele is often smaller and the gutter narrower than in a myelomeningocele, the membranous sac may be very large. It is often possible to exclude on ultrasound examination the presence of a neuroplaque and nerves crossing the cavity of the cyst. The legs should not be seen to have orthopaedic deformities.

The parents of a fetus with a meningocele need to have these facts explained so that they can decide how the pregnancy should be managed. A baby born with a meningocele will almost certainly require an operation to repair the back lesion shortly after birth, and if s/he develops hydrocephalus a ventriculo-peritoneal shunt will have to be inserted. But it must be emphasised to the parents that the prognosis from the point of view of mental and physical development is very favourable compared to that of a child with a myelomeningocele.

The future

In the last 50 years spectacular advances in the field of medicine have breached what were once thought to be impenetrable barriers. The heart and brain are no longer 'untouchable'. The fetus, wrapped up in the protective covering of the uterus, has resisted longer but is now yielding too. The first tentative steps in intrauterine intervention were rewarded with great success. Blood transfusions and the administration of medications have meant that fetuses once doomed to die are now born and go on to develop into fit and healthy children. Early achievements paved the way for bolder and more innovative procedures. So far only limited success has been achieved by treating CNS lesions, but it is hoped that hydrocephalus, spinal lesions and brain tumours among others will eventually be treated successfully. The answer may lie in transuterine laser surgery, remote-controlled computer-directed probes, or more likely in something not yet conceived.

REFERENCES

Awost, J., Levi, S. (1984) 'New aspects of fetal dynamics with a special emphasis on eye movements.' *Ultrasound in Medical Biology*, **10**, 107–116.

Bannister, C.M., Chapman, S.A. (1986) 'Response of the fetal rat brain to trauma during the 17th to 21st day of gestation.' *Developmental Medicine and Child Neurology*, **28**, 600–609.

—— —— (1987) 'Outcome of unilateral occipital lobectomy on the 100th day of gestation in fetal lambs.' *British Journal of Neurosurgery*, **1**, 353–358.

—— Cranley, J.J., Turnbull, I.W., Weller, J., Koutsoubelis, G. (1991) 'A comparison of healing of lesions in the calvarium of fetal lambs and young sheep.' *Neurological Research*, **13**, 107–112.

Barson, A.J. (1970) 'Spina bifida: the significance of the level and extent of the defect to the morphogenesis.' *Developmental Medicine and Child Neurology*, **12**, 129–144.

Berkowitz, R.L., Chitkara, U., Wilkins, I.A., Lynch, L., Mehalek, K.E. (1987) 'Technical aspects of intravascular intrauterine transfusions. Lessons learned from 33 procedures.' *American Journal of Obstetrics and Gynecology*, **157**, 4–9.

Bray, P.F. (1972) 'Mumps—a cause of hydrocephalus?' *Pediatrics*, **49**, 446–450.

Birnholtz, J.C., Frigoletto, F.D. (1981) 'Antenatal treatment of hydrocephalus.' *New England Journal of Medicine*, **303**, 1021–1023.

Campbell, S., Smith, P., Pearce, J.M. (1983) 'The ultra-sound diagnosis of neural tube defects and other cranio-spinal abnormalities.' *In* Rodeck, C.H., Nicolaides, K.H. (Eds) *Prenatal Diagnosis*. Chichester: Wiley. pp. 245–257.

Chapman, S.A., Bannister, C.M. (1989) 'Effect of excision of the occipital lobe on about the 70th day of gestation on the growth and development of the sheep's brain.' *Surgical Neurology*, **32**, 98–104.

Christie, A.D., Ivory, C.M. (1984) 'Fetal measurements.' *In* Bennett, M.J. (Ed.) *Ultrasound in Perinatal Care (Perinatal Practice, Vol. 1)*. Chichester: Wiley. pp. 35–48.

Clewell, W.H. (1988) 'Congenital hydrocephalus: treatment in utero.' *Fetal Therapy*, **3**, 89–97.

—— Johnson, M.L., Meier, P.R., Newkirk, J.B., Zide, S.L., Hendee, R.W., Bowes, W.A., Hecht, F., O'Keefe, D., Henry, G.P., Shikes, R.H. (1982) 'A surgical approach to the treatment of fetal hydrocephalus.' *New England Journal of Medicine*, **306**, 1820–1825.

Cosmi, E.V., Di Renzo, G.C. (1989) 'Prevention and treatment of fetal lung immaturity.' *Fetal Therapy*, **4** (Suppl. 1), 52–62.

Davis, L.E. (1981) 'Communicating hydrocephalus in newborn hamsters and cats following caccinia virus infections.' *Journal of Neurosurgery*, **54**, 767–772.

De Crespigny, L.C., Robinson, H.P., Quinn, M., Doyle, L., Ross, A., Cauchi, M. (1985) 'Ultrasound-guided fetal blood transfusion for severe Rhesus isoimmunization.' *Obstetrics and Gynecology*, **66**, 529–532.

Edwards, M.S.B., Harrison, M.R., Halks-Miller, M., Nakayama, D.K., Berger, M.S., Glick, P.L., Chinn, D.H. (1984) 'Kaolin-induced congenital hydrocephalus in utero in fetal lambs and rhesus monkeys.' *Journal of Neurosurgery*, **60**, 115–122.

Frigoletto, F.D., Birnholtz, J.C., Greene, M.F. (1982) 'Antenatal treatment of hydrocephalus by ventriculoamniotic shunting.' *Journal of the American Medical Association*, **248**, 2496–2499.

Glick, P.L., Harrison, M.R., Golbus, M.S., Adzick, N.S., Filly, R.A., Callen, P.W., Mahony, B.S., Anderson, R.L. (1985) 'Management of the fetus with congenital hydronephrosis. II. Prognostic criteria and selection for treatment.' *Journal of Pediatric Surgery*, **20**, 376–387.

Grannum, P.A.T., Copel, J.A., Moya, F.R., Scioscia, A.L., Robert, J.A., Winn, H.N., Cosier, B.C., Burdine, C.B., Hobbins, J.C. (1988) 'The reversal of hydrops fetalis by intravascular intrauterine transfusion in severe isoimmune fetal anemia.' *American Journal of Obstetrics*, **158**, 914–919.

Harrison, M.R., Golbus, M.S., Filly, R.A., Callen, P.W., Katz, M., De Lorimier, A.A., Rosen, M., Jonsen, A.R. (1982) 'Fetal surgery for congenital hydronephrosis.' *New England Journal of Medicine*, **306**, 591–593.

Hanigan, C.H., Gibson, J., Kleopoulos, N.J., Cusack, T., Zwicky, G., Wright, R.M. (1986) 'Medical imaging of fetal ventriculomegaly.' *Journal of Neurosurgery*, **64**, 575–580.

Hill, M.C., Lande, I.M., Larsen, J.W. (1988) 'Prenatal diagnosis of fetal anomalies using ultrasound and MRI.' *The Radiologic Clinics of North America, Vol. 26*. Philadelphia: W.B. Saunders. pp. 287–307.

Hoving, E.W. (1990) 'Separation of neural and surface ectoderm in relation to the pathogenesis of encephaloceles.' *Zeitschrift für Kinderchirurgie*, **45**, 40.

Ianniruberto, A., Tejani, E. (1981) 'Ultrasonographic study of fetal movements.' *Seminars in Perinatology*, **5**, 175–181.

Kirkinen, P., Suramo, I., Jouppila, P., Herua, R. (1982) 'Combined use of ultrasound and computed tomography in the evaluation of fetal intracranial abnormality.' *Journal of Perinatal Medicine*, **10**, 257–265.

Krummell, T.M., Nelson, J.M., Dieglemann, R.F., Lindblad, W.J., Salzberg, A.M., Greenfield, L.J., Cohen, I.K. (1982) 'Wound healing in fetal and neonatal rabbits.' *Surgical Forum*, **37**, 595–596.

Lemery, D., Urbain, M.-F., Micorek, J.-C., Jacquetin, B. (1988) 'Fetal umbilical cord catheterization under ultrasound guidance.' *Fetal Therapy*, **3**, 37–43.

Lipman, S.P., Pretorius, D.H., Rumack, C.M., Manco-Jonson, M.C. (1985) 'Fetal intracranial teratoma: US diagnosis of three cases and a review of the literature.' *Radiology*, **157**, 491–494.

Longaker, M.T., Chiu, E.S., Harrison, M.R., Crombleholme, T.M., Langer, J.C., Duncan, B.W., Adzick, N.S., Verrier, E.D., Stern, R. (1989) 'Studies in fetal wound healing. VI. Hyaluronic acid-stimulating activity distinguishes fetal wound fluid from adult fluid.' *Annals of Surgery*, **210**, 667–672.

—— Adzick, N.S., Hall, J.L., Stair, S.E., Crombleholme, T.M., Duncan, B.W., Bradley, S.M., Harrison, M.R., Stern, R. (1990) 'Studies in fetal wound healing. VII. Fetal wound healing may be modulated by hyaluronic acid stimulating activity in amniotic fluid.' *Journal of Pediatric Surgery*, **25**, 430–433.

Lorber, J., Bassi, U. (1965) 'The etiology of neonatal hydrocephalus (excluding cases with spina bifida).' *Developmental Medicine and Child Neurology*, **7**, 289–294.

Luthy, D.W., Wardinsky, T., Shurtleff, D.B., Hollenbach, K.A., Hickok, D.E., Nyberg, D.A., Benedetti, T.J. (1991) 'Cesarean section before the onset of labor and subsequent motor function in infants with meningomyelocele diagnosed antenatally.' *New England Journal of Medicine*, **324**, 662–666.

Manning, F.A., Harman, C.R., Lange, I.R. (1984) 'Experimental surgical ovine fetal neural tube defect: preliminary observation.' *Paper presented at the Annual Meeting of the Society of Obstetricians and Gynecologists, Montreal*.

—— Harrison, M.R., Rodeck, C. and Members of the International Fetal Medicine and Surgical Society (1986) 'Catheter shunts for fetal hydronephrosis and hydrocephalus. Report of the International Fetal Surgery Registry.' New England Journal of Medicine, **315**, 336–340.

McCullough, D.C. (1989) 'Hydrocephalus: etiology, pathologic effets, diagnosis, and natural history.' *In* McLaurin, R.L., Venes, J.L., Schut, L., Epstein, F. (Eds) *Pediatric Neurosurgery, 2nd Edn*. Philadelphia: W.B. Saunders. pp. 180–199.

Michejda, M., McCullough, D., Bacher, J., Queenan, J.T. (1983) 'Investigational approaches in fetal neurosurgery.' In Humphreys, R.P. (Ed.) *Concepts in Pediatric Neurosurgery 4*. Basel: Karger. pp. 44–54.

—— Petronas, N., DiCharo, G., Hogden, C. (1984) 'Amelioration of fetal porencephaly in utero therapy in nonhuman primates.' *Journal of the American Medical Association*, **251**, 2548–2558.

Nicolaides, K., Soothill, P., Rodeck, C., Clewell, W (1986a) 'Rh disease: intravascular fetal blood transfusion by cordocentesis.' *Fetal Therapy*, **1**, 185–192.

—— Campbell, S., Gabbe, S.G., Guidetti, R. (1986b) 'Ultrasound screening for spina bifida: cranial and cerebellar signs.' *Lancet*, **2**, 72–74.

Olund, A., Torell, S., Bistoletti, P., Kraepelien, T., Somell, C. (1983) 'Diagnosis in utero of congenital hydrocephalus by sonography and computerized tomography.' *Acta Obstetrica et Gynecologica Scandinavica*, **63**, 325–327.

Patterson, J.A., Gold, W.R., Sanz, L.E., McCullough, D.C. (1981) 'Antenatal evaluation of fetal hydrocephalus with computed tomography.' *American Journal of Obstetrics and Gynecology*, **140**, 344–345.

Pilu, G. (1986) 'Prenatal diagnosis of central nervous system abnormalities.' *Fetal Therapy*, **1**, 73–74.

Pretorius, D.H., Davis, K., Manco-Johnson, M.L. (1985) 'Clinical course of fetal hydrocephalus: 40 cases.' *American Journal of Neuroradiology*, **6**, 23–27.

Roberts, A.B., Clarkson, P.M., Pattison, N.S., Jamieson, M.G., Mok, P.M. (1986) 'Fetal hydrothorax in the second trimester of pregnancy: successful intra-uterine treatment at 24 weeks gestation.' *Fetal*

Therapy, **1**, 203–209.
Sainte-Rose, C., Hoffman, H.J., Hirsch, J.F. (1989) 'Shunt failure.' *In* Malin, A.E. (Ed.) *Concepts in Pediatric Neurosurgery 9*. Basel: Karger. pp. 7–20.
Sanders, R.C., James, A.E. (1985) *The Principles and Practice of Ultrasonography in Obstetrics and Gynecology. 3rd Edn.* New York: Appleton-Century-Crofts.
Shurtleff, D.B. (1986) 'Meningomyelocele: a new or a vanishing disease?' *Zeitschrift für Kinderchirurgie*, **41** (Suppl. I), 5–9.
Siebert, J.W., Burd, D.A., McCarthy, J.C., Weinzweig, J., Ehrlich, H.P. (1990) 'Fetal wound healing: a biochemical study of scarless healing.' *Plastic and Reconstructive Surgery*, **85**, 455–502.
Somasundaram, K., Prathap, K. (1972) 'The effect of exclusion of amniotic fluid on intra-uterine healing of skin wounds in rabbits.' *Journal of Pathology*, **107**, 127–130.
Stewart, P.A., Wladimiroff, J.W. (1987) 'Cardiac tachyarrythmia in the fetus: diagnosis, treatment and prognosis.' *Fetal Therapy*, **2**, 7–16.
Strauss, R.P., Davis, J.U. (1990) 'Prenatal detection and fetal surgery of clefts and craniofacial abnormalities in humans.' *Fetal Surgery*, **27**, 176–183.
Truccone, N.J., Mariona, F.D. (1986) 'Prenatal diagnosis and outcome of congenital complete heart block: the role of fetal echocardiography.' *Fetal Therapy*, **1**, 210–216.
Vitzileos, A.M., Ingardia, C.J., Nochimson, D.J. (1983) 'Congenital hydrocephalus: a review and protocol for perinatal management.' *Obstetrics and Gynecology*, **62**, 539–549.
Warsof, S.L., Griffin, D. (1984) 'The diagnosis of fetal anomalies.' *In* Bennett, M.J. (Ed.) *Ultrasound in Perinatal Care (Perinatal Practice: Vol. 1)*. Chichester: Wiley. pp. 75–102.
—— Abramowicz, J.S., Sayegh, S.K., Levy, D.L. (1988) 'Lower limb movements and urologic function in fetuses with neural tube defects.' Fetal Therapy, **3**, 129–134.
Williamson, R.A., Schauberger, C.W., Varner, M.W. (1981) 'Heterogeneity of prenatal onset of hydrocephalus: management and counselling implications.' *American Journal of Medical Genetics*, **18**, 105–110.

3
FETAL ABNORMALITY MANAGEMENT GROUPS

M. J. A. Maresh

All pregnant women are concerned about the possibility of their baby being abnormal. This is rarely expressed until delivery, when the mother asks the midwife whether her baby is all right. The woman who is found to have an abnormal fetus in pregnancy has extreme levels of anxiety. The average consultant obstetrician in a district general hospital can rarely assuage this anxiety, however, having limited knowledge about the current state of management of the wide range of fetal anomalies which are now being suggested by district ultrasound services. Accordingly there is a need for a regional referral unit—a fetal abnormality management group. Although sometimes the group can act as a telephone advisory service, more usually the woman needs to be seen by the group to give a definitive diagnosis. Once the diagnosis has been made, the various scenarios for outcome can be given and the couple can be offered support for the rest of pregnancy and afterwards. Since currently no fetal therapy is being offered in cases of spina bifida or hydrocephalus, the only options are termination of the pregnancy and planned delivery.

Assessment of a fetus with an abnormality can only be performed by a multidisciplinary group of senior clinicians who have built up expertise and knowledge which can be used for managing these cases. The main disciplines of the group include radiology, obstetrics, paediatric medicine, paediatric surgery and genetics. With certain fetal abnormalities subspecialists in specific paediatric aspects will be required and with spina bifida and hydrocephalus this will be the paediatric neurosurgeon. The service needs an efficient clerical administrator to ensure rapid appointments are made and that follow-up information is obtained. S/he may also be needed to locate the referring clinician by telephone to discuss management directly. A midwife is an asset to the group for a number of reasons. S/he can act as general counsellor, and can reiterate to the couple any aspects they did not manage to take in when first hearing of them from a clinician. S/he can discuss specific midwifery aspects, such as breast-feeding after surgery, and s/he can act as a nurse to help with invasive procedures. It is important for the group to have facilities for couples to be alone to think and talk between themselves in an unhurried way. Frequently they will have travelled some distance and may not feel like going home straight away.

Certain other facilities are required. A high-quality diagnostic ultrasound machine is essential. The addition of a duplex doppler facility, although helpful for some abnormalities, is of little benefit in spina bifida and hydrocephalus. The machine must be dedicated for the group's work during their sessions so that no pressure is put on hurrying through the diagnostic scanning, which may be lengthy since a full fetal anomaly scan must be performed to look for other abnormalities. The group also needs access to various laboratory services (*e.g.* cytogenetics for chromosomal analysis, and specialised biochemistry for the determination of the lecithin: sphingomyelin ratio to estimate lung maturity).

The majority of women will be confused when they arrive. It needs to be explained to them that the first stage is a detailed ultrasound scan to determine whether indeed there are any problems with the fetus and if so the extent of them. Cases of anencephaly are rarely seen, as there is not usually any doubt at the patient's own district hospital.

Karyotyping of the fetus is not usually necessary antenatally unless there is doubt about the ultrasound diagnosis. This may occasionally occur with differentiation between a cystic hygroma and an encephalocoele. Since amniocentesis takes about three weeks for the results from karyotyping the cultured fetal fibroblasts, an alternative method is necessary. A placental biopsy can be taken under direct ultrasound guidance. The standard method is to use a double needle technique with the outer (17 or 18g) sheath being placed into the placenta and the inner needle (19 or 20g) being moved in and out of the placenta with syringe suction aspiration. If sufficient chorionic villi are not obtained the first time, the inner needle is put back through the outer sheath and the procedure repeated. A direct preparation of the chorionic villi can give a result within 48 hours. These direct preparations are not always of a high quality and cytogeneticists prefer to confirm the result by culturing the cells, which will typically give a further week's delay. Placental preparations are time-consuming for the cytogeneticist so a fetal blood sample taken from the umbilical cord using ultrasound guidance has an advantage. This is more difficult to obtain than a placental biopsy and therefore is likely to put the fetus at more risk. However the obstetrician in a regional fetal management group should be able to offer this service. All these invasive techniques are associated with an increased risk of miscarriage. The procedure-related risk of amniocentesis is about 0.5 per cent and this rises to 1 to 2 per cent for fetal cord blood sampling. Accordingly if karyotyping is advised the couple need to be counselled about these risks and have time to think before making a decision.

Having made a diagnosis counselling must be given, with all the relevant specialties working together closely allows for the most knowledgeable to give the advice. With spina bifida and hydrocephalus the paediatric neurosurgeon, *i.e.* the person who operates and follows up these children, is in the best position to give unbiased information to the couple. The obstetrician needs to outline the two immediate management options, namely termination or continuation of the pregnancy, since in this area no specific fetal therapy is currently available. Again the couple will need time to be alone to consider the options and will want to ask further questions. Couples usually think that it was their fault that their baby had an abnormality. Accordingly they need to be reassured strongly that it was not. They may want to talk about implications for future pregnancies. If they wish to speak to a clinical geneticist this should be arranged, but in these conditions any discussion at this stage about recurrence and possible prevention can normally be with one of the other clinicians and a subsequent genetics consultation left as optional. Since most couples are already aware of a strong possibility of their baby having an abnormality and may already have had some counselling at their district hospital they may be able to make a decision straight away. Alternatively arrangements may need to be made for another appointment to answer further questions, and the couple can be given the telephone number of one of the team.

If pregnancy is to be terminated, it should be done without delay. A miscarriage is induced using prostaglandins. Vaginal pessaries appear best since they do not involve the immobility of an infusion pump or the nursing care involved in running it and yet are as effective as an extra-amniotic infusion. The abortion is usually completed within 24 hours, but may require a general anaesthetic to remove retained placental material. It is vital that the abortion is performed this way, rather than by a destructive method such as dilatation and evacuation, so that the fetus can be examined by a experienced pathologist to confirm the diagnosis. For this reason the abortions are often carried out at the regional unit to ensure that a thorough examination of the fetus takes place.

If the pregnancy is to continue, it should be managed in the most normal way possible. Regular ultrasound should be performed to monitor any development of hydrocephalus. Elective preterm delivery should be considered if hydrocephalus appears to be worsening. Fetal lung maturity may be accelerated by intramuscular maternal steroid injections. Lung maturity should be assessed by amniocentesis and measurement of the lecithin : sphingomyelin ratio before any intervention prior to 37 weeks gestation. Most women assume that if their baby has an abnormality it is best delivered by caesarean section. If the fetal head is significantly enlarged by hydrocephalus then a caesarean section will be required, but otherwise it is not specifically needed. Elective caesarean section or elective induction (provided the cervix is favourable) at 38 weeks may be performed for the convenience of the neurosurgeon.

One of the major roles of a fetal abnormality management group is to perform research and development in fetal medicine and surgery. Such work is aided by the multidisciplinary nature of the group. Others are needed such as an anaesthetist skilled in maternal and neonatal anaesthetic techniques. In addition animal work is necessary before introducing certain *in utero* fetal procedures, so members of the group need to have skills in this field or to have a collaborating experimental team.

Follow-up of all cases diagnosed antenatally by the fetal abnormality group is essential. A computerised system is ideal since this can generate reminders and produce reports by condition. However, whether a computerised or manual method is used, considerable effort is still needed to trace the outcome of all pregnancies. It is necessary to audit the accuracy of the initial diagnosis by clinical, diagnostic or pathological means. The grade of problem also needs confirmation to audit the predictive value of the ultrasound. If an invasive procedure such as cord sampling for fetal karyotyping has been performed, not only does an audit need to be performed of the cytogenetics service, but also of fetal, neonatal and maternal complications of the actual procedure. In such a field it is also wise to obtain some feedback via structured and unstructured response from the couples to look for ways to improve the sensitivity of the service.

In addition to regular group meetings to discuss results and review developments, members of the group need to meet groups in adjacent regions to review results. They need to compare their own audit results to ensure an acceptable service is being provided by all groups. They may need to pool the results of rarer conditions in order to gain more understanding of the natural history of the condition, and they may need to collaborate in order to obtain sufficient numbers for clinical trials. Finally, they may wish to collaborate about certain specific abnormalities so that the experimental work is all done by one group, and cases are transferred between groups where feasible.

In conclusion, fetal abnormality management groups are a way of ensuring that a comprehensive and caring service is provided and that research into reducing morbidity can develop further.

4
THE PSYCHOLOGICAL SEQUELAE AND MANAGEMENT OF PERINATAL DEATH AND FETAL MALFORMATION

Stanford Bourne and Emanuel Lewis

Mourning

After a perinatal death, mourning sometimes merges into persistent depression or various psychological problems like hypochondria or phobias (Giles 1970, Cullberg 1972). Some of the most important effects, however, are delayed and long-term. A subsequent normal pregnancy is reassuring, but people should be forewarned that complicated feelings may be reactivated, sometimes with unexpected severe puerperal disturbances. The wound may also be reopened at anniversaries or at any later bereavement or family crisis. Marriage and sexuality are strained by the climate of blame, anxiety and conflict. Fathers carry much of the distress, often unnoticed and unhelped, and are liable to become angry and touchy.

Children are stressed when the parents are least able to cope with it. As well as neurotic disturbances and behaviour disorders, there is the risk of profound effects upon the personality in surviving children. Paradoxically, child abuse is sometimes provoked (Lewis 1979a, Benedict *et al.* 1985). Often the next baby, conceived hastily as 'replacement child' (see p. 44) is born around the first anniversary. Some of the most important effects emerge when the children grow up and have their own children, to whom obscure images and fears are somehow conveyed.

There are also effects on doctors and nurses. The atmosphere of failure, blame and bewilderment involves staff as well as patients. The best intentions on all sides may capsize. People find themselves evasive, forgetful, clumsy and unappreciated. Contact can be most difficult when it is most needed (Bourne 1968). Ill health and absence from work are hazards for people carrying too much of the burden unsupported.

Childbirth is liable to be mysterious and painful even at the best of times. This complicates the mourning of any death in the family during pregnancy. Perinatal deaths are particularly bewildering as birth and death are fused into one experience. The situation is worse if there is also fetal abnormality.

It can help to consider theoretical aspects of normal and pathological mourning. Mourning involves coming to terms with what has happened and sorting out mixed feelings and lost hopes so that, eventually, memories of the death recede to a healthy perspective (Freud 1917). At first the bereaved person's inner world is occupied with conscious and unconscious images of the body and mind and illness of the dead, all of which contribute to the malaise. It is even more distressing to feel inhabited by a dead malformed fetus. Adversely, this may develop into hypochondria or psychosomatic illness. Eventually there will be normal forgetting and normal remembering but if mourning fails, a brittle type of forgetting belies a troubled preoccupation, a haunted state of mind. In an apparently easy recovery, there can remain a hidden vulnerability to subsequent traumas.

Difficulties arise when the loss is hard to comprehend because of uncertain and mystifying circumstances. Other difficulties arise from the confusion of good and bad feelings about the dead person and any unusual horror or revulsion concerned with the death (Parkes and Weiss 1983). Difficulty is caused by the reactivation of previous losses, just as later losses will be liable to reactivate this one. The unexpected re-emergence, in an adult, of long-forgotten infantile reactions to loss is particularly difficult to accommodate (Klein 1963).

Mourning is even more difficult around pregnancy than at other times. The complex motivation for pregnancy, together with the associated unconscious fantasies, collide with the mourning process (Bibring *et al.* 1961, Benedek 1970 1970, Kestenberg 1977, Blum 1980). This goes beyond the obvious problem of confronting death and birth at the same time. There are many reasons for becoming pregnant and the wish for pregnancy is not always the same as a wish to have a child. Some men repeatedly impregnate women yet have no interest in fatherhood. Some women are compulsively pregnant and become depressed when they have to stop, yet they may not be devoted mothers. Sometimes the addiction is to having a babe in arms, a baby at the breast, and interest is lost as the child grows up. The puerperium is generally psychiatrically hazardous (Kendell *et al.* 1987) and mild depression is very common—due probably to a mixture of physiological and psychological factors (the arguments remain inconclusive).

For those made vulnerable by ill health or previous losses, especially by loss in childhood or in the preceding generation, having a baby may be a source of reassurance and a healer of wounds. All may then be well if the baby is well, but if the baby is malformed and dies there is much else to contend with beside the immediate experience. Grave disturbance comes from the collapse of the hopes and ideas that the birth of the baby was conceived to sustain. Then, rather than just seeing a person mourning a death, we may be dealing with something more like a structure crumbling, the collapse of a personality and its defences.

A pregnancy is usually a happy event, but may also be tied up with primitive quasi-magical ideas of a life for a life. It is commonplace for any death in the family to be followed by a replacement pregnancy. So if the baby dies, it is as if the recent dead have died over again. It can be felt that a dead malformed baby is mocking procreation and defiling sexuality. Insofar as a replacement pregnancy tends to involve a facile belief in renewal rather than a secure sense of hard-earned careful reparation, a further failure can have an exacerbated effect on the bereaved parents. There is fury at the failure of magical hopes as well as guilt at having aspired to them.

A supervening pregnancy tends to cut mourning short. A death occurring during pregnancy is harder to mourn than at other times. The normal healing process of mourning is impeded and then depression and other symptoms can result (Lewis 1979b). Expectation of a new baby collides with the stance necessary for preoccupation with a death, necessary for healthy mourning to develop. However, the clash between mourning and expecting a baby is only one side of the problem. The other side involves paradoxical similarities between mourning and the state of 'primary maternal preoccupation' in expectation of a new baby (Winnicott 1958). Thoughts are turned towards an inner world, occupied in one case by the new baby developing, and in the other by a death. Primary maternal preoccupation moves towards the state of devotion in which a mother will normally receive her new baby at the end of pregnancy; whereas the mourning process enables us to lay to rest and relinquish someone who has gone. It can seem impossible to cope with both processes at once, and normally the new baby receives priority; mourning may be postponed, to be reactivated by some later crisis.

All this suggests that after any perinatal death the next pregnancy should be postponed until mourning has been completed, and in particular the conception of a baby to be born near the first anniversary should be avoided. Puerperal disturbances in the next pregnancies may be severe and unexpected (Bourne and Lewis 1984).

Children's perceptions

Infantile fantasy-life has a powerful bearing on the psychopathology around fetal malformation. Even in happy families, it is quite normal for children to envy the mother's baby-making capacity, to resent siblings and to imagine harming rival babies inside the mother: anxious thoughts which may seem to be confirmed by a stillbirth happening (Leon 1990). Normally, good feelings and successful childbirth are adequate antidotes to the darker side of us (Klein 1932, Segal 1973).

Young children are deeply curious about how to make a baby and have theories, fantasies and dreams about it. When parents are devastated by fetal loss, they may find it difficult to cope with their child's state of mind, questions and fears. Indeed most adults have great difficulty in talking to young children about such a death. Children rarely see the body of the dead baby and this makes it harder to correct disturbing fantasies and misconceptions. The secrecy and mystery about the making of a baby is intensified by the sudden disappearance of the body from inside the mother. A child may imagine that it has been stolen. These ideas are magnified by the mother's own fears and conflicts. Some children run away from home, others become intensely clinging.

Children know that babies grow in their mother's tummy and small babies begin with no knowledge of any world other than the mother's body. The ingredients for baby-making in the infant's world are the only ingredients s/he knows much about—food, drink, excreta and body parts. Babies are made from substances and those likely to be of use are food, the products of digestion and body substances in general. The infantile suspicion that babies are made of faeces is 'supported' by learning or guessing where a baby comes out of the mother's body, with similarities to defaecation. Such ideas persist and inform the anxieties and symptoms of children (and even adults) trying to digest the experience of a malformed baby born and dying, and can lead to constipation, soiling, stomach ache and other hypochondriacal symptoms.

Children envy the mother's baby-making capacity. Unable to make their own baby, infants may imagine stealing their mother's baby. This urge is also mixed up with unconscious fantasies of jealous attacks on the rival baby inside the mother. A tiny child's conscious and unconscious ideas about stealing babies may be imagined as a piecemeal dismembering of the fetus inside the mother, to be rebuilt inside the child himself. In fetal abnormality it is as if the reconstructions go awry.

When an abnormal baby is unlikely to have a good independent life, few people could avoid thoughts and wishes that it might die. It may make it easier to accept the death on a rational basis if it is thought that this baby is better off dead. Nevertheless, such thoughts feel wrong and carry an undercurrent of intense unease, with the risk of a guilty depressive reaction, especially when entangled with unconscious conflict and infantile fantasy. Such reactions may go underground and await reactivation at some later loss, or perhaps at a subsequent birth.

Adult ideas and emotions about the possible real reasons for a malformed baby are mixed up with unconscious residual memories from childhood fantasy about how babies are made and destroyed. We do not totally grow out of infantile ideas of babies stolen, babies made of faeces, babies endangered or even killed from envy and jealousy. All these ideas are a potential source of guilty anguish when a pregnancy has gone wrong and they generate some of the irrational and exaggerated responses that are so common.

Such unconscious fantasies, incredible in daylight, are common to us all and the Frankenstein story may have such fascination because it makes play with these frightening ideas. Doctor Frankenstein built his monster from parts of bodies stolen from a graveyard. The mother's womb has become a graveyard and robbed, but the reconstruction has gone wrong. Mary Shelley, who created the Frankenstein story, had the desperate experience of her own mother dying in childbirth with another baby.

Management

Coping with emotions

Although there is no panacea, it may be easier to contain the most troublesome reactions if they can be recognised clearly. In addition to the bewildering collision of birth and death, the feelings of unreality and perplexity are aggravated by the strangeness of congenital malformation itself and by the abnormal circumstances of general anaesthetics, caesarean section—and by staff embarrassment, evasiveness and other mismanagement.

Anger and quarrelsomeness are features of mourning, often unreasonable, with old grievances being reactivated. As with all obstetric abnormalities, matters easily escalate into fruitless recrimination and litigation. Marriages break up. There is understandable envy of more fortunate people with healthy babies. It may be less easy to spot envy disguised as futile spitefulness. A great danger is the destructive aspect of envy, the urge to spoil what somebody else has, and it may then feel like revenge or punishment when a person's own baby is malformed and dies.

Then there is jealousy, the possessive feeling about somebody or something loved. Parents of a malformed or dead baby can feel as if they have been robbed or betrayed. They may be puzzled at their own seemingly irrational anger with the dead baby. Jealous possessiveness causes clinging, and may have something to do with the dreadful syndromes of relentless clinging to a loss and to grievances. Shame is the feeling of an outcast, the person who cannot show his face from feelings of humiliation and degradation. Space and privacy are needed for normal mourning but shame can lead to exaggerated withdrawal. The well known dilemma about offering a side room is connected with this. It may be a relief to hide, but feeling shut away from everybody else may also add to the humiliation. The problem may later escalate into agoraphobia.

Guilt and shame are often entangled, but guilt has more to do with ideas of wrong-doing and punishment whereas shame is connected with feelings of being inferior and unacceptable to everybody else. Shame leads to hiding whereas guilt may invite punishment—sometimes leading to such delinquent behaviour as shoplifting and getting caught and punished. Guilt and self-reproach are prominent features of such depressive states. Less obviously, feelings may be reversed and channelled into complaints about other 'guilty' people.

Support groups
Beyond concern and compassion, the aim must be to minimise the inevitable bewilderment and confusion. It may be hard to stay in contact, especially since the bereft parents may feel inclined to withdraw, uncertain whether they feel diseased, ashamed, guilty or angry. Self-help groups such as the Stillbirth and Neonatal Death Society (SANDS) and Support After Termination for Fetal Abnormality (SATFA) may be invaluable. Every person involved in this field should obtain a copy of their guidelines for professionals (SANDS 1991). This indispensable 80-page booklet discusses management options and dilemmas at every stage from diagnosis in early pregnancy to the provision and use of photographs, books of remembrance and support for professional staff. Although many details of funeral procedure and documentation are specific to the UK, most of the guidelines would be applicable everywhere; and, indeed, religious and ethnic differences are discussed, including problems of language difficulties and the use of interpreters.

There is no single right way of going about this, and staff require as much mutual support as possible to cope with their own feelings of pain and failure, as well as the feelings of the patients. Most staff are unlikely to have enough experience of dealing with fatal congenital abnormalities, and shared experience and support is vital. Staff dysfunction often leads to fragmentation of care and responsibility which is liable to exacerbate the problems, especially the tendency to cover up (Menzies 1960).

Disclosing the death is grim work but women carrying a dead baby often know before the doctors. It is sensible to share information as soon as possible without evasiveness, but tact and decorum are necessary. It may be better to delay a little, rather than blurt things out, if it conveys thoughtfulness and care. The exact manner of breaking the bad news may be less important than the way staff stay with it and remain accessible. It is seldom a good idea to designate one person in the unit who is 'good at talking to patients who are upset'. It overburdens the individual and leaves something wrong with the position of everybody else. (Specialist counselling or psychotherapy later on, if necessary, is quite another matter.)

Effects on the family
An awareness of different options and a sense of what is not being done may be more helpful than the vain hope of getting it right. Delaying the news, while the father arrives, may be misunderstood as devaluing of the mother or being afraid of facing her on her own. Yet telling the mother by herself inevitably causes the father to feel 'left out', and the mother may feel that she has been caught at a weak moment. Nobody has yet solved the problem of exactly what or when to tell the other children, but at the very least they should be kept in mind. They will often avoid asking, and the parents should be warned against the temptation to turn a blind eye. Children must get some adequate explanation and optimal opportunity to return with their questions. It is also important to help the family to share things. Making a mystery will not successfully protect the children from a disaster. The primary care team must be involved so that there is no gap in the support.

The frequent tendency for fathers to be excluded from the delivery room when things are going wrong, when their wives need them most, should be resisted. Nowadays there is widespread agreement on management designed to make the events as clear as possible and to avoid aggravating the dangerous sense of residual bewilderment following stillbirth as a 'non-event'. Even in cases of severe fetal abnormality, staff are now learning not to shuffle the corpse away in secret, out of the misconceived idea of sparing the mother her grief (Lewis 1976). Such behaviour usually has more to do with our wish to avoid pain and embarrassment when communicating our own revulsion to the patient. Of course parents should not be forced to see what they do not wish to look at, but there is growing experience that parents of dead babies can find something good to hang onto from moments captured in the face of even great anguish. The parents of an anencephalic child expect to see a headless monster, whereas usually the reality is not as ghastly as they might imagine (Shokeir 1979). Patients who have at first been afraid to look at the dead baby are often permanently grateful if they have been successfully supported and encouraged to seize the chance. Those who never see or hold their dead baby are liable to remain tantalised and regretful. These matters should not become rigid and institutionalised, but if there is no prepared procedure, the busy atmosphere of the delivery room may leave people without space to think. Midwives have learned to wrap the dead malformed baby so that some of the most distressing features may be screened until the parents may or may not decide to see every detail as it really is. Feeling normal limbs through the wraps has often been found to provide the basis for some comforting memories. Frequently this leads parents to hold the whole uncovered baby. We hear repeatedly of mothers who gratefully exclaim 'What lovely fingers and toes' (Klaus and Kennell 1982). Professional staff are also important for their own role in looking and remembering, provided they remain available to talk later. Parents may be overwhelmed in the delivery room but may take up the option to see their baby later, and this should be facilitated. Rather than sending vulnerable people to the mortuary, the dead child can be brought to the parents in a Moses basket.

Photographs and mementoes
Mementoes are helpful on many levels. Photographs and post-mortem x-ray pictures are helpful in the diagnosis of congenital abnormality, and the recording of scientific data is more likely to be done than in the case of stillbirth in general. Such records are of further value as aids to discussion later with the parents, not only for genetic counselling but also in order to provide them with mementoes. All this aids reality testing in the mourning process as well as giving comfort. Unfortunately, the photographs prepared by the pathology department to record post-mortem specimens are often grotesquely unsuitable to give to the parents, who may be outraged by what they see as a further insult. Photographs of several kinds should be kept as an available record and these should include photographs of the baby naked, and dressed or wrapped to present an acceptable appearance. Labour wards often possess an instant camera so that it is possible to verify that satisfactory photographs are available before it is too late to take them. Black-and-white photographs may also be more acceptable than coloured ones in the case of a damaged or macerated fetus.

As well as the post-mortem photograph, some units try to assemble an envelope of mementoes such as ultrasound pictures, a lock of hair, the name band, the hand print or a foot print. Parents have sometimes been induced to 'steal' such items when they have not been provided by the hospitals. Some hospitals keep a memory book, and families may appreciate this option for recording the brief existence of their dead baby.

Hospital procedure
Space and privacy are essential for the family to share their grief and to bring in the other surviving children. A side ward should be available for privacy but these people should not become isolated or feel ostracised. Sometimes these parents are moved to a ward away from the other mothers with live babies, but our impression is that this solves no problems and may exacerbate them. In spite of the pain, bereft

mothers will often find it helpful to confront and test some of their complicated feelings about other women with live babies and it is reassuring to find themselves trusted to be near them or even to hold them. This could help to prevent the phobia of live babies and the fear of harming or stealing them.

Certification and registration of death are not entirely a nuisance. In addition to legal requirements, these procedures may be useful to clarify the events and the diagnosis. Staff should help parents with these matters but avoid taking over and bypassing their role. Parents should be given copies of any certificates or letters to keep as mementoes of their baby's existence. There is no legal requirement for a certificate or registration of the death of a baby before the legal age of viability. However, rather than consign the body to the hospital incinerator, parents may choose to have a seemly burial or cremation: in which case they will need a certificate or letter from the doctor or registered midwife in attendance, stating that the baby was born before the legal age of viability and showed no signs of life, to enable funeral directors to arrange cremation or burial. This is very appropriate for mid-trimester deaths but the current tendency to encourage funerals for very early miscarriages must remain debatable. Psychologically, there is an important and helpful hiatus between early miscarriage (very frequent and somewhat private) and perinatal death in advanced pregnancy (much less common and almost inevitably involving the parents with the medical services and statutory considerations, perhaps causing great anguish).

Termination of pregnancy
We have mainly been considering the unavoidable perinatal death of a malformed baby, but the problem is often anticipated by a decision to terminate pregnancy early. Parents are usually more troubled by choosing to have an abnormal fetus aborted when they wanted the baby, than after termination of a normal one for social reasons. In termination of a normal pregnancy for social reasons, the element of personal choice is much more clear, and feelings of responsibility and guilt are largely conscious and straightforward. This is painful but not so pathogenic as the unconscious tangle of more complex feelings about termination for fetal abnormality. A termination for malformation can have difficult emotional sequelae precisely because mixed feelings and doubts about the pregnancy are complicated and less available for thinking through. Because of the disappointment and distress it causes, the abnormal fetus is itself a source of resentment, most of which will be repressed from consciousness. When mixed feelings are denied, thinking about an abortion is impeded and the processes of mourning will be impaired. Unbearable guilt is repressed from awareness but can remain pathogenic; and such guilt may be worse if the termination is perceived as for the parents' sake, to ease their own lot, rather than as protecting the unborn child from a wretched life.

The ethical problems exercise theologians, philosophers and jurists, yet those on the spot have to make their choices. Religious beliefs and the customs of society exert an obvious influence upon guilt, not always in accord with rational judgement but often deeply rooted in the mind. The more 'rational' viewpoint is liberating from superstition but can be worryingly tainted with unpleasant associations and echoes from the repugnant principles of Nazi eugenics, the idealisation of imaginary perfect people and the hatred of anybody who is different. The reasonable, open-minded approach to termination for fetal abnormality, fully justified at one level of thought, may feel unpardonable at another.

Failure to make a perfect baby gives rise to worse shame if there was previously undue pride or triumph over other childless people. A malformed fetus may then be felt as divine retribution, but particularly if it was preceded by a termination of a normal pregnancy for social reasons, or by a baby given away for adoption.

Elective termination of pregnancy stirs up considerable anxiety and crises of conscience in doctors and nurses, which have sometimes led to an unfeeling management of women who have had an early miscarriage. An overreaction (a recent pattern, possibly iatrogenic) is to treat an early miscarriage as being 'exactly the same' as a stillbirth. This is unhelpful, since a stillbirth in late pregnancy is very different, in most aspects of the experience and its scale, from the loss of a tiny fetus that might have become a baby. To obscure this difference, in order to pay due attention to the miscarriage, may lead to neglect of the need to understand and work through the emotional significance of the loss of the ability to make a baby, especially poignant after termination for malformation.

Terminations in late pregnancy are especially distressing. The psychological pros and cons about the different methods must be considered: induction of labour and vaginal delivery, or dilatation, dismemberment and evacuation under general anaesthesia. As well as obstetric considerations, the feelings of differing members of the hospital team may affect the choice of the method used, and the parents' views should also be clarified if possible. Going through labour, and seeing and handling an intact fetus, may not be pleasant but will probably make the experience more understandable to the mother and her family, and so facilitate grieving. Pathological examination of the intact fetus is also a more reliable way of diagnosing the abnormality. Residual uncertainty generates untold pain and everything should be done to avoid it.

Multiple pregnancy

Modern technology can prevent the birth of an abnormal baby in multiple pregnancy by the selective killing of a malformed fetus, although it may also stir up many disturbing emotional and ethical questions in us all. In addition to the soul-searching and guilt that occur in these cases there are other disturbing ideas. There will be thoughts of the live baby lying for many weeks by the side of the dead twin. With the survival of the live baby, it is not as easy to forget and forgive oneself as it is after a simple termination of pregnancy. The remainder is always there. The fate of the dead fetus is worrying and puzzling, whether relics persist and are delivered as a fetus papyraceous or whether it vanishes altogether. Maternity ward staff will also be inclined to forget the dead twin if they can, and this failure to acknowledge and respect the dead baby may cause distress to the parents. On the other hand, a photograph of the ultrasound scan showing both babies may be a precious and unique proof for parents to keep (Bryan 1989).

The normal mourning processes for the lost baby tend to be blocked by the continuing pregnancy, and later the natural preoccupation with the care of the new live baby (who should have been a twin) tends to inhibit grieving in the puerperium still further. A residual sign of the unresolved mourning can be that parents are sometimes plagued with grievances (often with the hospital) but find it harder to grieve. The remaining baby is susceptible to all the problems of surviving twins and replacement children, and the parents may be bewildered by their own peculiar feelings and by difficulties in rearing.

When one twin dies, or after selective feticide, the survivor has parents who are bereft at the birth. The mother has the very difficult and contradictory task of celebrating and nurturing the newborn child while being preoccupied with thoughts and feelings about the dead baby (Lewis and Bryan 1988). The worried look in the mother's eyes, and the depressed mother's inability to be sufficiently devoted to the surviving baby, can disturb the child's emotional and cognitive development. After selective feticide, the grief about the loss of the baby that might-have-been may be suppressed by the inhibiting effect of pregnancy on mourning; but the buried feelings, partly remembered, may trouble the surviving child as s/he grows up. Vague hints, difficult to comprehend, may be picked up in family conversation, and the child remains mystified by the feeling that the family has bad secrets in the closet.

Conclusions

The 'replacement child' is one born after any bereavement but especially after the death of another child or fetus (Cain and Cain 1964). Mourning may have been interrupted by the pregnancy and the new baby is only precariously differentiated from the dead one. This can entail a tangle of confused feelings and expectations, which go far beyond the mere hope that the new child will make up for the loss. Unresolved mixed feelings about the dead are carried over, and parents may be taken by surprise at their sense of hostility, disappointment, sadness or bewilderment. The replacement child may later have severe uncertainty about his or her identity, destiny or right to be alive. Doctors and midwives sometimes have the chance of picking up these dangers early, if only to protect the new baby from being given the dead one's name. Parents expect to be overanxious if they have lost a previous baby but may be helped by being warned of sadness and other feelings which could take them by surprise. They may need 'permission' to be confused or frightened to help them not to be overwhelmed.

Follow-up and counselling should always be available in these cases. We have focused intentionally on the prime importance of the roles of the obstetric and paediatric teams and the primary caregivers, but specialised psychotherapy may be necessary for problem causes and self-help groups are also very valuable. However, a reliable system of follow-up is vital and there is evidence that it helps if counselling is routinely available in all cases (Morris *et al.* 1984, Elder and Laurence 1991).

REFERENCES

Benedek, T. (1970) 'The psychobiology of pregnancy.' *In* Anthony, E.J. Benedek, T. (Eds) *Parenthood: Its Psychology and Psychopathology.* Boston: Little Brown. pp. 137–152.

Benedict, M.I., White, R.B., Cornely, D.A. (1985) 'Maternal perinatal risk factors and child abuse.' *Child Abuse and Neglect*, **9**, 217–224.

Bibring, G.L., Dwyer, T.F., Huntington, D.S., Valenstein, A.F. (1961) 'A study of the psycho-social processes in pregnancy and of the earliest mother-child relationship.' *Psychoanalytic Study of the Child*, **16**, 9–24.

Blum, H. (1980) 'The maternal ego ideal and the regulation of maternal qualities.' *In* Greenspan, S., Pollock, G.H. (Eds) *The Course of Life: Psychoanalytic Contributions Toward Understanding Personality Development, Vol. III: Adulthood and the Ageing Process.* Washington, DC: US Government Printing Office. pp. 91–141.

Bourne, S. (1968) 'The psychological effects of stillbirth on women and their doctors.' *Journal of the Royal College of General Practitioners*, **16**, 103–112.

—— Lewis, E. (1984) 'Pregnancy after stillbirth or neonatal death.' *Lancet*, **2**, 31–33.

Bryan, E. (1989) 'The response of mothers to selective feticide; ethical problems.' *Reproductive Medicine*, **1**, 28–30.

Cain, A.C., Cain, P.C. (1964) 'On replacing a child.' *Journal of the American Academy of Child Psychiatry*, **3**, 443–455.

Cullberg, J. (1972) 'Mental reactions of women to perinatal death.' *In* Morris, N. (Ed.) *Psychosomatic Medicine in Obstetrics and Gynaecology.* Basel: Karger. pp. 326–329.

Elder, S.H., Laurence, K.M. (1991) 'The impact of supportive intervention after second trimester termination of pregnancy for fetal abnormality.' *Prenatal Diagnosis*, **11**, 47–54.

Freud, S. (1917) *Mourning and Melancholia.* London: Hogarth Press and Institute of Psychoanalysis.

Giles, P.F.H. (1970) 'Reactions of women to perinatal death.' *Australian and New Zealand Journal of Obstetrics and Gynaecology*, **10**, 207–210.

Kendell, R.E., Chalmers, J.C., Platz, C. (1987) 'Epidemiology of puerperal psychoses.' *British Journal of Psychiatry*, **150**, 662–673.

Kestenberg, J.S. (1977) 'Regression and reintegration in pregnancy.' *In* Blum, H.P. (Ed.) *Female Psychology: Contemporary Psychoanalytic Views.* New York: International Universities Press. pp. 213–250.

Klaus, M.H., Kennell, J.H. (1982) *Parent-Infant Bonding, 2nd Edn.* St Louis: C.V. Mosby.

Klein, M. (1932) *The Psychoanalysis of Children.* London: Hogarth Press.

—— (1963) *Our Adult World and Other Essays.* London: Heinemann.

Leon, I.G. (1990) *When a Baby Dies: Psychotherapy for Pregnancy and Newborn Loss.* New Haven: Yale University Press.

Lewis, E. (1976) 'The management of stillbirth: coping with unreality.' *Lancet*, **2**, 619–620.

—— (1979*a*) 'Two hidden predisposing factors in child abuse.' *International Journal of Child Abuse*, **3**, 327–330.

—— (1979*b*) 'Inhibition of mourning by pregnancy: psychopathology and management.' *British Medical Journal*, **2**, 27–28.

—— Bryan, E. (1988) 'Management of perinatal loss of a twin.' *British Medical Journal*, **297**, 1321–1323.

Menzies, I.E.P. (1960) 'A case study in the functioning of social systems as a defence against anxiety.' *Human Relations*, **13**, 95–121.

Morris, J., Tew, B., Laurence, K.M. (1984) 'Long-term reactions following a stillbirth with a congenital abnormality: a preliminary report.' *Zeitschrift für Kinderchirurgie*, **39** (Suppl. 2), 117–119.

Parkes, C.M., Weiss, R.S. (1983) *Recovery from Bereavement.* New York: Basic Books.

SANDS (1991) *Miscarriage, Stillbirth and Neonatal Death: Guidelines for Professionals.* London: Stillbirth and Neonatal Death Society.

Segal, H. (1973) *Introduction to the Work of Melanie Klein.* London: Hogarth Press.

Shokeir, M. (1979) 'Managing the family of the abnormal newborn.' *In* Hall, B.D. (Ed.) *Proceedings of the 1978 Birth Defects Conference, National Foundation.* New York: March of Dimes.

Winnicott, D.W. (1958) *Collected Papers: Through Paediatrics to Psycho-Analysis.* London: Tavistock. pp. 300–305.

5
PATHOLOGY OF HYDROCEPHALUS

Keasley Welch and Antonio V. Lorenzo

In hydrocephalus the brain is under stress. The corresponding strain, deformation or compression in which the liquid compartments intrude upon the solid, is what is known as hydrocephalus. Thus the pathology falls into two parts, antecedent and consecutive to the disorder. In the first, consideration is given to insults to the brain, either developmental or acquired, leading to hydrocephalus; in the second the focus is on the converse, harm resulting from the compression.

Antecedents to hydrocephalus
Malformations
Malformations of the brain accounted for just over half of 100 cases of hydrocephalus counted by Welch (1980), but geographic and secular factors, and varying patterns of referral, may lead to different distributions. An extensive review of the aetiology of malformations by Kalter and Warkany (1983) showed the majority to be without known cause; inheritance and chromosomal abnormalities accounted for 7½ and 6 per cent, maternal infection for 2 per cent, and drugs for a lower figure. Multifactorial influences, especially in relation to neural tube defects, accounted for 20 per cent. Maternal diabetes doubled or trebled the incidence, but according to Barr *et al.* (1983) magnified by many times the occurrence of holoprosencephaly, caudal regression syndrome and heart defects. Each of the malformations to be described may comprise a number of separate elements, and those may be shared between malformation complexes. The multiplicity and the crossover show that it would be naive, as indicated by Andersson and Carlson (1966) in relation to spina bifida, 'to base a theory of pathogenesis upon a single primary error of development'.

Spina bifida
This malformation complex involves all parts of the nervous system and, either directly or indirectly, all other systems as well. It is generally conceded to be multifactorial in origin (Carter 1974); among the known factors are maternal diabetes (Myrianthopoulos and Melnick 1986) and diet (Smithells *et al.* 1981, 1983), and elevation of maternal core temperature early in pregnancy has recently been cited as a risk (Milunsky *et al.* 1991). Valproate has been suggested as a ter-atogen (MMWR 1982). But x-linked transmission has been observed (Baraitser and Burn 1984, Toriello 1984). Also two types have been identified, 'singles' and 'multiples' (Khoury *et al.* 1982, Windham and Bjerkedal 1982). The former make up the majority of cases with white female preponderance, geographic gradients

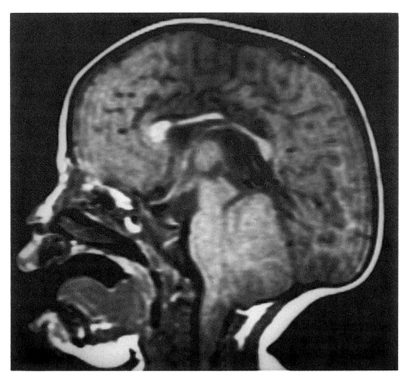

Fig. 5.1. A midline sagittal MR image of the head of an infant with spina bifida. There is agenesis of the corpus callosum, a large massa intermedia, beaking of the mesencephalic tectum, dilatation of the subarachnoid space above the cerebellum and of the ambiens cistern and vellum interpositum, and caudal ectopia of the hindbrain (Chiari II). The signal arising from the motion of fluid is cut off at or near the foramen magnum. (Courtesy of Dr Roy Strand.)

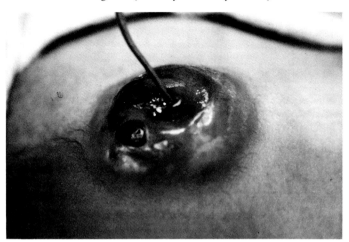

Fig. 5.2. Myelomeningocele. A probe has been placed in the ostium of the central canal of the spinal cord. The dark area represents the area medullovasculosa (from Welch and Winston 1987, by permission).

TABLE 5.I
Distribution of spina bifida aperta by level

	Doran and Guthkelch 1961	Ingraham and Swan 1943	Welch and Winston 1987	Total	%
Cervical	12	23	3	38	4.1
Thoracic	20	39	4	63	6.8
Thoracolumbar	32	43	28	103	11.1
Thoraco-lumbosacral	10	10	3	23	2.5
Lumbar	100	205	55	360	39.0
Lumbosacral	96	87	48	231	25.0
Sacral	38	46	9	93	10.1
Unknown		8	1	9	1.0
Pelvic		1		1	0.1
Total	308	462	151	921	

and secular changes; 'multiples' show separate malformations outside the nervous system and do not share in the above characteristics. Almost all studies in many countries have shown a decrease in incidence over the last decade or two; the east to west gradient in Britain is matched by a west to east gradient in the United States.

Virtually all features of the anatomical pathology of spina bifida were described many years ago (Cleland 1883, Marsh *et al.* 1885, Von Recklinghausen 1886, Chiari 1891) (Fig. 5.1). There have been many inconclusive attempts to understand the pathogenesis of the malformation complex.

THE SPINAL LESION

The spinal lesion is usually a cystic protrusion with walls consisting of thinned out meninges and skin excepting at its apex. There the spinal cord, having emerged from the spinal canal beneath the last intact vertebral lamina, is attached in a flattened placode. Frequently there is a small angioma, the area medullovasculosa, on its outside surface. There is also a pit, the ostium of the central canal of the spinal cord (Fig. 5.2), which is in communication with the ventricular system (Andersson *et al.* 1967). Following the same general pattern there is a sessile form, rachischisis, which may occupy a greater length than the cystic. Lesser degrees are also seen; hydrocephalus does not occur in concealed forms, but open and occult spina bifida share familial recurrence risks (Carter *et al.* 1976). The distribution of levels is shown in Table 5.I.

THE FOREBRAIN

There is an overabundance of cortical sulci, and as a result the gyri are thin and numerous. This malformation was described by Ingraham and Scott (1943): they characterised its appearance as 'wormy' and named it microgyria, later changed to polymicrogyria. An enlarged massa intermedia is a regular feature. Agenesis of the corpus callosum, cysts of the cava and various other deformities are sometimes seen.

The mesencephalic tectum is deformed into a pyramidal shape. The hindbrain is displaced caudally, the vermis of the cerebellum in the lead, the Chiari II malformation.* The vermis and the medulla (including the fourth ventricle) intrude into the upper cervical spinal canal, making a very tight fit. It has been suggested that the caudal ectopia is due to low spinal pressure because of loss of CSF through the central canal (Cameron 1957).

HYDROCEPHALUS

The hydrocephalus is usually attenuated before birth by leakage of fluid through the central canal of the cord (Andersson *et al.* 1967), but grows worse after that conduit is closed by surgical repair. Blockage to the flow of fluid may be at the Sylvian aqueduct and/or in the posterior fossa.

OTHER

Hydromyelia occurs in about half the cases. Thinned areas of the skull (craniolacunae), and changes in the configuration of the posterior fossa and its dura occur.

Cranium bifidum

This condition is known also as encephalocele, cephalocele and exencephaly. Its essence is a protrusion of brain through a defect in the skull. Anteriorly situated lesions are not associated with hydrocephalus, but those located posteriorly are frequently so complicated. Females are more often affected than males, the ratio being between two and three to one (Mealey *et al.* 1970, Lorber and Schofield 1979). Eighteen instances were examined post mortem by Emery and Kalhan (1970). Sixteen showed low occipital exencephaly of extreme degree, involving cerebellum and brainstem, but only nine of 74 infants seen in life by Guthkelch (1970) were not viable because of massive exencephaly. Parietal lesions may be less severe; of 13 described by McLaurin (1964) five were simple meningoceles or heterotopic glial rests, but beneath four of the remaining eight there was agenesis of the corpus callosum. Even seemingly trivial lesions may be accompanied by hydrocephalus (Yamada *et al.* 1979).

The great variety of accompanying malformations of the nervous system was emphasised by Karch and Urich (1972), who examined five examples at autopsy; all were female, four had defective regulation of body temperature during life. (A similar defect in hypothalamic function has been described in connection with agenesis of the corpus callosum, see below.) Another five autopsied cases were studied by Leong and Shaw (1979) who pointed out the great assortment of associated lesions. One had the Meckel-Gruber syndrome; this and other named syndromes may include cranium bifidum.

---

*In the Chiari I deformity, the tonsils of the cerebellum are herniated. It is indistinguishable from foraminal herniation of the brain due to pressure differences.

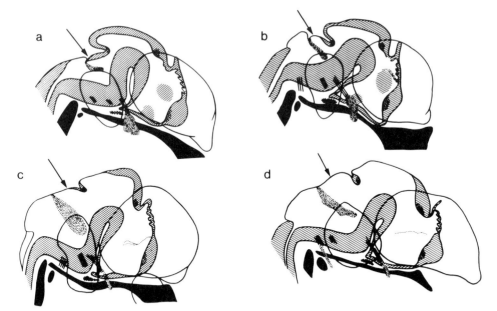

Fig. 5.3. In the hy-1 mouse (now extinct), a lesion similar to the Dandy-Walker cyst occurred as a recessive trait. *a:* the cerebellar anlage has replaced the area membranacea superior. *b–d:* progressive bulging with hydrocephalus and failure of cerebellar development in affected mice (redrawn from Bonnevie 1943, by permission).

The Dandy-Walker syndrome

The rhombencephalic roof plate normally differentiates into two parts (Weed 1917): the caudal (the area membranacea inferior) becomes the lining of the tela choroidea; the rostral (the area membranacea superior) is assimilated in advance of the development of the cerebellar anlage (Fig. 5.3*a*). The Dandy-Walker cyst occurs with the persistence of the area membranacea superior, which bulges out to form a great cyst (Fig. 5.3 *b–d*). There is asplasia or hypoplasia of the cerebellar vermis, and the posterior rotation and descent of the tentorium of the cerebellum, with its sinuses and the torcular Herophili, is prevented by the increased volume of the posterior fossa (Fig. 5.4).

The malformation was described by Dandy and Blackfan (1914) and ascribed (incorrectly, as it proved) to obstruction of the outlets of the fourth ventricle, which may be present, but is not essential (Hart *et al.* 1972). An obstruction of the CSF may occur at the aqueduct of Sylvius as well as in the posterior fossa (Raimondi *et al.* 1969). Associated anomalies may include agenesis of the corpus callosum, cortical dysplasia, dysmorphia of the brainstem and deformity of the skeletal system. Congenital heart disease (Huong *et al.* 1975) and ocular and renal abnormalities have been recorded. The associated lesions of the brain may account for a poor outlook for intellectual development (Raimondi and Soare 1974).

The anomaly has been observed in siblings (Benda 1954, D'Agostino *et al.* 1963, Nova 1979), including identical twins (Jenkyn *et al.* 1981).

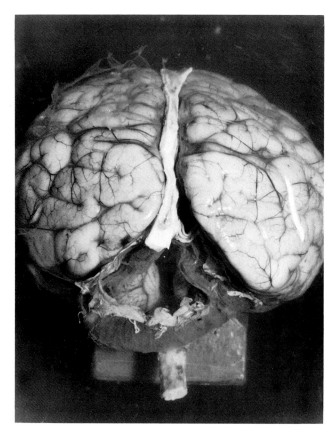

Fig. 5.4 (*left*). The brain in Dandy-Walker syndrome. The torcular Herophili is high, the cerebellar hemispheres can be seen through the open dura, but the vermis is absent (from Davson *et al.* 1987, by permission).

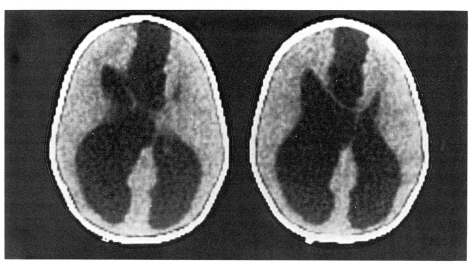

Fig. 5.5. Agenesis of the corpus callosum with paramedian cyst. Seizures began at 10 months of age and an enlarged head was noted (from Davson *et al.* 1987, by permission).

Malformations in the midline
Because of shared features in development (Rakic and Yakovlev 1968), agenesis of the corpus callosum and cysts of the cavum septi pellucidi and cavum Vergae are considered under one heading.

AGENESIS OF THE CORPUS CALLOSUM
Callosal defects occur because of a failure of fusion of the cerebral hemispheres; without a glial bridge to guide the intended commissural fibres they are thwarted from crossing and grow to form tangles (Probst bundles), which are responsible for the characteristic rounded impressions on the medial walls of the adjacent lateral ventricles. The defect may be partial or complete, isolated or accompanied by other anomalies. Among the latter are neural tube defects, Dandy-Walker syndrome, cortical abnormalities and others. The association of hypothalamic lesions leading to periodic hypothermia, described by Shapiro *et al.* (1969), was reviewed by Summers *et al.* (1981). The median and paramedian cysts and clefts that occur with callosal defect (Fig. 5.5) are porencephalies, formally speaking, but have been given special attention in their own right (Foerster 1939, Swett and Nixon 1975) and have been observed to underlie encephaloceles (McLauren 1964).

Autosomal recessive inheritance has been suggested in a small minority of instances, but most are sporadic. Specially named inherited syndromes may be interesting, but not in relation to hydrocephalus.

CYSTS OF THE CAVUM SEPTI PELLUCIDI AND CAVUM VERGAE
The cavum septi pellucidi, a fluid-filled space between the leaves of the septum pellucidum, is prominent in the brains of the very young (Shaw and Alvord 1969); it communicates with a potential space, the cavum Vergae, which is bordered above by the corpus callosum, laterally by the fornices and below by the hippocampal commissure. Very occasionally one or other of these cava becomes distended, blocking the foramina of Monro or the posterior third ventricle (Dandy 1931).

Holoprosencephaly
Failure of evagination of the telencephalic vesicles and of cleavage of the prosencephalon underlie the basic malformation in holoprosencephaly (Yakovlev 1959). The degree of deformity varies; at its greatest there is a spherical brain with a single ventricle and a large dorsal cyst (Fig. 5.6); at its least there is a well formed brain with hemispheres joined frontally. These have been called alobar and lobar, intermediate forms, semilobar (DeMyer *et al.* 1964). Facial malformations are frequent.

The incidence is 1 per 19–20,000 births, but is much greater in the offspring of diabetic mothers (Barr *et al.* 1983). Half are due to trisomy 13 (Hintz 1979), but other karyotypes occur, as do dominant and autosomal recessive patterns of inheritance (Cohen *et al.* 1971). According to Osaka and Matsumoto (1978), hydrocephalus occurs in 40 per cent of those affected and is more often present in those without facial deformity.

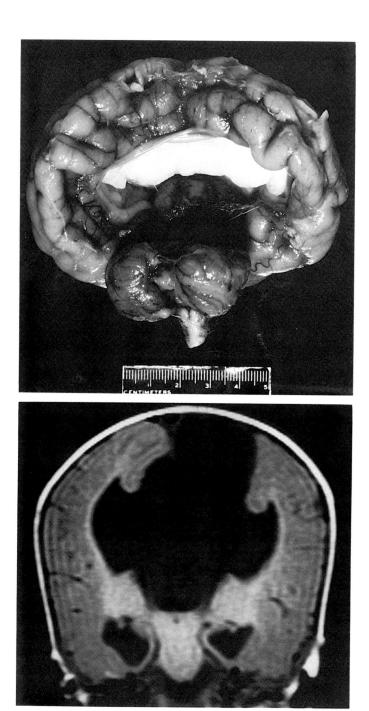

Fig. 5.6. *Top:* alobar holoprosencephaly with trisomy 13. The view through the large posterior cyst reveals the monoventricle. Cotton has been placed in the ventricle to hold it open (from Davson *et al.* 1987, by permission). *Bottom:* MR image in a comparable case. (Courtesy of Dr Roy Strand.)

Hydranencephaly and porencephaly
Porencephaly was named by Heschl (1859)* and described as a defect through the
entire thickness of the brain; hydranencephaly qualifies under that definition
because most of the telencephalon is missing, only some posterior and basal
remnants being spared. Both conditions are thought to be encephaloclastic;
vascular, infectious, traumatic and other agents are suspected. Because of the
thorough cleansing of distinctive marks of injury to the fetal brain (Spatz 1920), the
cause is hidden. Aicardi *et al.* (1972) suggested autotransfusion between twins,
leading to death in one and hydranencephaly in the other. Hydranencephaly has
been found in siblings (Hamby *et al.* 1950).

Stenosis of the aqueduct of Sylvius
Bickers and Adams (1949*b*) reviewed the literature in relation to autopsy findings
in this condition. Of 21 subjects under the age of one, spina bifida was present in
six; there were three instances of meningitis and four of gross malformation of the
brain. In the other half there were no distinguishing features, suggesting that the
condition may occur as an independent malformation. In the older group of 19
cases, ependymitis and gliosis predominated; there were only two gross malformations and one instance of glial heterotopia. In the same year gliosis and forking
of the aqueduct were described by Russell (1949).

SEX-LINKED STENOSIS (BICKERS-ADAMS SYNDROME)
A male baby with aqueduct stenosis whose three brothers were similarly affected,
but whose two sisters were not, was encountered by Bickers and Adams (1949*a,b*).
In the preceding generation on the maternal side four males were affected, but two
male and four female siblings were not. Other families with this rare condition have
been reported. The full syndrome includes spasticity, wasting and contracture of
the legs, flexion deformity of the thumb and curious facies.

Arachnoid cysts
An arachnoid cyst was defined by Scherer (1935) as a fluid-filled space confined by
two layers of arachnoid membrane. For the most part, so-called 'arachnoid' cysts
are in fact lined by glial and secretory elements (Gilles and Rockett 1971, Walsh *et
al.* 1978, Go *et al.* 1984). Such cysts may occur on the surface of the brain (Fig. 5.7),
or occupy any of the major cisterns, blocking the flow of CSF.† Two kinds deserve
special mention. Suprasellar cysts may be accompanied by sexual precocity; and
cysts of the middle fossa, which have been described as 'relapsing juvenile chronic
subdural hematoma' (Davidoff and Dyke 1938), are frequently complicated by
bleeding into the subdural space.

*Heschl named the condition so that it would not be called Heschl's idiocy.

†Because a retrocerebellar cyst displaces the cerebellum it is distinguished from a large cistern. The
literature reveals that the distinction has not always been made.

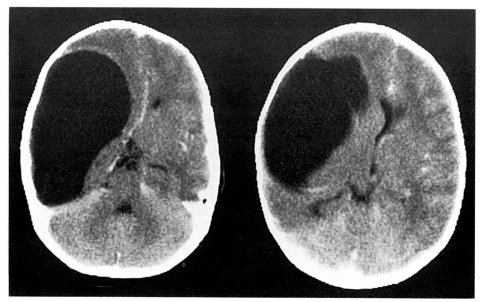

Fig. 5.7. A large arachnoid cyst involving the surface of the brain in a child. Attention was drawn to the lesion at 14 months because of a seizure and an enlarged head (from Davson *et al.* 1987, by permission).

Achondroplasia

Achondroplasia is due to a defect in the formation of enchondral bone. It is inherited as a dominant feature, but most cases arise from a new mutation. The basal (enchondral) portion of the skull is foreshortened, and the foramen magnum is small. The circumference of the head is large by ordinary criteria. It exceeded the 90th centile on standard charts in all but two of the 15 cases studied by Cohen *et al.* (1967); the charts published by Horton *et al.* (1978) show the mean circumference of the head to exceed that for unaffected children by more than 2 SD. Dennis *et al.* (1961) found a large brain and corresponding head size to be characteristic and encountered five consecutive cases showing megalencephaly and mild ventricular enlargement, but not hydrocephalus. Hydrocephalus is unusual, but children have been unnecessarily treated for it, based on head size.

Craniosynostosis

Fishman *et al.* (1971) reported the coexistence of craniosynostosis and hydrocephalus in 14 patients, eight females and six males. Apert's syndrome (eight instances) was most common; the others were of mixed variety. Accompanying malformation of the brain was thought responsible.

Meningeal accumulations

HURLER'S DISEASE

This fatal disease is characterised by the accumulation of mucopolysaccharides due to want of α-L iduronidase; the inheritance is recessive. Russell (1949) described a case of gargoylism with hydrocephalus due to the accumulation of storage material in the meninges. Hydrocephalus and dilatation of basal cisterns characterised six cases described by Newhauser *et al.* (1968), but were found only in patients with corneal opacity.

Intrauterine infection

Toxoplasma gondii is a coccidian parasite in Felidae (Hutchison *et al.* 1970, 1971), widely distributed in secondary hosts. The uncooked meat of such a host is the usual vehicle for transmission to man; ingestion of material containing oocysts in cat faeces is less often responsible. Transplacental infection occurs from a newly infected woman. The fetal disease may be a rampant, necrotising and granulomatous process leading to fetal death, hydranencephaly or severe permanent cerebral injury (Wolff and Cowen 1937). A miliary form may yield stenosis of the aqueduct of Sylvius, choroidoretinal scarring and punctate calcification of the brain. Hydrocephalus may present early or after many years.

OTHER FETAL INFECTIONS

Hydrocephalus rarely occurs with congenital rubella infection (Swan 1949) or cytomegalovirus disease (McCracken *et al.* 1969).

Acquired forms

The borderline between congenital and acquired forms is not always clear. For example, intraventricular haemorrhage may occur *in utero*, certain tumours are congenital and some postnatal events may be determined before birth.

Neonatal intraventricular haemorrhage

When Gilles and Shillito (1970) examined 1050 autopsies in children to identify causes of hydrocephalus, not one case of ventricular haemorrhage was included. Many had been encountered, but the process was considered to be agonal, or fatal, and of interest only to pathologists. Now, because of available methods of diagnosis, this form of bleeding in preterm babies is known not just as a common complication of preterm birth (Papile *et al.* 1978) and an important cause of neonatal death (Fedrick and Butler 1970) but also as the cause of the most frequent form of acquired infantile hydrocephalus. The cause is unknown, but contributing factors are the same as those for preterm birth—maternal youth, poverty and want of prenatal care. There is an association with the occurrence of pneumothorax. The bleeding usually comes from vessels within the germinal matrix, often the ganglionic eminence; when the haemorrhage occurs in babies born at term, vessels of the choroid plexus are usually responsible.

The ultrastructure of vessels of the human germinal matrix was examined by Povlishock *et al.* (1977) to 23 weeks gestation and by Larroche (1982) to 26. In each case the endothelium was intact, the vessels were invested by basement membrane

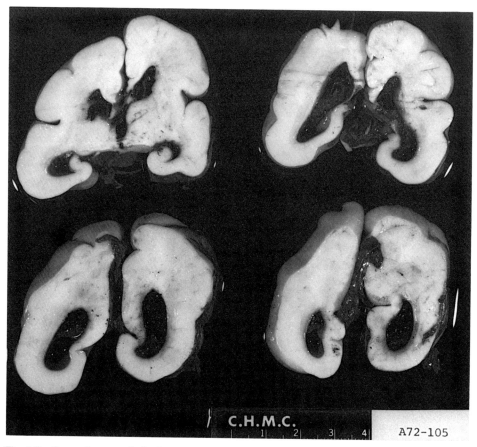

Fig. 5.8. Severe intraventricular haemorrhage in an infant born weighing 1kg. The clotted blood forms a cast of the distended ventricular system (from Davson *et al.* 1987, by permission).

and glial attachment was present. Similar observations were made by Nelson *et al.* (1982) in beagle pups in which vessels of the matrix were similar to those of the cerebral cortex; such also was the finding in 26-day rabbit pups, but not at 28 days when involutional change involved discontinuity of endothelium and of basement membrane with haemorrhage (Welch and Lorenzo 1984).

Spillage of blood may be severe, with casts of clotted blood filling the ventricles and subarachnoid spaces (Fig. 5.8); in milder cases there are varying degrees of staining of the fluid. The mechanical blocking of the system by blood is succeeded by a chemical meningitis and ependymitis. In the end there is scarring of the leptomeninges and sometimes blocking of the iter.

Haemorrhage due to injury at birth
There persists the suspicion that obstetrical injury may contribute significantly to the incidence of hydrocephalus. That idea was fuelled by Fraser and Dott (1922),

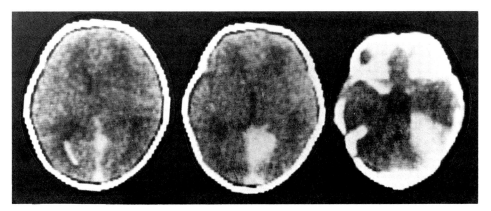

Fig. 5.9. Parturitional haemorrhage in the posterior fossa. The blood occupies the subdural space on the right and the cerebellar parenchyma (from Davson *et al.* 1987, by permission).

who found that seven of 21 infants with hydrocephalus had had a difficult birth and showed a bloody effusion at the base of the brain. Similarly, half of a group of children examined by Granholm and Rådberg (1963) because of communicating hydrocephalus had a history of difficult birth. These findings may indicate that birth was difficult because of congenital hydrocephalus. Neither Ford (1926) nor Russell (1949) could confirm or establish a close relationship. Retrocerebellar haematoma accounted for three of 97 instances of hydrocephalus encountered at autopsy by Gilles and Shillito (1970); one of 100 cases examined in life by Welch (1980) was due to birth injury.

Risk factors include pre-eclampsia, primiparous birth, the birth of the second of twins and high birthweight. Hurried delivery because of fetal distress poses a hazard.

The pathology was first elucidated by Beneke (1910) as based upon a tear at the free edge of the tentorium of the cerebellum. During birth the head becomes foreshortened while its height increases. Stress on the tentorium at that time may cause the tear. The medial tentorial artery courses near that edge and is thus subject to injury (Welch and Strand 1986). Bleeding may extend below or above the tentorium, the former being more dangerous because of the small size of the posterior fossa (Fig. 5.9).

Hydrocephalus complicated five of 35 instances of parturitional haemorrhage seen by Munro (1928) and three of 25 reported by Welch and Strand (1986). Thus there is a significant risk of hydrocephalus after birth injury, but its overall contribution to hydrocephalus is not great.

Infections, infestations and granulomas
The likelihood of hydrocephalus following purulent meningitis is roughly proportional to the duration of the process. The organisms that are difficult to eradicate and take some time to respond to therapy, as do the common causes of

TABLE 5.II

Oversecretion of CSF by papilloma of choroid plexus

Author	Measured rate	Method
Vigouroux 1908	0.56 ml/min., 800 ml/da	Collected fluid from fistula
Johnson 1958	0.75 ml/min.	Ventricular drainage at 450mm H_2O
Fairburn 1960	400, 500, 900 ml/da	Ventricular drainage at 50mm H_2O dehydrated terminally ill infant
Eisenberg *et al.* 1974	1.45 ml/min.	Ventriculo-spinal perfusion
Milhorat *et al.* 1976	1.05 ml/min.	Ventriculo-spinal perfusion
Sahar *et al.* 1980	0.35 ml/min.*	Method of Portnoy and Croissant (1976)

*This measurement was made in a patient with a fourth ventricular papilloma and is not different from a postoperative measurement.

neonatal meningitis—enteric organisms and Group B *Streptococcus*—may cause sufficient scarring to lead to hydrocephalus. Moreover, ependymitis resulting from the infection may cause multilocular hydrocephalus (Albanese *et al.* 1981). In communicating hydrocephalus, the fourth ventricle does not generally play a large part in the ventricular dilatation; because of the open foramina of Luschka and Magendie, only a small difference in pressure can be sustained between the ventricle and the surface of the cerebellum. But when scarring closes its outlets, the fourth ventricle participates fully in the distention of the ventricles, and a large fourth ventricle is almost indicative of a meningitic cause of the disorder. The dilatation of the fourth ventricle is shared by the central canal of the spinal cord, and if the aqueduct is closed as well, the distended fourth may be isolated (De Feo *et al.* 1975). Vasculitis with infarction sometimes results from meningitis; the end result is a porencephaly.

Tuberculous and fungal meningitis (the latter due usually to an opportunistic invader) provoke meningeal desmoplasia, as does sarcoid. In the racemose form of cysticercosis there are many grape-like cysts in the ventricles and leptomeninges with scarring.

Johnson *et al.* (1967) showed that ependymitis occurred following cerebral inoculation of mumps virus in suckling hamsters. This led to stenosis of the Sylvian aqueduct, with no trace of the earlier inflammation. There have been several subsequent reports of closure of the iter consecutive to mumps in humans (Timmons and Johnson 1970).

Tumours

CHOROID PLEXUS

It has been shown repeatedly that there is an excessive secretion of CSF by choroid plexus papillomas (Table 5.II), but those in the third and fourth ventricles block the flow of fluid as well. Villous hypertrophy of the plexuses (Davis 1924), in which the plexuses of several ventricles are greatly enlarged, has also been found to be associated with excessive fluid production (Gudeman *et al.* 1979, Welch *et al.* 1983).

Russell (1949) pointed out that tectal tumours may have a very indolent course and be difficult to distinguish from gliosis, even at autopsy. The onset of stenosis of the aqueduct in late childhood usually signals a tumour.

GIANT HAIRY NAEVUS

This birthmark is itself benign, but is associated with malignant melanomatosis of the meninges (Hoffman and Freeman 1967).

Effects of hydrocephalic compression

Assessment of the pathological reactions of the brain and spinal cord in human hydrocephalus is confounded by various factors. In the newborn infant and the young child, when the cranial sutures are open and the brain is developing and undergoing rapid growth, the effects of raised ICP and ventricular compression are different from those that occur later. The problem is further complicated by the chronicity of the hydrocephalic process, and the inability to discriminate between the brain pathology that can reasonably be attributed to compression of the brain and that which might be superimposed by ventricular or meningeal infection, haemorrhage, or the lesion responsible for the hindrance of normal flow. The relative paucity of human material at known stages of hydrocephalus, free of pathology attributable to factors other than raised ICP and ventricular expansion, has led to dependence on pathological material obtained from animals with hereditary or experimentally induced hydrocephalus.

At a microscopic level interest has centred on the ependyma, choroid plexuses and white matter. Certain gross features—stretching and fenestration of the septum pellucidum, and herniations of the brain—will not be given further consideration here.

Secondary block

AQUEDUCT STENOSIS IN COMMUNICATION HYDROCEPHALUS

Dandy (1932) recognised that a double block might occur in hydrocephalus, but the literature was silent on the subject until Woollam and Millen (1953) observed the development of aqueductal block in rabbit pups with communication hydrocephalus due to vitamin A deficiency in the dams. This sequence was observed in a number of animal models (Borit and Sidman 1972). Raimondi *et al.* (1976) suggested that the cause was periaqueductal oedema; others have blamed supratentorial expansion with midbrain distortion. Secondary obstruction of the aqueduct has also been found to occur in human hydrocephalus (Williams 1973). Nugent *et al.* (1979) observed widening of the affected iter after diversion of fluid.

SUBARACHNOID BLOCK IN OBSTRUCTIVE HYDROCEPHALUS

The reverse situation, the superimposition of a subarachnoid block in the setting of obstructive hydrocephalus, was noted by Sayers (1966, 1971) in human hydrocephalus. The observation was confirmed in monkeys by Milhorat and Clark (1970), who showed impaired access of dye to the surface of the brain after ventricular obstruction; Milhorat *et al.* (1971) found, by cisternography, that the subarachnoid space had reopened after shunting. The obstruction occurs because of ironing out of the subarachnoid space against the bone of the skull.

Diverticulation

As first pointed out by Magendie (1842), a cerebral ventricle expands to take the space of lost cerebral substance: a passive process of space replacement unlike the space-consuming diverticulation that may occur in hydrocephalus.

INTRUSION INTO VULNERABLE BRAIN

Perhaps the most striking instance is the encroachment of the ventricle into a needle track left after puncture of the ventricle, leading to the formation of a cyst or porencephaly (Salmon 1967). Adams (1975) recorded several instances of encephalopathy due to expansion of a hydrocephalic ventricle into brain rendered vulnerable by earlier processes.

PULSION (PENFIELD'S) DIVERTICULUM OF THE LATERAL VENTRICLE

Penfield (1929) described a diverticulum from a lateral ventricle into the posterior fossa in the setting of a block at the aqueduct or above. The site of election for the failure of the ventricular wall is the fornix at the trigone; the path is through the transverse fissure and into the posterior fossa. Russell (1949) described a dimple in the ventricular wall as a precursor. It may occur on both sides. Nowadays it is rarely seen because hydrocephalus is treated before the development of such an extreme state.

Anterior and posterior diverticula of the third ventricle have been described.

FALSE DIVERTICULA

Northfield and Russell (1939) described two instances in which there was an apparent dissection and accumulation of fluid exterior to the ependyma; in each there developed a hemiparesis.* Ependymal separation and ventricular synechiae are characteristic in ventriculitis and the resulting hydrocephalus.

Hydromyelia

Adams (1975) considered that distention of the spinal cord's central canal, in the setting of hydrocephalus, was another example of diverticulation. Formally, this is true, but it will be remembered (p. 68) that the fourth ventricle does not participate proportionately in ventricular enlargement, nor does the central canal of the spinal cord become distended unless there is outlet obstruction of the fourth ventricle. Camus and Roussy (1914) found hydromyelia due to basal meningitis after the

---

*Such subependymal accumulations of fluid may be akin to those seen in severe oedema in rodent hydrocephalus (p. 73).

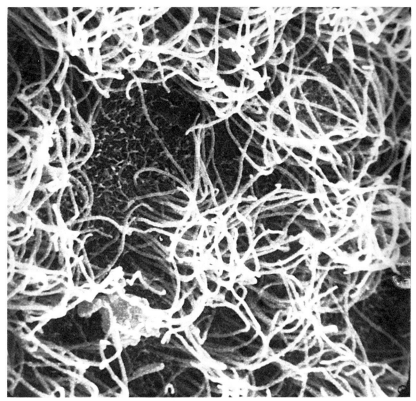

Fig. 5.10. Scanning electron micrograph of cilia on the lateral wall of the lateral venticle of a rat. Microvilli are also seen arising from the ependymal surface. A white blood cell is entangled in the cilia in the lower left corner. Mag × 5500. (Micrograph supplied by C. M. Bannister).

cisternal injection of an irritant, and that observation has been repeated many times after instillation of various materials into the subarachnoid space; clinically, meningitis has figured as a forerunner in the formation of syringomyelia (Appleby *et al.* 1969).

CEREBROSPINAL FLUID FISTULA

Chronically raised ICP may erode the base of the skull giving rise to an external fistula. The literature was reviewed by Walker (1949) in connection with a report of three new cases. As recorded in Table 5.II, the first measurement of overproduction of CSF was based on measurement of fluid outflow from the nose.

Ependyma

Normally, as shown in rabbits (Page 1975, Page *et al.* 1979*a*), the ependyma over the grey matter is cuboidal and rich in cilia, while over the white matter it is squamous and less heavily ciliated (Fig. 5.10). The changes with hydrocephalus

71

respect this difference, the degree of change being greater adjacent to the white matter where the wall of the ventricle is more stretched, and worse in proportion to the severity of the hydrocephalus. The examination of brains of newborn rabbits and cats with acute hydrocephalus may reveal only flattening and stretching of ependymal epithelial cells with little or no evidence of separation or desquamation of the ependymal layer (Ogata *et al.* 1972); but more extensive damage, such as widening of the interependymal space together with a separation of the entire ependymal layer from the underlying tissue, has been detected in experimentally induced hydrocephalus in monkeys (Milhorat *et al.* 1970). In more chronic stages of hydrocephalus, destruction of ependymal cells has been noted as well as partial multifocal separation (Ogata *et al.* 1972, Strecker *et al.* 1974). Attempts to avoid the possible effects of inflammation by the use of substances which produce little or no inflammatory response, such as silicone oil (Wisniewski *et al.* 1969) or silastic materials (James *et al.* 1974), have indicated that the ependymal changes are not dependent on the cause of the hydrocephalus. Rabbits (Page 1979*b*) and rats (Go *et al.* 1976), made hydrocephalic by intracisternal silicone oil, showed flattened and attenuated ependymal cells, and loss of cilia, but no breaks or desquamation of the ependymal layer. Similar results have been reported following kaolin adminis-tration to rabbits (Torvik *et al.* 1981) and rats (Go *et al.* 1976, Weller *et al.* 1978). Moreover, the infusion of silicone oil into the spinal subarachnoid space of two-week-old puppies, leading to elevation of CSF pressure and ventricular enlarge-ment, resulted within 20 days in severe ependymal damage (Weller *et al.* 1971). Ependymal damage and desquamation has also been reported in adult dogs, cats and primates following the introduction of silastic material into the baṣal cisterns (James *et al.* 1977). A further complication is that in infants the absence of ependymal lining along focal areas of the ventricular wall is thought to be a feature of normal development (Gilles *et al.* 1983, Gilles 1986).

Change in cilia (initially clumping, and later loss) parallels the topographic distribution of cell change (Lindberg 1977, Bannister and Chapman 1980). Increased numbers of subependymal cells have been observed (Clark and Milhorat 1970, Weller *et al.* 1978), as well as an increase in Kolmer cells on the ventricular walls. Separation of the ependyma, with cavitation and pooling of fluid outside the subependymal glia, is described in two strains of hereditary hydrocephalus in rodents (Lawson and Raimondi 1973, Jones *et al.* 1987).

Choroid plexus
The epithelium of the choroid plexus was not affected by the viral ependymitis described by Johnson *et al.* (1967) in suckling hamsters; in the subsequent hydrocephalus those authors described the plexuses as somewhat atrophic. Scanning electron microscopy (Nielsen and Gauger 1974) revealed some separation of cells, alterations in microvilli and an increased number of Kolmer cells. The latter finding was common to many observers. In kaolin hydrocephalus the changes were atrophic (Hochwald *et al.* 1969): flattened epithelium with fewer villi and

fibrosis of the tela choroidea. Such flattening of the epithelium with an increase in numbers of vacuoles was described by Dohrmann (1971) in dogs. In hereditary hydrocephalus in mice there was accumulation of fluid between epithelial cells, which spread apart so that they were held together only by their apical junctions. There was oedema of the stroma as well (Lawson and Raimondi 1973). In the acute phase of hydrocephalus brought on by kaolin or silicone, Go *et al.* (1976) found debris on the epithelial surface, thought to be due to impaired function of cilia. Later the surface had cleared. It is likely that the differences in pathology—mild or severe—are related to the severity of the compression.

White matter

Most of the injury to the brain in hydrocephalus is to the white matter. The changes were summarised by Rubin *et al.* (1976*a*), who suggested on the basis of light and electron microscopy in cats with craniectomies (which allow for greater distention of the brain) and kaolin- or silicone-induced hydrocephalus, that there was 'a sequence of events consisting of ventriculomegaly, disruption of the periventricular ependyma, periventricular edema, axonal destruction, secondary myelin disintegration and finally reactive astrocytosis. The damage to axons and myelin and resulting gliosis is irreversible'.

The particulars must be considered in some detail.

Oedema

MORPHOLOGY

Oedema of the white matter adjoining the ventricles was observed microscopically by De (1950) in rats rendered hydrocephalic by intracisternal lamp black. Since then, the microscopic identification of oedema has been demonstrated repeatedly. Weller and Wisniewski (1969) studied the olfactory tract by light and electron microscopy in seven rabbits with artificial hydrocephalus due to silicone, and found varying degrees of oedema with tissue disruption in the most severe. In puppies with hydrocephalus of the same aetiology, Weller *et al.* (1971) found oedema with tissue destruction at 20 and 40 days, but with some improvement at 80 days. In dogs and monkeys with surgically produced obstructive hydrocephalus, Clark and Milhorat (1970) found increased fluid in white matter adjacent to the ventricles with disruption of tissue; further study (Milhorat and Clark 1970), including electron microscopy, elaborated on the description. In hereditary hydrocephalus in mice (McLone *et al.* 1971) the oedema may be severe and subependymal pooling of fluid is observed. James *et al.* (1977) summarised a number of studies from their laboratory.

WATER CONTENT

In keeping with the Monro-Kelley doctrine it was widely believed that the reduced or apparently reduced volume of the brain in hydrocephalus was based upon the squeezing of water out of the brain due to its compression. But Fishman and Greer

(1963) studied the composition of the brain in nine dogs with kaolin hydrocephalus. They found water, Na^+ and Cl^- to be increased in the white matter and to be accompanied by a loss of solids, compared to the grey matter and to parallel measurements in nine control animals. Increased water content of the hydrocephalic brain has been documented also in hydrocephalic cats (Lux *et al.* 1970), and a preserved dry and increased wet weight has been found by others including Rubin *et al.* (1976*a*).

PERMEATION OF MATERIALS

As expected, the larger volume of extracellular fluid in the oedematous region, and perhaps the passage of ventricular fluid into that space, allow an increased penetration of extracellular markers into the swollen brain. Such observations are numerous. The markers varied; phenosulphonphthalein (Milhorat and Clark 1970), radiopharmaceuticals (Strecker *et al.* 1974, James *et al.* 1977), inulin (Lux *et al.* 1970) and other materials, after introduction into the ventricular system, were found to move into the region of oedema. These observations were mistakenly taken as evidence for transfer of CSF by the brain into the blood.

Myelin and axons

Demyelination in the white matter has long been recognised in hydrocephalus (Penfield and Elvidge 1932, Yakovlev 1947). Penfield and Elvidge speculated that collateral fibres might be lost; Yakovlev proposed that the paraplegia of hydrocephalus (then much more severe than it is now) was due to stretching of motor fibres as they passed around the distended ventricles. Demyelination as shown by microscopic and ultramicroscopic study (Rubin *et al.* 1976*c*, James *et al.* 1977, Gadson *et al.* 1979) is confirmed by loss of galactolipids from the brain (Rubin *et al.* 1976*b*). Secondary degeneration in corticospinal fibres was seen by James *et al.* (1977). Elevated levels of myelin basic protein, characteristic in other types of brain damage, have been found in the CSF of children and adults with hydrocephalus (Sutton *et al.* 1983, Levin *et al.* 1985).

Blood vessels

In the past, when angiography was sometimes used for the study of the brain in hydrocephalus, it was apparent that in severe hydrocephalus there was stretching of arteries and veins on the cerebral surface. That observation has also been made in hereditary murine hydrocephalus (Wozniak *et al.* 1975, McLone and Raimondi 1984). The finer vessels were less densely distributed than normal; sometimes they were not filled with injectate and were probably gone. Whether this was cause or effect of cerebral destruction is unclear. In dogs with acute kaolin hydrocephalus, studied by Sato *et al.* (1984), the filling of vessels by an injectate (carbon black) was inhomogeneous compared with controls, especially in the periventricular areas. In later stages microvascular perfusion was more even, but there were multiple small areas of infarction, principally in the regions near the ventricles. Regional CBF, measured by hydrogen clearance, was reduced in both grey and white matter, compared to measurements in normal animals.

Cerebral cortex
VESSELS

Glees and Voth (1988) and Glees *et al.* (1989) studied biopsies of the cerebral cortex in connection with shunt revisions and described pinocytotic vesicles in the capillaries, hypertrophic pericytes and swelling of astrocytic end feet.

NEURONS

It has generally been conceded that injury to nerve cells is a late phenomenon. Rubin *et al.* (1972, 1976*b*) did craniectomies in cats in order to worsen the hydrocephalus subsequently induced by kaolin or silicone. They attempted to estimate the number of nerve cells by measuring DNA, RNA and protein, and found the values to be a little higher than normal. They thought that this was due to the proliferation of reactive cells. Similarly negative findings were recorded by Edwards *et al.* (1984) in the brains of lambs and monkeys in which hydrocephalus had been induced *in utero* by kaolin injection. The cortex was thinned, but the neuronal architecture was preserved, and the neurons and their processes seemed normal. Newborn rats made hydrocephalic by kaolin were studied by McAllister *et al.* (1985); the nerve cell bodies were unaffected, but the basilar dendrites showed many abnormalities including fewer branches, reduction in dendritic spines and the occurrence of dendritic varicosities. The injury to the cortex thus appears to be a subtle one.

REFERENCES

Adams, R.D. (1975) 'Diverticulation of the cerebral ventricles: a cause of progressive focal encephalopathy.' *Developmental Medicine and Child Neurology*, **17** (Suppl. 35), 135–137.
Aicardi, J., Goutières, F., De Verbois, A.H. (1972) 'Multicystic encephalomalacia of infants and its relation to abnormal gestation and hydranencephaly.' *Journal of the Neurological Sciences*, **15,** 357–373.
Albanese, V., Tomasello, F., Sampaolo, S. (1981) 'Multiloculated hydrocephalus in infants.' *Neurosurgery*, **8**, 641–646.
Andersson, H., Carlsson, C.-A. (1966) 'The surgical management of myelomeningocele with a preliminary report of 31 cases.' *Acta Paediatrica Scandinavica*, **55**, 626–635.
—— —— Rosengren, K. (1967) 'A radiological study of the central canal in myelomeningocele.' *Developmental Medicine and Child Neurology*, **9**, (Suppl. 13), 96–102.
Appleby, A., Bradley, W.G., Foster, J.B., Hankinson, J., Hudgson, P. (1969) 'Syringomyelia due to chronic arachnoiditis at the foramen magnum.' *Journal of the Neurological Sciences*, **8**, 451–464.
Bannister, C.M., Chapman, S.A. (1980) 'Ventricular ependyma of normal and hydrocephalic subjects: a scanning electronmicroscopic study.' *Developmental Medicine and Child Neurology*, **22**, 725–735.
Baraitser, M., Burn, J. (1984) 'Neural tube defects as an X-linked condition.' *American Journal of Medical Genetics*, **17**, 383–385.
Barr, M. Jr., Hanson, J.W., Currey, K., Sharp, S., Toriello, H., Schmickel, R.D., Wilson, G.N. (1983) 'Holoprosencephaly in infants of diabetic mothers.' *Journal of Paediatrics*, **102**, 565–568.
Benda, C.E. (1954) 'The Dandy-Walker syndrome or the so-called atresia of the foramen of Magendie.' *Journal of Neuropathology and Experimental Neurology*, **13**, 14–29.
Beneke, R. (1910) 'Über Tentoriumzerreissungen bei der Geburt, sowie die Bedeutung der

Duraspannung für chronische Gehirnerkrankungen.' *Münchener Medizinische Wochenschrift*, **57**, 2125–2127.

Bickers, D.S., Adams, R.D. (1949*a*) 'Hereditary stenosis of the aqueduct of Sylvius.' *Journal of Neuropathology and Experimental Neurology*, **8**, 104–105.

—— —— (1949*b*) 'Hereditary stenosis of the aqueduct of Sylvius as a cause of congenital hydrocephalus.' *Brain*, **72**, 246–262.

Bonnevie, K. (1943) 'Hereditary hydrocephalus in the house mouse. I. Manifestation of the hy-mutation after birth and in embryos 12 days old or more.' *Norske Vid-Akademie Oslo Skr I Mat-Naturv Klinik*, **1**, 32P.

Borit, A., Sidman, R.L. (1972) 'New mutant mouse with communicating hydrocephalus and secondary aqueductal stenosis.' *Acta Neuropathologica*, **21**, 316–331.

Cameron, A.H. (1957) 'The Arnold-Chiari and other neuroanatomical malformations associated with spina bifida.' *Journal of Pathology and Bacteriology*, **73**, 195–211.

Camus, J., Roussy, G. (1914) 'Cavités médullaires et méningites cervicales.' *Révue Neurologique*, **27**, 213–225.

Carter, C.O. (1974) 'Clues to the aetiology of neural tube malformations.' *Developmental Medicine and Child Neurology*, **16** (Suppl. 32), 3–15.

—— Evans, K.A., Till, K. (1976) 'Spinal dysraphism: genetic relation to neural tube malformations.' *Journal of Medical Genetics*, **13**, 343–350.

Chiari, H. (1891) 'Über Veränderungen des Kleinhirns infolge von Hydrocephalie des Grosshirns.' *Deutsche Medizinische Wochenschrift*, **17**, 1172–1175.

Clark, R.G., Milhorat, T.H. (1970) 'Experimental hydrocephalus. Part 3: Light microscopic findings in acute and subacute obstructive hydrocephalus in the monkey.' *Journal of Neurosurgery*, **32**, 400–413.

Cleland, J. (1883) 'Contribution to the study of spina bifida, encephalocele, and anencephalus.' *Journal of Anatomy and Physiology*, **17**, 257–292.

Cohen, M.E., Rosenthal, A.D., Matson, D.D. (1967) 'Neurological abnormalities in achondroplastic children.' *Journal of Pediatrics*, **71**, 367–376.

Cohen, M.M. Jr., Jirasek, J.E., Guzman, R.T., Gorlin, R.J., Peterson, M.Q. (1971) 'Holoprosencephaly and facial dysmorphia: nosology, etiology and pathogenesis.' *Birth Defects*, **7**, 125–135.

D'Agostino, A.N., Kernohan, J.W., Brown, J.R. (1963) 'The Dandy-Walker syndrome.' *Journal of Neuropathology and Experimental Neurology*, **22**, 450–470.

Dandy, W.E. (1931) 'Congenital cerebral cysts of the cavum septi pellucidi (fifth ventricle) and cavum Vergae (sixth ventricle). Diagnosis and treatment.' *Archives of Neurology and Psychiatry*, **25**, 44–66.

—— (1932) 'The brain.' *In* Lewis, D. (Ed.) *Practice of Surgery*. Hagerstown: W. F. Prior.

—— Blackfan, K.D. (1914) 'Internal hydrocephalus. An experimental, clinical and pathological study.' *American Journal of Diseases of Children*, **8**, 406–482.

Davidoff, L.M., Dyke, C.G. (1938) 'Relapsing juvenile chronic subdural hematoma. A clinical and roentgenographic study.' *Neurological Institute of New York Bulletin*, **8**, 95–111.

Davis, L.E. (1924) 'A physio-pathologic study of the choroid plexus with the report of a case of villous hypertrophy.' *Journal of Medical Research*, **44**, 521–534.

Davson, H., Welch, K., Segal, M.B. (1987) *Physiology and Pathophysiology of the Cerebrospinal Fluid*. Edinburgh, New York: Churchill Livingstone.

De, S.N. (1950) 'A study of the changes in the brain in experimental internal hydrocephalus.' *Journal of Pathology and Bacteriology*, **62**, 197–208.

DeFeo, D., Foltz, E.L., Hamilton, A.E. (1975) 'Double compartment hydrocephalus in a patient with cysticercosis meningitis.' *Surgical Neurology*, **4**, 247–251.

DeMyer, W., Zeman, W., Palmer, C.G. (1964) 'The face predicts the brain: diagnostic significance of median facial anomalies for holoprosencephaly (arhinencephaly).' *Pediatrics*, **34**, 256–263.

Dennis, J.P., Rosenberg, H.S., Alvord, E.C. Jr. (1961) 'Megalencephaly, internal hydrocephalus and other neurological aspects of achondroplasia.' *Brain*, **84**, 427–445.

Dohrmann, G.J. (1971) 'The choroid plexus in experimental hydrocephalus. A light and electron microoscopic study in normal, hydrocephalic, and shunted hydrocephalic dogs.' *Journal of Neurosurgery*, **34**, 56–69.

Doran, P.A., Guthkelch, A.N. (1961) 'Studies in spina bifida cystica. I. General survey and reassessment of the problem.' *Journal of Neurology, Neurosurgery and Psychiatry*, **24**, 331–345.

Edwards, M.S.B., Harrison, M.R., Halks-Miller, M., Nakayana, D.K., Berger, M.S., Glick, P.L., Chinn, D.H. (1984) 'A model of congenital hydrocephalus *in utero* in fetal lambs and Rhesus monkeys produced by the intracisternal injection of kaolin.' *In* Shapiro, K., Marmarou, A., Portnoy, H. (Eds) *Hydrocephalus*. New York: Raven.

Eisenberg, H.M., McComb, J.G., Lorenzo, A.V. (1974) 'Cerebrospinal fluid overproduction and hydrocephalus associated with choroid plexus papilloma.' *Journal of Neurosurgery*, **40**, 381–385.

Emery, J.L., Kalhan, S.C. (1970) 'The pathology of exencephalus.' *Developmental Medicine and Child Neurology*, **12** (Suppl. 22), 51–64.

Fairburn, B. (1960) 'Choroid plexus papilloma and its relation to hydrocephalus.' *Journal of Neurosurgery*, **17**, 166–171.

Fedrick, J., Butler, N.R. (1970) 'Certain causes of neonatal death. II. Intraventricular haemorrhage.' *Biology of the Neonate*, **15**, 257–290.

Fishman, R.A., Greer, M. (1963) 'Experimental obstructive hydrocephalus. Changes in the cerebrum.' *Archives of Neurology*, **8**, 156–161.

Fishman, M.A., Hogan, G.R., Dodge, P.R. (1971) 'The concurrence of hydrocephalus and craniosynostosis.' *Journal of Neurosurgery*, **34**, 621–629.

Foerster, O. (1939) 'Ein Fall von Agenesie des Corpus callosum verbunden mit einem Diverticulum paraphysarium des Ventriculus tertius.' *Zeitschrift für Gesamte Neurologie und Psychiatrie*, **164**, 380–391.

Ford, F.R. (1926) 'Cerebral birth injuries and their results.' *Medicine*, **5**, 121–194.

Fraser, J., Dott, N.M. (1922) 'Hydrocephalus.' *British Journal of Surgery*, **10**, 165–191.

Gadsdon, D.R., Variend, S., Emery, J.L. (1979) 'Myelination of the corpus callosum. II. The effect of relief of hydrocephalus upon the processes of myelination.' *Zeitschrift für Kinderchirurgie und Grenzgebiete*, **28**, 314–321.

Gilles, F.H. (1986) 'Hydrocephalus in the neonate, infant and child.' *In* Hoffman, H.J., Epstein, F. (Eds) *Disorders of the Developing Nervous System: Diagnosis and Treatment*. Boston: Blackwell Scientific. pp. 541–572.

—— Shillito, J. Jr. (1970) 'Infantile hydrocephalus: retrocerebellar subdural hematoma.' *Journal of Pediatrics*, **76**, 529–537.

—— Rockett, F.X. (1971) 'Infantile hydrocephalus: retrocerebellar "arachnoidal" cyst.' *Journal of Pediatrics*, **79**, 436–443.

—— Leviton, A., Dooling, E. C. (1983) *The Developing Human Brain*. Boston: John Wright.

Glees, P., Voth, D. (1988) 'Clinical and ultrastructural observations of maturing human frontal cortex. Part I (Biopsy material of hydrocephalic infants).' *Neurosurgical Review*, **11**, 273–278.

—— Hasan, M., Voth, D., Schwarz, M. (1989) 'Fine structural features of the cerebral microvasculature in hydrocephalic human infants: correlated clinical observations.' *Neurosurgical Review*, **12**, 315–321.

Go, K.G., Stokroos, I., Blaauw, E.H., Zuiderveen, F., Molenaar, I. (1976) 'Changes of ventricular ependyma and choroid plexus in experimental hydrocephalus, as observed by scanning electron microscopy.' *Acta Neuropathologica*, **34**, 55–64.

—— Houthoff, H-J., Blaauw, E.H., Havinga, P., Hartsuiker, J. (1984) 'Arachnoid cysts of the Sylvian fissure. Evidence of fluid secretion.' *Journal of Neurosurgery*, **60**, 803–813.

Granholm, L., Rådberg, C. (1963) 'Congenital communicating hydrocephalus.' *Journal of Neurosurgery*, **20**, 338–343.

Gudeman, S.K., Sullivan, H.G., Rosner, M.J., Becker, D.P. (1979) 'Surgical removal of bilateral papillomas of the choroid plexus of the lateral ventricles with resolution of hydrocephalus.' *Journal of Neurosurgery*, **50**, 677–681.

Guthkelch, A.N. (1970) 'Occipital cranium bifidum.' *Archives of Disease in Childhood*, **45**, 104–109.

Hamby, W.B., Krauss, R.F., Beswick, W.F. (1950) 'Hydranencephaly: clinical diagnosis. Presentation of seven cases.' *Pediatrics*, **6**, 371–383.

Hart, M.N., Malamud, N., Ellis, W.G. (1972) 'The Dandy-Walker syndrome. A clinicopathological study based on 28 cases.' *Neurology*, **22**, 771–780.

Heschl, R. (1859) 'Gehirndefect und Hydrocephalus.' *Vierteljahrschrift für die Praktische Heilkunde*, **61**, 59–74.

Hintz, R.L. (1979) 'Holoprosencephaly.' *In* Bergsma, D. (Ed.) *Birth Defects Compendium. National*

Foundation March of Dimes, 2nd Edn. New York: Alan R. Liss. pp. 526–527.

Hochwald, G.M., Sahar, A., Sadik, A.R., Ransohoff, J. (1969) 'Cerebrospinal fluid production and histological observations in animals with experimental obstructive hydrocephalus.' *Experimental Neurology*, **25**, 190–199.

Hoffman, H.J., Freeman, A. (1967) 'Primary malignant leptomeningeal melanoma in association with giant hairy nevi.' *Journal of Neurosurgery*, **26**, 62–71.

Horton, W.A., Rotter, J.I., Rimoin, D.L., Scott, C.I., Hall, J.G. (1978) 'Standard growth curves for achondroplasia.' *Journal of Pediatrics*, **93**, 435–438.

Huong, T.T., Goldbatt, E., Simpson, D.A. (1975) 'Dandy-Walker syndrome associated with congenital heart defects: report of three cases.' *Developmental Medicine and Child Neurology*, **17** (Suppl. 35), 35–41.

Hutchison, W.M., Dunachie, J.F., Siim, J.C., Work, K. (1970) 'Coccidian-like nature of *Toxoplasma gondii*.' *British Medical Journal*, **1**, 142–144.

—— —— Work, K., Siim, J.C. (1971) 'The life cycle of the coccidian parasite, *Toxoplasma gondii*, in the domestic cat.' *Transactions of the Royal Society of Tropical Medicine and Hygiene*, **65**, 380–399.

Ingraham, F.D., Scott, H.W. Jr. (1943) 'Spina bifida and cranium bifidum. V. The Arnold-Chiari malformation: a study of 20 cases.' *New England Journal of Medicine*, **229**, 108–114.

—— Swan, H. (1943) 'Spina bifida and cranium bifidum. I. A survey of five hundred and forty-six cases.' *New England Journal of Medicine*, **228**, 559–563.

James, A.E. Jr., Strecker, E-P. (1974) 'Use of silastic to produce communicating hydrocephalus.' *Investigative Radiology*, **8**, 105–110.

—— Flor, W.J., Novak, G.R., Strecker, E-P., Burns, B., Epstein, M. (1977) 'Experimental hydrocephalus.' *Experimental Eye Research*, **25** (Suppl.), 435–459.

Jenkyn, L.R., Roberts, D.W., Merlis, A.L., Rozycki, A.A., Nordgren, R.E. (1981) 'Dandy-Walker malformation in identical twins.' *Neurology*, **31**, 337–341.

Johnson, R.P. (1958) 'Clinicopathological aspects of the cerebrospinal fluid circulation.' *In* Wolstenholme, G.E.W., O'Connor, C.M. (Eds) *Ciba Foundation Symposium on Production, Circulation and Absorption of the Cerebrospinal Fluid*. Boston: Little Brown.

—— Johnson, K.J., Edmonds, C.J. (1967) 'Virus induced hydrocephalus: development of aqueductal stenosis after mumps infection.' *Science*, **157**, 1066–1067.

Jones, H.C., Dack, S., Ellis, C. (1987) 'Morphological aspects of the development of hydrocephalus in a mouse mutant (SUMS/NP).' *Acta Neuropathologica*, **72**, 268–276.

Kalter, H., Warkany, J. (1983) 'Congenital malformations. Etiologic factors and their role in prevention.' *New England Journal of Medicine*, **308**, 424–431; 491–497.

Karch, S.B., Urich, H. (1972) 'Occipital encephalocele: a morphological study.' *Journal of the Neurological Sciences*, **15**, 89–112.

Khoury, M.J., Erickson, J.D., James, L.M. (1982) 'Etiologic heterogeneity of neural tube defects: clues from epidemiology.' *American Journal of Epidemiology*, **115**, 538–548.

Larroche, J.-C. (1982) 'The fine structure of matrix capillaries in human embryos and young fetuses.' *In The Second Special Ross Laboratories Conference on Perinatal Intracranial Haemorrhage, December 2–4, 1982*. Washington, DC. pp. 2–5.

Lawson, R.F., Raimondi, A.J. (1973) 'Hydrocephalus-3, a murine mutant: I. Alterations in fine structure of choroid plexus and ependyma.' *Surgical Neurology*, **1**, 115–128.

Leong, A.S.Y., Shaw, C.M. (1979) 'The pathology of occipital encephalocele and a discussion of pathogenesis.' *Pathology*, **11**, 223–234.

Levin, S.D., Hoyle, N.R., Brown, J.K., Thomas, D.G.T. (1985) 'Cerebrospinal fluid myelin basic protein immunoreactivity as an indicator of brain damage in children.' *Developmental Medicine and Child Neurology*, **27**, 807–813.

Lindberg, L.A., Vasenius, L., Talanti, S. (1977) 'The surface fine structure of the ependymal lining of the lateral ventricle in rats with hereditary hydrocephalus.' *Cell and Tissue Research*, **179**, 121–129.

Lorber, J., Schofield, J.K. (1979) 'The prognosis of occipital encephalocele.' *Zeitschrift für Kinderchirurgie und Grenzgebiete*, **28**, 347–351.

Lux, W.E. Jr., Hochwald, G.M., Sahar, A., Ransohoff, J. (1970) 'Periventricular water content. Effect of pressure in experimental chronic hydrocephalus.' *Archives of Neurology*, **23**, 475–479.

Magendie, F. (1842) *Recherches Philosophiques et Cliniques sur le Liquide Céphalo-rachidien ou Cérébro-spinal*. Paris: Librairie Médicale de Mequignon-Marvis Fils.

78

Marsh, H., Gould, A.P., Clutton, H.H., Parker, R.W. (1885) 'Report of a committee of the society nominated November 10, 1882 to investigate spina bifida and its treatment by the injection of Dr Morton's Iodoglycerine solution.' *Transactions of the Clinical Society of London*, **18**, 339–418.

McAllister, J.P., Maugans, T.A., Shah, M.V., Truex, R.C. Jr. (1985) 'Neuronal effects of experimentally induced hydrocephalus in newborn rats.' *Journal of Neurosurgery*, **63**, 776–783.

McLaurin, R.L. (1964) 'Parietal encephaloceles.' *Neurology*, **14**, 764–772.

McLone, D.G., Bondareff, W., Raimondi, A.J. (1971) 'Brain edema in the hydrocephalic hy-3 mouse: submicroscopic morphology.' *Journal of Neuropathology and Experimental Neurology*, **30**, 627–637.

—— Raimondi, A.J. (1984) 'The hydrocephalic-3 house mouse.' *In* Shapiro, A., Marmarou, A., Portnoy, H. (Eds) *Hydrocephalus*. New York: Raven.

Mealey, J. Jr., Dezenitis, A.J., Hockey, A.A. (1970) 'The prognosis of encephaloceles.' *Journal of Neurosurgery*, **32**, 209–218.

Milhorat, T.H., Clark, R.G. (1970) 'Some observations on the circulation of phenosulfonphthalein in cerebrospinal fluid: normal flow and the flow in hydrocephalus.' *Journal of Neurosurgery*, **32**, 522–528.

—— Clark, R.G., Hammock, M.K., McGrath, P.P. (1970) 'Structural, ultrastructural, and permeability changes in the ependyma and surrounding brain favoring equilibration in progressive hydrocephalus.' *Archives of Neurology*, **22**, 397–407.

—— Hammock, M.K., DeChiro, G. (1971) 'The subarachnoid space in congenital obstructive hydrocephalus. Part 1. Cisternographic findings.' *Journal of Neurosurgery*, **35**, 1–6.

—— —— Davis, D.A., Fenstermacher, J.D. (1976) 'Choroid plexus papilloma. I. Proof of cerebrospinal fluid overproduction.' *Childs Brain*, **2**, 273–289.

Milunsky, A., Ulcickas, M.E., Willett, W., Rothman, K., Jick, S., Jick, H. (1991) 'Hyperthermia and neural tube defects (NTD).' *Pediatric Research*, **29**, 71A.

MMWR (1982) 'Valproic acid and spina bifida: a preliminary report.' (France.) *Centre for Disease Control Morbidity and Mortality Weekly Report*, **31**, 565–566.

Munro, D. (1928) 'Cranial and intracranial damage in the newborn. An end-result study of one hundred seventeen cases.' *Surgery, Gynecology and Obstetrics*, **47**, 622–630.

Myrianthopoulos, N.C., Melnick, M. (1986) 'Studies in neural tube defects. I. Epidemiologic and etiologic aspects.' *American Journal of Medical Genetics*, **26**, 783–796.

Nelson, R.M. Jr., Leuschen, M.P., Shuman, R.M. (1982) 'A morphometric analysis of germinal matrix and cortical capillaries in beagle pups.' *In The Second Special Ross Laboratories Conference on Perinatal Intracranial Haemorrhage, December 2–4, 1982*. Washington DC. pp. 6–18.

Neuhauser, E.B.D., Griscom, N.T., Gilles, F.H., Crocker, A.C. (1968) 'Arachnoid cysts in the Hurler-Hunter syndrome. (Kystes arachnoïdiens dans le syndrome de Hurler-Hunter.)' *Annales de Radiologie (Paris)*, **11**, 453–469.

Nielsen, S.L., Gauger, G.E. (1974) 'Experimental hydrocephalus: surface alterations of the lateral ventricle. Scanning electron microscopic studies.' *Laboratory Investigation*, **30**, 618–625.

Northfield, D.W.C., Russell, D.S. (1939) 'False diverticulum of a lateral ventricle causing hemiplegia in chronic internal hydrocephalus.' *Brain*, **62**, 311–320.

Nova, H.R. (1979) 'Familial communicating hydrocephalus, posterior cerebellar agenesis, mega cisterna magna, and port-wine nevi. Report on five members of one family.' *Journal of Neurosurgery*, **51**, 862–865.

Nugent, G.R., Al-Mefty, O., Chou, S. (1979) 'Communicating hydrocephalus as a cause of aqueductal stenosis.' *Journal of Neurosurgery*, **51**, 812–818.

Ogata, J., Hochwald, G.M., Cravioto, H., Ransohoff, J. (1972) 'Light and electron microscopic studies of experimental hydrocephalus. Ependymal and subependymal areas.' *Acta Neuropathologica*, **21**, 213–223.

Osaka, K., Matsumoto, S. (1978) 'Holoprosencephaly in neurosurgical practice.' *Journal of Neurosurgery*, **48**, 787–803.

Page, R.B. (1975) 'Scanning electron microscopy of the ventricular system in normal and hydrocephalic rabbits. Preliminary report and atlas.' *Journal of Neurosurgery*, **42**, 646–664.

—— Rosenstein, J.M., Leure-duPree, A.E. (1979*a*) 'The morphology of extrachoroidal ependyma overlying gray and white matter in the rabbit lateral ventricle.' *Anatomical Record*, **194**, 67–81.

—— —— Dovey, B.J., Leure-duPree, A.E. (1979*b*) 'Ependymal changes in experimental hydrocephalus.' *Anatomical Record*, **194**, 83–103.

Papile, L.-A., Burstein, J., Burstein, R., Koffler, H. (1978) 'Incidence and evolution of subependymal and intraventricular haemorrhage: a study of infants with birth weights of less than 1,500 gm.' *Journal of Pediatrics*, **92**, 529–534.

Penfield, W. (1929) 'Diencephalic autonomic epilepsy.' *Archives of Neurology and Psychiatry*, **22**, 358–374.

—— Elvidge, A.R. (1932) 'Hydrocephalus and the atrophy of cerebral compression.' *In* Penfield, W. (Ed.) *Cytology and Cellular Pathology of the Nervous System, Section XXVII, Vol. 3*. New York: Paul R. Hoeber.

Portnoy, H.D., Croissant, P.D. (1976) 'A practical method for measuring hydrodynamics of cerebrospinal fluid.' *Surgical Neurology*, **5**, 273–277.

Povlishock, J.T., Martinez, A.J., Moossy, J. (1977) 'The fine structure of blood vessels of the telencephalic germinal matrix in the human fetus.' *American Journal of Anatomy*, **149**, 439–452.

Raimondi, A.J., Clark, S.J., McLone, D.G. (1976) 'Pathogenesis of aqueductal occlusion in congenital murine hydrocephalus.' *Journal of Neurosurgery*, **45**, 66–77.

—— Samuelson, G., Yarzagaray, L., Norton, T. (1969) 'Atresia of the foramina of Luschka and Magendie: the Dandy-Walker cyst.' *Journal of Neurosurgery*, **31**, 202–216.

—— Soare, P. (1974) 'Intellectual development in shunted hydrocephalic children.' *American Journal of Diseases of Children*, **127**, 664–671.

Rakic, P., Yakovlev, P.I. (1968) 'The development of corpus callosum and cavum septi in man.' *Journal of Comparative Neurology*, **132**, 45–72.

Rubin, R.C., Hochwald, G.M., Liwnicz, B., Tiell, M., Mizutani, H., Shulman, K. (1972) 'The effect of severe hydrocephalus on size and number of brain cells.' *Developmental Medicine and Child Neurology*, **14**, 112–117.

—— Hochwald, G.M., Tiell, M., Mizutani, H., Ghatak, N. (1976a) 'Hydrocephalus: I. Histological and ultrastructural changes in the pre-shunted cortical mantle.' *Surgical Neurology*, **5**, 109–114.

—— —— Liwnicz, B.H. (1976b) 'Hydrocephalus: II. Cell number and size, and myelin content of the pre-shunted cerebral cortical mantle.' *Surgical Neurology*, **5**, 115–118.

—— —— —— Epstein, F., Ghatak, N., Wisniewski, H. (1976c) 'Hydrocephalus: III. Reconstitution of the cerebral cortical mantle following ventricular shunting.' *Surgical Neurology*, **5**, 179–183.

Russell, D.S. (1949) 'Observation on the pathology of hydrocephalus.' *Special Report Series No. 265. Medical Research Council*. London: HMSO.

Sahar, A., Feinsod, M., Beller, A.J. (1980) 'Choroid plexus papilloma: hydrocephalus and cerebrospinal fluid dynamics.' *Surgical Neurology*, **13**, 476–478.

Salmon, J.H. (1967) 'Puncture porencephaly. Pathogenesis and prevention.' *American Journal of Diseases of Children*, **114**, 72–79.

Sato, O., Ohya, M., Nojiri, K., Tsugane, R. (1984) 'Microcirculatory changes in experimental hydrocephalus: morphological and physiological studies.' *In* Shapiro, A., Marmarou, A., Portnoy, H. (Eds) *Hydrocephalus*. New York: Raven.

Sayers, M.P. (1966) 'Discussion.' *In* Shulman, K. (Ed.) *Workshop in Hydrocephalus*. Philadelphia: Children's Hospital of Philadelphia.

—— (1971) 'Surgery for obstructive hydrocephalus.' *Acta Neurologica Latinoamericana*, **17** (Suppl. 1), 245–254.

Scherer, E. (1935) 'Über Cystenbildung der weichen Hirnhäute im Liquorraum der Sylvischen Furche mit hochgradiger Deformierung des Gehirns.' *Zeitschrift für die Gesamte Neurologie und Psychiatrie*, **152**, 787–799.

Shapiro, W.R., Williams, G.H., Plum, F. (1969) 'Spontaneous recurrent hypothermia accompanying agenesis of the corpus callosum.' *Brain*, **92**, 423–436.

Shaw, C.-M., Alvord, E.C. Jr. (1969) 'Cava septi pellucidi et Vergae: their normal and pathological states.' *Brain*, **92**, 213–224.

Smithells, R.W., Sheppard, S., Schorah, C.J. (1976) 'Vitamin deficiencies and neural tube defects.' *Archives of Disease in Childhood*, **51**, 944–950.

—— —— —— Seller, M.J., Nevin, C., Harris, R., Read, A.P., Fielding, D.W. (1981) 'Apparent prevention of neural tube defects by periconceptional vitamin supplementation.' *Archives of Disease in Childhood*, **56**, 911–918.

—— Seller, M.J., Harris, R., Fielding, D.W., Schorah, C.J., Nevin, N.C., Sheppard, S., Read,

A.P., Walker, S., Wild, J. (1983) 'Further experience of vitamin supplementation for prevention of neural tube defect recurrences.' *Lancet*, **1**, 1027–1031.

Spatz, H. (1920) 'Über eine besondere Reaktionweise des unreifen Zentralnervengewebes.' *Zeitschrift für Gesamte Neurologie und Psychiatrie*, **53**, 363–394.

Strecker, E.-P., James, A.E. Jr, Kelley, J.E., Merz, T. (1974) 'Semiquantitative studies of transependymal albumin movement in communicating hydrocephalus.' *Radiology*, **111**, 341–346.

Summers, G.D., Young, A.C., Little, R.A., Stoner, H.B., Forbes, W.S. T.C., Jones, R.A.C. (1981) 'Spontaneous periodic hypothermia with lipoma of the corpus callosum.' *Journal of Neurology, Neurosurgery and Psychiatry*, **44**, 1094–1099.

Sutton, L.N., Wood, J.H., Brooks, B.R., Barrer, S.J., Kline, M., Cohen, S.R. (1983) 'Cerebrospinal fluid myelin basic protein in hydrocephalus.' *Journal of Neurosurgery*, **59**, 467–470.

Swan, C. (1949) 'Rubella in pregnancy as an aetiological factor in congenital malformation, still birth, miscarriage and abortion.' *Journal of Obstetrics and Gynaecology of the British Empire*, **56**, 341–363; 591–605.

Swett, H.A., Nixon, G.W. (1975) 'Agenesis of the corpus callosum with interhemispheric cyst.' *Radiology*, **114**, 641–645.

Timmons, G.D., Johnson, K.P. (1970) 'Aqueductal stenosis and hydrocephalus after mumps encephalitis.' *New England Journal of Medicine*, **283**, 1505–1507.

Toriello, H.V. (1984) 'Report of a third kindred with X-linked anencephaly/spina bifida.' (Letter.) *American Journal of Medical Genetics*, **19**, 411–412.

Torvik, A., Stenwig, A.E., Finseth, I. (1981) 'The pathology of experimental obstructive hydrocephalus. A scanning electron microscopic study.' *Acta Neuropathologica*, **54**, 143–147.

Vigouroux, A. (1908) 'Écoulement de liquide céphalo-rachidien. Hydrocéphalie papillome des plexus choroïdes du IVᶜ ventricule.' *Révue Neurologique*, **16**, 281–285.

Von Recklinghausen, E. (1886) 'Untersuchungen über die Spina bifida.' *Virchows Archiv für Pathologische Anatomie und Physiologie und für Klinische Medizin*, **105**, 243–330; 373–455.

Walker, A.E. (1949) 'Spontaneous ventricular rhinorrhea and otorrhea.' *Journal of Neuropathology and Experimental Neurology*, **8**, 171–183.

Walsh, J., Gilles, F.H., Welch, K. (1978) 'Infantile retrocerebellar cyst with immature neural tissue.' *Journal of Neurosurgery*, **48**, 628–631.

Weed, L.H. (1917) 'The development of the cerebro-spinal spaces in pig and in man.' *Carnegie Institution of Washington, Publication 225, No. 14, Washington DC. Contributions to Embryology*, **5**, 41–52.

Welch, K. (1980) 'The etiology and classification of hydrocephalus in childhood.' *Zeitschrift für Kinderchirurgie*, **31**, 331–335.

—— Strand, R., Bresnan, M., Cavazzuti, V. (1983) 'Congenital hydrocephalus due to villous hypertrophy of the telencephalic choroid plexuses.' *Journal of Neurosurgery*, **59**, 172–175.

—— Lorenzo, A.V. (1984) 'Germinal matrix and ventricular hemorrhage in the lagomorph.' *In* Shapiro, K., Marmarou, A., Portnoy, H. (Eds) *Hydrocephalus*. New York: Raven.

—— Strand, R. (1986) 'Traumatic parturitional intracranial hemorrhage.' *Developmental Medicine and Child Neurology*, **28**, 156–159.

—— Winston, K.R. (1987) 'Spina bifida.' *In* Vinken, P.J., Bruyn, G.W., Klawans, H.L. (Eds) *Congenital malformations of the spine and spinal cord. Handbook of Clinical Neurology*, **6** (50). Amsterdam, New York: Elsevier.

Weller, R.O., Wisniewski, H. (1969) 'Histological and ultrastructural changes with experimental hydrocephalus in adult rabbits.' *Brain*, **92**, 819–828.

—— —— Shulman, K., Terry, R.D. (1971) 'Experimental hydrocephalus in young dogs: histological and ultrastructural study of the brain tissue damage.' *Journal of Neuropathology and Experimental Neurology*, **30**, 613–626.

—— Mitchell, J., Griffin, R.L., Gardner, M.J. (1978) 'The effects of hydrocephalus upon the developing brain. Histological and quantitative studies of the ependyma and subependyma in hydrocephalic rats.' *Journal of the Neurological Sciencies*, **36**, 383–402.

Williams, B. (1973) 'Is aqueduct stenosis a result of hydrocephalus?' *Brain*, **96**, 399–412.

Windham, G.C., Bjerkedal, T. (1982) 'Secular trends of neural tube defects by demographic subgroups in Norway, 1967–1981.' *NIPH Annals* (Oslo), **5**, 57–67.

Wisniewski, H., Weller, R.O., Terry, R.D. (1969) 'Experimental hydrocephalus produced by the subarachnoid infusion of silicone oil.' *Journal of Neurosurgery*, **31**, 10–14.

Wolff, A., Cowen, D. (1937) 'Granulomatous encephalomyelitis due to an encephalitozoon (Encephalitozoic encephalomyelitis).' *Neurological Institute of New York Bulletin*, **6**, 306–371.

Woollam, D.H.M., Millen, J.W. (1953) 'Anatomical considerations in the pathology of stenosis of the cerebral aqueduct.' *Brain*, **76**, 104–112.

Wozniak, M., McLone, D.G., Raimondi, A.J. (1975) 'Micro- and macrovascular changes as the direct cause of parenchymal destruction in congenital murine hydrocephalus.' *Journal of Neurosurgery*, **43**, 535–545.

Yakovlev, P.I. (1947) 'Paraplegias of hydrocephalus.' *American Journal of Mental Deficiency*, **51**, 561–576.

—— (1959) 'Pathoarchitectonic studies of cerebral malformations. III. Arhinencephalies (holo-telencephalies).' *Journal of Neuropathology and Experimental Neurology*, **18**, 22–55.

Yamada, H., Sakata, K., Kashiki, Y., Okuma, A., Takada, M. (1979) 'Peculiar congenital parieto-occipital head tumor. Report of 3 cases.' *Childs Brain*, **5**, 426–432.

6
DIAGNOSTIC IMAGING IN SPINA BIFIDA AND HYDROCEPHALUS

Jane M. Hawnaur

Prenatal diagnosis of congenital intracranial and spinal malformation has become possible in recent years with routine screening for elevated levels of maternal serum alpha-fetoprotein and the widespread availability of high-resolution realtime ultrasound scanning. The ability to assess the severity of fetal abnormality at an early stage of gestation enables the prospective parents and their doctor to discuss prognosis and make an informed decision regarding termination of the affected pregnancy. Gowland (1988) identified the problems which may be created by false-positive, false-negative or equivocal ultrasound findings in a low-risk population.

Ultrasound imaging of the brain is restricted to the first few months of postnatal life while the fontanelles and sutures remain open. Computed x-ray tomography (CT) or magnetic resonance imaging (MRI) are necessary for subsequent cranial imaging. In infants under one year of age, ultrasound can be used to screen for intraspinal pathology (Naidich *et al.* 1984). In later childhood, more complex radiological investigations may be required. Until recently, the possible benefit of demonstrating a significant neural lesion had to be balanced against the necessity for myelography and/or CT, techniques which are invasive, employ ionising radiation and are often poorly tolerated by children. MRI has revolutionised assessment of the spine, and can display the entire range of abnormalities associated with spinal dysraphism with minimal risk or trauma to the patient (Barnes *et al.* 1986, Altman and Altman 1987, Szalay *et al.* 1987). This chapter describes imaging techniques for congenital abnormalities of the brain and spine, and reviews recent applications to obtain functional information.

Imaging techniques
Ultrasound
Ultrasound is relatively cheap and portable, and does not use ionising radiation. There is no evidence of hazard to the fetus or neonate from the degree of ultrasound exposure used in diagnostic imaging. A beam of high-frequency soundwaves is produced by applying short electrical impulses to piezo-electric material in the imaging transducer. The higher the frequency of ultrasound used (typically 2.0 to 10.0MHz in diagnostic imaging) the greater the spatial resolution, but also the more rapid the attenuation in tissue, limiting the depth of penetration of the ultrasound beam. Ultrasound reflected back from tissue interfaces within the patient physically deforms the lattice of the piezo-electric crystal, generating an

electrical signal. An image can be produced by calculating the distance of the reflective tissue interface from the transducer. Rapid display of successive images on a monitor creates realtime images on which vascular pulsation and other physiological motion can be appreciated. Routine antenatal scans are usually performed at around 16 weeks of gestation by specialist radiographers. Given good quality equipment, successful screeening depends on a systematic approach and a high degree of experience on the part of the operator. Axial views at the level of the thalami, lateral ventricles and cerebellum enable most significant intracranial lesions to be identified, and allow cranial abnormalities associated with spinal dysraphism to be sought.

Postnatal cranial ultrasound examinations are performed in the radiology department or at the bedside using portable equipment with minimal disturbance of the infant. Transfontanellar coronal and sagittal sections are obtained routinely, supplemented if necessary by transaxial views via the thin temporoparietal squama. Serial measurement of ventricular size can be used to monitor progression of hydrocephalus following periventricular haemorrhage and to identify infants for whom insertion of a ventricular shunt becomes desirable (Holt 1989).

The use of ultrasound for antenatal detection of spina bifida was first suggested by Campbell *et al.* (1975). Marked improvements in sensitivity and specificity have occurred subsequently due to increased operator experience and technological advances (Roberts *et al.* 1983, Pearce *et al.* 1985). Adequate assessment of the spine may be difficult in breech presentation, twin pregnancy, fetal lie with the spine posteriorly, or oligohydramnios. The longitudinal plane is ideal for displaying the extent of spina bifida while the transverse view is more sensitive for detection of small dysraphic defects. Absence of active movement of the lower limbs can be observed in the fetus with severe spina bifida using realtime ultrasound.

In infants up to one year of age, the bony structures of the posterior neural arch are small and poorly ossified and the interlaminar spaces can be used as acoustic windows. An acoustic window is also created by surgical laminectomy or dysraphic defects. A high-frequency transducer (up to 10MHz) is used in conjunction with a water path or stand-off device. Normal appearances have been well described (Raghavendra and Epstein 1985).

Computed tomography

CT images are produced by detecting the amount of radiation transmitted when a narrow beam of x-rays passes through the patient from multiple points around the circumference of a body 'slice'. A grey-scale image is produced in which each picture element or pixel represents the linear attenuation value for x-rays of the tissue within the volume element scanned. Each CT slice takes approximately two seconds to acquire and the radiation dose is related to the number and thickness of image slices, the radiographic technique and the particular CT equipment used. An interslice gap reduces the total radiation dose, and angulation of the scan plane to 20° above the orbitomeatal line avoids scanning directly through the lens of the eye.

Direct scanning is virtually limited to the transaxial plane; production of sagittal or coronal images usually requires computer reconstruction of multiple contiguous thin transaxial scans. Administration of intravenous iodinated contrast medium is rarely indicated except in the evaluation of congenital tumours. Artefacts due to beam hardening are produced from dense material such as metal clips or dental amalgam. Soft-tissue detail is limited adjacent to dense cortical bone in the cranial vault, posterior fossa and at the craniocervical junction.

Neonates can be transported to the CT room in a portable incubator. During scanning, babies must be kept warm and subjected to as little handling as possible. Sedation is rarely required in infants if advantage is taken of postprandial drowsiness. Sedation or a general anaesthetic may be necessary in older children in order to obtain images of diagnostic quality.

In the spine, CT allows detailed cross-sectional display of bony abnormalities in spinal dysraphism and, in combination with intrathecal contrast medium, can show morphological changes in soft-tissue structures. The ability to demonstrate the substance of the spinal cord is limited. For example, demonstration of syringomyelia requires myelography to identify the degree and extent of the spinal-cord expansion, and CT scanning should be delayed for 18 to 24 hours to show diffusion of contrast media from cerebrospinal fluid (CSF) into the cavity. Many transaxial CT slices may be necessary to demonstrate the full extent of the syringomyelic cavity, involving a prohibitive radiation dose.

Myelography

Myelography is an invasive procedure which requires general anaesthesia in the young child, is unpleasant and traumatic for the older child, uses ionising radiation and has a small but significant morbidity and mortality. The technique involves injection of water-soluble contrast medium, with an iodine content of approximately 200mg/ml, into the thecal sac. In children with suspected spinal dysraphism, the usual practice of injection at the L3/L4 level requires particular caution because of the danger of damage to a tethered cord. Radiographs are routinely obtained with the patient prone, but supine films may be necessary to exclude meningocele or an intradural tumour. Intrathecal injection of contrast medium is associated with convulsions, particularly if it is run up to the skull base to examine the cervical region.

Magnetic resonance imaging

Image production in MRI depends on generation of signals from atomic nuclei with an intrinsic magnetism and nuclear spin. MRI is approved for imaging after the first trimester of pregnancy and there is no known biological hazard at field strengths of less than 2 Tesla. Hydrogen nuclei (protons) are used in imaging because of their abundance in body water and fat. Repetitive pulses of radiofrequency (RF) radiation in a uniform magnetic field induce alternate absorption and release of RF energy (resonance) by protons. Signals emitted are detected by head or spine receiver coils, and the source from within the body is localised by superimposing magnetic gradients across the main field and taking advantage of the fact that the frequency at which protons resonate depends on the magnetic field strength. Image contrast is related to the proton density, flow, and relaxation times of the tissues, and pulse sequences can be designed to reflect one or more of these parameters. T1 and T2 relaxation times describe the changes in magnetisation which occur respectively in planes parallel and perpendicular to the main magnetic field when the excitational RF pulses are removed and protons return to the equilibrium state. On T1-weighted scans, CSF has a low signal intensity, neural and other soft tissue is of medium signal intensity, and fat has a high signal intensity. Evaluation of morphological abnormalities such as hydrocephalus or Arnold-Chiari malformation can be accomplished by using relatively short T1-weighted spin echo (SE) or gradient echo (GE) sequences. Inversion recovery (IR) sequences have a superior grey/white-matter contrast and may be useful in assessment of brain maturation and dysmyelination. On T2-weighted scans, CSF and fat have a relatively high signal intensity and pathological tissues are usually brighter than normal because of increased water content. T2-weighted sequences are valuable for detecting white-matter abnormalities, grey-matter heterotopias, tumours and inflammation. Imaging time depends on the pulse sequences used and various technical parameters relating to the spatial resolution required: around five minutes or less for T1-weighted SE and GE sequences, and 10 minutes or more for IR and T2-weighted SE sequences. Although relatively lengthy compared to CT, up to 16 separate images can be obtained during this acquisition time. Alternatively three-dimensional scanning allows thin sections from a block of tissue to be viewed from any angle. The multiplanar imaging facility of MRI is a major advantage over CT. Sagittal imaging is useful to evaluate the corpus callosum, brainstem, fourth ventricle and craniospinal junction. The coronal plane is useful to assess the interhemispheric fissure, the sella and suprasellar regions, and the middle and posterior cranial fossae.

In the spine, T1-weighted sequences in the sagittal plane are usually adequate to assess morphological abnormality but T2-weighted images may be necessary in a spinal tumour. Assessment of the entire spinal column and the skull base may require several repositions on the surface coil. Because sequences should be obtained in more than one plane, examination may take 30 minutes or more. Fast scanning techniques and motion compensating sequences may be helpful. The coronal plane is useful for demonstrating diastematomyelia and spinal curvature. Oblique scanning can be used to compensate for spinal curvature.

Many of the practical problems in MRI scanning of infants and children are similar to those that apply to CT. Care is necessary in neonates and small children to maintain body temperature in the cool environment of the MRI scan room. The longer acquisition time for MRI scans is a particular drawback in children. Each set of images takes minutes rather than seconds to acquire, and patient movement during this time is a major source of image degradation. Entering the scanner itself can be a daunting experience for children. The scanner gantry resembles a tunnel and restricts visual and aural contact with parents and nursing staff. Gradient switching during scanning creates a disturbing level of noise, particularly at high field strengths. The reassuring presence of a parent or nurse at the mouth of the magnet, maintaining physical contact and talking to the child, provides valuable support and encouragement. Cassette tapes of suitable music or nursery rhymes help to keep cooperative but easily bored children quiet and entertained. Babies and young infants can usually be scanned during their postprandial nap, and rarely require sedation. Children over the age of five or six years can usually be persuaded to keep still long enough for a diagnostic scan to be performed. A light general anaesthetic or sedative is necessary in mentally retarded or uncooperative children between the ages of one and six years. Ferro-magnetic life-support equipment cannot be used in close proximity to the magnet, resulting in difficulty monitoring vital signs in sedated or clinically unstable patients. Monitoring of heart rate can be achieved by modified electrocardiogram equipment with fibreoptic connections. Electronic equipment may malfunction in the magnetic field and, if generating RF pulses, can interfere with the RF signal of the scanner, resulting in image degradation. Small ferro-magnetic objects may be pulled at high velocity into the magnet, potentially injuring the patient. Metallic objects at a safe distance from the magnetic pull may still distort the magnetic field and degrade the image.

Intracranial abnormalities
Hydrocephalus
Non-communicating hydrocephalus results from obstruction to the flow of CSF between the choroid plexuses and the foramina of Luschka and Magendie at the outlet of the fourth ventricle. There is dilatation of the ventricular system proximal to the obstruction with normal ventricular size distally.

In communicating hydrocephalus there is obstruction to CSF flow within the subarachnoid space between the outlet of the fourth ventricle and the arachnoid granulations, leading to failure of reabsorption of CSF. The most common causes are haemorrhage and infection with adhesions and scarring of the meninges and subarachnoid spaces. There is usually a moderate degree of enlargement of the lateral ventricles and mild dilatation of the third and fourth ventricles. Radiological studies have shown that, in the early stages, enlargement is confined to the subarachnoid channels overlying the cerebral hemispheres (Robertson and Gomez 1978). Simultaneous dilatation of the subarachnoid spaces and ventricles then occurs until eventually only ventriculomegaly can be demonstrated.

Cardiac pulsation and respiratory movements are superimposed on the CSF flow. Studies using MRI have postulated pulsatile flow of CSF at the foramen of Monro and the aqueduct with antegrade flow during systole and a smaller retrograde flow during diastole giving net forward flow of CSF into the basal cisterns (Mark *et al.* 1987).

A classification of hydrocephalus is given in Table 6.I. Most patients with

TABLE 6.I

Classification of hydrocephalus

Congenital malformation	Aqueduct stenosis
	Dandy-Walker syndromes
	Arnold-Chiari malformation
	Encephalocele
	Other major cerebral malformation
	Skull deformity
Acquired lesions	Sequelae of haemorrhage
	Sequelae of infection
	Tumour
	Other obstructive lesions

congenital hydrocephalus have aqueduct stenosis (43 per cent), communicating hydrocephalus (38 per cent) or Dandy-Walker malformation (13 per cent) (Burton 1979).

Prenatal ultrasound diagnosis

Enlargement of the head occurs late in hydrocephalus, making measurement of the biparietal diameter alone unreliable for early detection. Identification of hydro-cephalus *in utero* depends upon the direct demonstration of ventricular dilatation. The ventricles are relatively large up to 18 to 20 weeks of gestation but as the cerebral tissue grows they occupy proportionally less of the cranium and the ratio of ventricular volume to brain falls. The lateral ventricle-to-hemisphere ratios are accurate predictors of fetal hydrocephalus over a wide range of gestational ages, including less than 24 weeks (Chervenak *et al.* 1984). This ratio is normally up to 70 per cent at 16 weeks, reducing to 40 per cent by 23 weeks. Measurement of the atria, which undergo the earliest and most pronounced changes, is probably the most sensitive method (Pearce *et al.* 1985). The normal third ventricle appears as a midline slit on axial images and is triangular in sagittal sections. It communicates with the fourth ventricle via the aqueduct of Sylvius, which is not usually visible on ultrasound. The underlying cause can often be inferred from the level of ventricular obstruction or by demonstrating specific lesions such as the Dandy-Walker malformation or spina bifida.

Prenatal ventricular drainage

Prenatal drainage of hydrocephalus by intrauterine ventriculo-atrial shunt place-ment, or serial ventricular puncture under ultrasound control, has yielded disappointing results (Manning *et al.* 1986). Although 29 of 32 fetuses survived, over half were moderately to severely disabled.

Diagnostic imaging of specific lesions associated with hydrocephalus

Aqueduct stenosis

Aqueduct stenosis accounts for about two thirds of cases of hydrocephalus, including those associated with dysraphism. Intrauterine infection such as toxoplasmosis or cytomegalovirus may result in gliotic stenosis of the aqueduct. True malformations include narrowing, forking (associated with Arnold-Chiari II malformation), an obstructing transverse septum and gliotic narrowing. Congenital tumours such as pinealoma may cause external compression of the aqueduct.

Diagnostic imaging shows moderate to severe dilatation of the lateral and third ventricles. The size of the fourth ventricle is usually normal if the Chiari malformation is absent; but otherwise it is small. Extrinsic causes of aqueduct stenosis can be shown on CT; intravenous contrast administration is mandatory to exclude both inflammatory and neoplastic lesions. MRI can directly demonstrate the aqueductal region on midline sagittal T1-weighted images and is more sensitive than CT for detection of mass lesions compressing the aqueduct and periaqueductal gliosis.

The patency of the cerebral aqueduct can be assessed using flow-sensitive MRI sequences. Atlas *et al.* (1988) examined 20 patients with aqueduct obstruction: lack of CSF flow through the aqueduct was established using gradient echo sequences on which stationary CSF had a low signal intensity and flowing CSF showed high signal.

The Dandy-Walker malformation
The Dandy-Walker malformation is characterised by cystic dilatation of the fourth ventricle, hypoplastic cerebellar hemispheres and absence of the vermis. The underlying cause is thought to be failure of regression of the posterior medullary velum and atresia of the foramina of Luschka and Magendie. Associated malformations include agenesis of the corpus callosum, abnormal cerebral gyri, heterotopias, holoprosencephaly and encephaloceles.

The retrocerebellar cyst and deficiency of the cerebellar vermis may be demonstrated by ultrasound *in utero* but hydrocephalus is an inconstant finding, developing months or years after birth (Hirsch *et al.* 1984). The CT appearance is of a large low-attenuation cyst in the posterior fossa, with no fourth ventricle visualised. The cerebellar hemispheres are hypoplastic and displaced by the dilated fourth ventricle and retrocerebellar cyst against the petrous pyramids. There is high insertion of the tentorium above the lambda and the hypoplastic superior vermis may be displaced through the incisura by the posterior fossa cyst. Downward herniation of the cyst may also occur through the foramen magnum. The lack of artefact from bone and the multiplanar facility of MRI is advantageous for imaging of the posterior fossa (Fig. 6.1).

The Dandy-Walker variant consists of hypoplasia of the inferior vermis with outpouching of the fourth ventricle. It has to be differentiated from other cystic lesions in the posterior fossa such as a large cisterna magna, trapped fourth ventricle or retrocerebellar arachnoid cyst.

The Arnold-Chiari malformations
The type I malformation consists of herniation of the inferior cerebellar tonsils

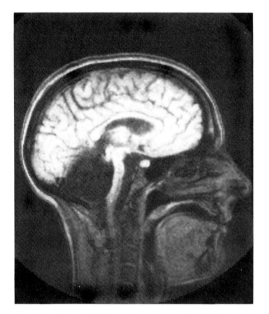
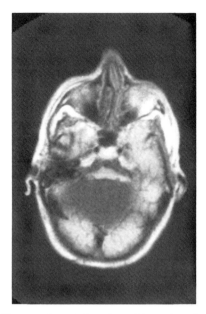

Fig. 6.1. Sagittal (*left*) and transverse (*right*) T1-weighted MR scans of an adult patient with ataxia and mild mental retardation. There is a large posterior fossa cyst contiguous with the fourth ventricle, absence of the cerebellar vermis and hypoplastic cerebellar hemispheres consistent with Dandy-Walker syndrome. There was no hydrocephalus in this patient.

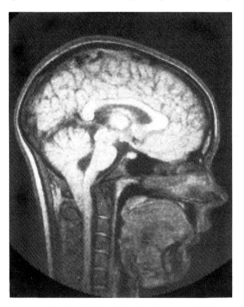
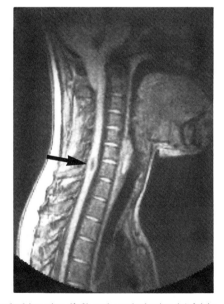

Fig. 6.2. Sagittal T1-weighted MR scans of the craniocervical junction (*left*) and cervical spine (*right*) in a teenage girl with neck pain and nystagmus. There is an Arnold-Chiari malformation with compression of the medulla and herniated tonsils at the foramen magnum, and a localised syrinx cavity at C6/C7 level (*arrow*).

through the foramen magnum ('tonsillar ectopia') without displacement of the fourth ventricle or medulla. There is no association with myelomeningocele but syringomyelia is present in approximately two thirds of patients. There may be skull-base deformities such as platybasia, Klippel-Feil anomaly or assimilation of the c1 vertebra to the occiput. The configuration of the craniocervical junction and the presence and degree of tonsillar herniation and syringomyelia are readily demonstrated on sagittal T1-weighted MR images (Fig. 6.2).

In Arnold-Chiari II malformation there is a hindbrain dysgenesis, almost invariably associated with myelomeningocele. Hydrocephalus is probably related to obstruction at the level of the aqueduct or fourth ventricle. The third ventricle is usually mildly dilated and the massa intermedia is prominent. Dilatation of the lateral ventricles is greatest at the level of the atria and occipital horns. Areas of cranial thinning are shown on skull radiographs or CT scans displayed at bone settings. Other radiological features include displacement of the inferior vermis of the cerebellum into the cervical canal, elongation and inferior displacement of the brainstem, aqueduct and fourth ventricle, and enlargement of the foramen magnum. The medulla may be kinked at the cervico-medullary junction. The pons is often flattened and the midbrain beaked due to fusion of the colliculi. On CT the apparent degree of tectal beaking depends on the angle of the scan plane; the configuration of the midbrain is better visualised on sagittal MRI (El Gammal *et al.* 1988). The cerebellum may enclose the brainstem or expand into the cerebellopontine angles. Poor development of the tentorium results in a wide incisura elongated in the sagittal plane. Wide separation of the left and right tentorial blushes may be demonstrated on contrast-enhanced CT but the malformation is more readily appreciated on sagittal MRI images which show the low insertion of the tentorial leaves and a small posterior fossa. Elevation of the cerebellum through the widened incisura results in the formation of a 'mass' which may be mistaken for a neoplasm on transaxial CT scans.

In Arnold-Chiari III malformation there is an occipital encephalocele or high cervical encephalocele associated with hindbrain herniation. Arnold-Chiari IV malformation consists of cerebellar hypoplasia without displacement.

Encephalocele

An encephalocele is a protrusion of brain and meninges through a defect in the skull (cranium bifidum). Herniation of CSF-containing meninges alone is more correctly termed a meningocele, and is less frequent. A midline occipital location is commonest (70 per cent), but encephaloceles may also occur in the parietal, fronto-ethmoidal or basal regions of the skull. Most occipital encephaloceles are associated with Arnold-Chiari II malformation. Other associations include agenesis of the corpus callosum, abnormalities of gyral and sulcal pattern and schizencephaly. Hydrocephalus may result from abnormal CSF circulation.

Ultrasound demonstrates a swelling adjacent to the calvarium with herniated brain appearing as solid tissue within the meningeal sac. Differentiation of a low occipital encephalocele from cystic hygroma or hydropic oedema of the neck may be a problem (Nicolini *et al.* 1983). Although ultrasound may demonstrate the defect in the calvarium, bony detail prior to reconstructive surgery is best demonstrated by CT. The amount of brain within the encephalocele can usually be determined on CT, but angiography may be required in some cases to demonstrate which part. The lack of bone artefact on MRI is of particular benefit when assessing the contents of basal and fronto-ethmoidal encephaloceles, but the size of the bony defect has to be inferred from the diameter of the neck of the herniated meninges. Dural venuous sinuses related to the encephalocele can be localised preoperatively by MRI, appearing as curvilinear tubular structures with variable signal intensity depending on the rate of bloodflow within them.

Holoprosencephaly
Holoprosencephaly is due to incomplete diverticulation of the developing forebrain and is categorised as alobar, semilobar or lobar depending on the degree of forebrain cleavage. It is associated with midline facial dysmorphism with manifestations such as cyclopia, hypotelorism and cleft palate. In alobar holoprosencephaly there is a single horseshoe-shaped cerebral ventricle incorporating the lateral and third ventricles, surrounded by a thin mantle of cortical tissue. The thalami are fused and the septum pellucidum and interhemispheric fissure are absent. The posterior fossa structures are usually intact. In the semilobar form there is partial cleavage of the thalamus and attempted formation of the third ventricle. The falx is partly present with some formation of the interhemispheric fissure and corpus callosum. Prenatal ultrasound diagnosis has been reported (Cayea *et al.* 1984, Filly *et al.* 1984, Hoffman-Tretin *et al.* 1986). Few neonates with alobar or semilobar holoprosencephaly survive, but children with the lobar type may require further cranial imaging by CT or MRI. The parietal, temporal and occipital lobes are formed but the frontal lobes are fused anteriorly. The septum pellucidum is absent and the corpus callosum may be underdeveloped anteriorly. The third ventricle is normal without thalamic fusion.

Septo-optic dysplasia can be considered as a mild form of holoprosencephaly and findings on prenatal ultrasound may be similar to those of lobar holoprosencephaly (Williams and Faerber 1985). Associated maldevelopment of the optic nerves and chiasm can be visualised by postnatal CT and MRI (Manelfe and Rochiccioli 1979).

Iniencephaly
Iniencephaly is a rare malformation comprising severe retroflexion of the head, an occipital defect with or without an encephalocele and cervical spinal dysraphism. Hydrocephalus and more extensive dysraphic lesions may be associated.

Agenesis of the corpus callosum
Agenesis of the corpus callosum may be an isolated finding but is usually associated

with other CNS anomalies (Byrd *et al.* 1990). Common associations include interhemispheric cysts, hydrocephalus, Dandy-Walker syndromes, Chiari II malformation, migrational disorders, interhemispheric lipoma, encephaloceles and septo-optic dysplasia.

The lateral ventricles are widely separated and abnormally shaped with a large and high third ventricle. The abnormal ventricular configuration can be recognised on fetal ultrasound scans (Comstock *et al.* 1985). Postnatally, absence of the corpus callosum—an echolucent structure on ultrasound—can be recognised on transfontanellar scans. The MRI and CT appearances have been described; MRI has the advantage over CT because of its multiplanar imaging facility (Byrd *et al.* 1990). MRI features are best evaluated on midline sagittal T1-weighted scans where the myelinated corpus callosum is normally visible as a hyperintense structure. In children with true agenesis, collateral callosal bundles known as Probst's bundles may be demonstrated in the medial wall of the lateral ventricles on coronal T1-weighted images. Lipomas of the corpus callosum are highly echogenic on ultrasound, of low attenuation on CT and of high signal intensity on MRI scans. They are usually situated in the region of the genu but may extend around the splenium and along interhemispheric vessels.

Choroid plexus papilloma may cause hydrocephalus by secreting large amounts of CSF, at rates greater than can be reabsorbed. Intraventricular haemorrhage or mechanical obstruction by the tumour may exacerbate ventricular dilatation. Prenatal ultrasound diagnosis has been described (Pilu *et al.* 1986).

Other intracranial mass lesions that may be associated with hydrocephalus include arachnoid cysts, aneurysm of the vein of Galen and tumours. Doppler ultrasound has been used to demonstrate turbulent bloodflow in a vein of Galen aneurysm *in utero* (Hirsch *et al.* 1983).

Diagnostic imaging in treated hydrocephalus
Intraoperative ultrasound can be used to guide catheter placement into the anterior horn of a lateral ventricle. Adequate shunt function or complications such as subdural haemorrhage or slit ventricle syndrome following rapid ventricular decompression can be assessed by ultrasound if the fontanelles are patent. If there is no acoustic window, CT or MRI can be used. Skull radiographs may be used to exclude disconnection of shunt components. In some patients, CT ventriculography may be useful following shunt insertion for hydrocephalus to demonstrate any communication with intracranial cysts. CT shuntography can also be used to provide functional information: the rate of dissipation of intraventricular contrast medium allows differentiation between physiological undershunting and normal shunt function when both limbs of the shunt are anatomically patent (Benzel *et al.* 1990). The technique of radioisotope shuntography provides similar functional information, but is less quantifiable and has poorer anatomic resolution for identifying the level of shunt obstruction. Problems involving the distal shunt such as fluid loculation around the tip of an intraperitoneal catheter can be assessed using

abdominal ultrasound. Patency of the distal catheter can be tested by contrast injection into the reservoir. CSF shunt patency can be monitored using flow-sensitive MRI sequences (Martin *et al.* 1989). Flow rates can be accurately assessed down to 0.5mm/s.

Spinal abnormalities
Prenatal diagnosis: cranial signs
The fetal biparietal diameter is below the fifth centile for gestational age in open spina bifida (Nicolaides and Campbell 1989). The 'lemon sign', first reported by Nicolaides *et al.* (1986), consists of bilateral scalloping of the frontal bones at the level of the ventricles and is associated with spina bifida. Its positive predictive value ranges from 81 per cent in a high-risk population to 6 per cent in a low-risk population (Filly 1988); nevertheless it is a valuable prompt for careful evaluation of the spine. Associated ventricular dilatation increases the likelihood of myelomeningocele. The lemon sign becomes less consistently visible after 24 weeks (Nyberg *et al.* 1988). The 'banana sign'—absence or anterior curvature of the cerebellar hemispheres associated with obliteration of the cisterna magna—is also a reliable pointer to the diagnosis of spina bifida (Nicolaides and Campbell 1989).

Ultrasound assessment of the fetal spine
In open spina bifida, the normal echogenic ring of ossified posterior elements is U-shaped, deficient posteriorly, and with bulging soft tissue due to associated meningocele, myelomeningocele or lipomyelomeningocele. In longitudinal sections the level and extent of the defect can be assessed. A meningocele containing CSF only appears as a cystic, echolucent sac, while strands or plaques of echogenic neural tissue may be visible in myelomeningocele. Associated lipomatous masses are highly echogenic.

Postnatal diagnosis of spinal dysraphism
Spinal dysraphism encompasses a wide spectrum of abnormalities resulting from incomplete or disordered closure of the neural tube. Spinal imaging rarely plays a role in the preoperative evaluation of neonates with myelomeningocele in whom immediate closure of the defect is indicated to prevent infection. Imaging may subsequently be required for identification of associated developmental anomalies or postoperative complications. Ultrasound can be used to examine the cord and conus in infants with unossified posterior arches in whom cutaneous abnormalities are suggestive of spina bifida (Scheible *et al.* 1983). Older children with neural arch defects at more than one vertebral level on spine radiographs have a high incidence of anomalies such as diastematomyelia, syringomyelia, tethered cord and sacral lipoma (Altman and Altman 1987). CT myelography has been the gold standard for investigation of spinal dysraphism in recent years (Harwood-Nash *et al.* 1978, Rothwell *et al.* 1987). MRI is increasingly being used in paediatric spinal imaging in preference to X-ray techniques; in addition to the lack of ionising radiation, it has

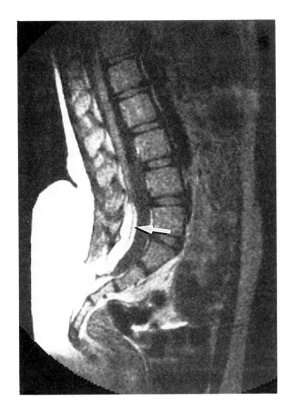

Fig. 6.3. Sagittal T1-weighted MR scan demonstrating a low tethered cord associated with an extradural lipoma extending through the dysraphic defect to the subcutaneous tissues. Linear low signal intensity within the lipoma (*arrow*) may represent fibrous or neural elements.

the advantage of multiplanar imaging and high intrinsic soft-tissue contrast, obviating the need for intrathecal contrast administration. Comparative studies suggest that the diagnostic accuracy of MRI in spinal dysraphism is at least as good as CT myelography (Davis *et al.* 1988, Jaspan *et al.* 1988).

Lipoma and lipomyelomeningocele

Lipomas may be isolated, but more commonly form part of a dysraphic complex, tethering the spinal cord or conus or forming part of a lipomyelomeningocele. The latter consists of a complex mass formed by the open spinal cord (neural placode), herniated subarachnoid space and meninges and a fatty tumour often extending subcutaneously and containing fibrovascular bands (Naidich *et al.* 1983). Plain radiographs demonstrate a relatively radiolucent soft-tissue mass in addition to neural arch defects and expansion of the spinal canal. On CT a low-attenuation mass is seen to extend between subcutaneous tissues and the dorsal neural arch defect. On MRI, fat has a high signal intensity on both T1- and T2-weighted sequences. Low signal bands of fibrous tissue and neural elements can be identified extending from the neural placode into the lipoma (Fig. 6.3). The lipoma may extend into the spinal canal forming an extradural or intradural tumour (Fig. 6.4).

95

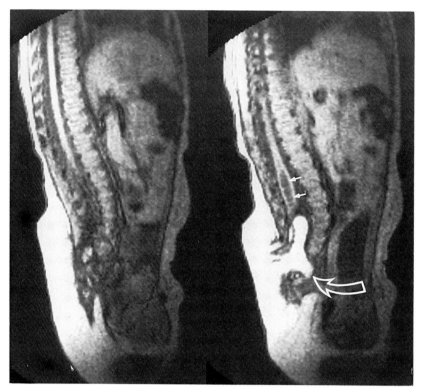

Fig. 6.4. Sagittal T1-weighted MR scans of a four-month-old infant with an enlarging sacral lipoma. T1-weighted MR scans demonstrate a low tethered cord, expanded distally by a loculated syrinx (*arrows*). The large subcutaneous lipoma extends into the spine and anteriorly through the sacrum (*open arrows*).

Tethered cord

Textbooks often state that the normal conus ascends throughout infancy to adult life; a recent study using MRI showed that in fullterm neonates, the conus lies at or above the L2/L3 interspace and does not change during growth (Wilson and Prince 1989).

CSF and neural tissue are virtually isodense on CT and demonstration of spinal-cord morphology requires intrathecal contrast injection. Lumbar puncture may be difficult because of intrathecal tumour and hazardous in the presence of tethered neural tissue. On MRI the position of the cord down to its distal placode can be shown on sagittal T1-weighted images with good contrast between neural tissue, CSF and fat. Thickening and fatty infiltration of the filum terminale may occur in association with tethering (Nokes *et al.* 1987, Raghavan *et al.* 1989). Both the thickened filum terminale and tethered spinal cord may terminate in a lipoma or dermal sinus.

Cord tethering postoperatively may be due to adherence of the placode to dura, dural graft or adjacent subcutaneous tissues at the repair site (Heinz *et al.*

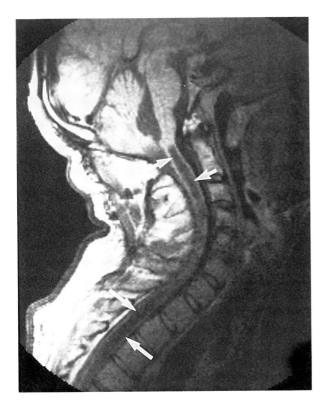

Fig. 6.5. Sagittal T1-weighted MR scan of the craniocervical region in a patient with persistent symptoms following posterior fossa decompression and shunt insertion for syringomyelia. A persistent low signal intensity syrinx cavity was demonstrated (*arrows*), which extended down to D12 level on thoracic MR scans.

1979). MRI often shows the cord at the same vertebral level as preoperatively and lack of retethering is inferred if a CSF space can be demonstrated between the released cord and the operative site. Phase imaging using MRI has shown pulsatile motion to be reduced in tethered cords (Samuelsson *et al.* 1987).

Syringomyelia
In syringomyelia there is cavitation of the spinal cord with gliotic walls, which may extend up or down the spinal cord. There is an association with spina bifida and Arnold-Chiari malformation. Syringomyelia was present in 40 per cent of patients with myelomeningocele and scoliosis examined by MRI, all of whom had Chiari malformations (type II in 93 per cent and type I in 7 per cent) (Samuelsson *et al.* 1987). The presence and extent of syringomyelic cavities is best assessed on sagittal T1-weighted MR scans. The entire cord should be imaged as there may be multiple cavities. High signal intensity surrounding the cyst cavity on T2-weighted MR scans may be due to gliosis, oedema or tumour. Differentiation of benign and neoplastic causes is an indication for administration of the MRI contrast agent gadolinium-DTPA. Signal voids within the syrinx cavity on T2-weighted sequences are due to CSF pulsation and imply communication with the subarachnoid space at the obex (Sherman *et al.* 1987). Following shunt insertion, MRI can be used to demonstrate

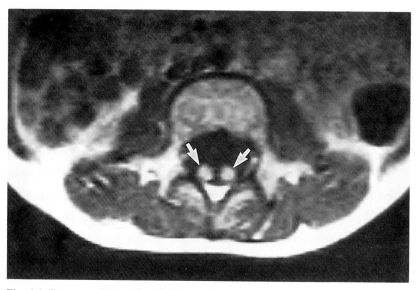

Fig. 6.6. Transverse T1-weighted MR scan through the lumbar spinal canal of a seven-year-old child with back and leg pain. There is diastematomyelia with two hemicords (*arrows*) occupying the same subarachnoid space. No dividing bony or fibrous spur is identified.

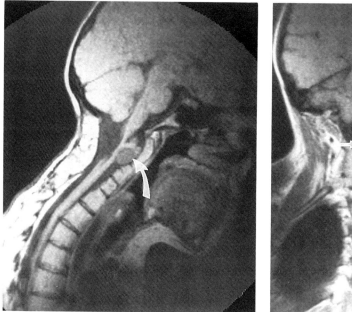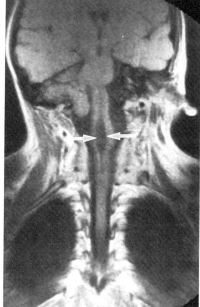

Fig. 6.7. Sagittal (*left*) and coronal (*right*) MR scans of the craniocervical region in an adult patient with recent onset of symptoms suggestive of cervical spondylosis. There is a capacious foramen magnum associated with diastematomyelia of the spinal cord (*straight arrows*) and an intraspinal dermoid tumour which contained cystic and fatty elements (*curved arrow*). Extensive segmentation anomalies of the cervical spine are also present.

reduction in size of the syrinx and identify causes for inadequate drainage, such as displaced shunts or septations within the cavity (Fig. 6.5).

Diastematomyelia
In diastematomyelia there is longitudinal splitting of the spinal cord with each half having its own dorsal and ventral nerve roots. True duplication of the spinal cord (diplomyelia) is extremely rare. There may be duplication of the thecal sac, or the hemicords may lie within the same subarachnoid space (Fig. 6.6). The latter is more common when the division is produced by a fibrous septum. The conus is low-lying and often tethered. Impingement of tethered neural tissue against a bony or fibrous spur as growth proceeds is associated with back pain, lower-limb spasticity and scoliosis. Syringomyelia of the hemicords may be seen. Lipomas, dermal sinuses and cutaneous stigmata are common. Vertebral anomalies associated with diastematomyelia include segmentation anomalies, butterfly vertebrae, hemiver-tebrae, and widening of the interpedicular distance (Fig. 6.7).

Features of diastematomyelia on prenatal ultrasound include localised widening of the posterior ossification centres on coronal views with a central echogenic focus at the site of the median septum (Winter *et al.* 1989). Associated vertebral body anomalies may be apparent, such as the double ossification centres in butterfly vertebrae. The absence of a posterior bony defect or soft-tissue mass and the lack of cranial ultrasound signs help to exclude associated open spina bifida.

The diagnostic feature on the spinal radiograph is the presence of a midline bony spur. CT with intrathecal contrast may show the divided thecal sac containing two hemicords. Coronal and axial T1-weighted MR images best display the site and extent of the cord division, the presence of syrinx cavities and the nature of the tethering. Division of the cord may be difficult to appreciate on sagittal images alone. A well developed bony spur may be identified by virtue of the marrow within it, but spurs consisting of compact bone and fibrous bands both show a low signal intensity on T1-weighted sequences, difficult to discern against the low signal intensity of CSF. Transverse T2-weighted sequences may be helpful to demonstrate the median bony spur or fibrous band but cannot always distinguish between them. CT may be necessary to define the detailed bony architecture of the malformation.

Scoliosis
There is an association between congenital scoliosis and spinal dysraphism. An underlying lesion was demonstrated in 15 out of 28 scoliotic children studied using MRI (Nokes *et al.* 1987). Findings included tethering of the cord, syringomyelia, Arnold-Chiari I and II malformations, spinal-cord tumour and diastematomyelia.

Congenital tumours
Spinal teratomas may occur in childhood in association with spinal anomalies and frequently have a complex appearance due to the mixture of soft tissue, fat, keratin

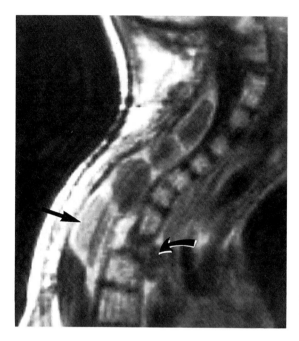

Fig. 6.8. Sagittal T1-weighted MR scan of a child with a neuroenteric cyst of the cervicodorsal spine. The relatively high signal intensity within the lowest cystic loculation (*arrow*) implies a high protein content or the presence of blood. Extensive segmentation anomalies and an anterior meningocele (*curved arrow*) are also demonstrated.

and calcification. Dermoid tumours characteristically contain a high proportion of fat resulting in low density on CT scans and high signal intensity on MRI, but they may be predominantly cystic. Approximately 25 per cent of spinal dermoids are associated with dermal sinus tracts and 50 per cent of patients with dermal sinuses have an underlying congenital dermoid or epidermoid tumour, usually at the termination of the tract (Barkovich *et al.* 1991). The subcutaneous and intramedullary portions of dermal sinuses can be readily identified on T1-weighted MR scans. The intraspinal component may be difficult to see because of its isointensity with CSF, unless lined by fat. A neuroenteric cyst is a congenital cyst of foregut origin which connects with the spinal canal through an anterior spina bifida (Fig. 6.8). A paraspinal location is usual although intraspinal cysts may occur.

New developments in imaging and functional assessment
Fetal Doppler
Assessment of high-risk pregnancies by Doppler ultrasound can improve detection of complications such as fetal hypoxia and intrauterine growth retardation. The anterior fontanelle can be used as an acoustic window in neonates for imaging the circle of Willis. The pattern of arterial cerebral flow in normal neonates is characterised by relatively low resistance and continuous forward flow throughout diastole. The resistance index may be elevated in several neonatal abnormalities including hydrocephalus (Hill and Volpe 1982). Correlation between resistance index, cerebral perfusion pressure and raised intracranial pressure has been demonstrated in longitudinal studies (Siebert *et al.* 1989).

Echo-planar imaging

Realtime images of the fetus can be obtained in the second and third trimesters using echo-planar imaging (Mansfield *et al.* 1990). Image quality is degraded by fetal movement during the relatively long acquisition times of conventional MRI. By using an ultra-high-speed MRI technique, fetal motion is frozen and snapshot images are obtained. Because of the lack of myelin within the fetal brain, internal structure is difficult to evalute; but in later gestation, the structure of the ventricles, basal ganglia and gyri are seen. Echo-planar imaging has also been applied to the study of flow patterns in CSF pathways (Stehling *et al.* 1991). Results indicate that the technique can provide quantifiable data on CSF flow dynamics in both normal and pathological conditions.

Assessment of myelination by MRI

The neonatal brain has a high water content with little contrast between grey and white matter. As myelination proceeds, relative signal intensities of grey and white matter change as proportionally more water is lost from the white matter. Delayed myelination is demonstrated on MRI scans of asphyxiated infants (Johnson *et al.* 1983). There is good correlation between MRI assessment of the stage of myelination and neurodevelopmental outcome in preterm infants; demonstration of periventricular leukomalacia on ultrasound, however, is of greater predictive value (Guit *et al.* 1990).

Magnetic resonance spectroscopy

Magnetic resonance spectroscopy uses high field strength magnets to generate a spectrum of different frequency signals which reflect the chemical composition of the tissue. Using the atomic nucleus of ^{31}P, rather than hydrogen, allows changes in concentration of different phosphorus compounds involved in energy metabolism to be quantified. Abnormal spectra have been demonstrated in birth-asphyxiated infants (Hope *et al.* 1984).

REFERENCES

Altman, N.R., Altman, D.H. (1987) 'MR imaging of spinal dysraphism.' *American Journal of Neuroradiology*, **8**, 533–538.

Atlas, S.W., Mark, A.S., Fram, E.K. (1988) 'Aqueduct stenosis: evaluation with Gradient-Echo rapid MR imaging.' *Radiology*, **169**, 449–453.

Barkovich, A.J., Edwards, M.S.B., Cogen, P.H. (1991) 'MR evaluation of spinal dermal sinus tracts in children.' *American Journal of Roentgenology*, **156**, 791–797.

Barnes, P.D., Lester, P.D., Yamanashi, W.S., Prince, J.R. (1986) 'Magnetic resonance imaging in infants and children with spinal dysraphism.' *American Journal of Roentgenology*, **147**, 339–346.

Benzel, E.C. Mirfakhraee, M., Hadden, T.A. (1990) 'Evaluation of CSF shunt function: value of functional examination with contrast material.' *American Journal of Roentgenology*, **156**, 801–805.

Burton, B.K. (1979) 'Recurrence risks in congenital hydrocephalus.' *Clinical Genetics*, **16**, 47–53.

Byrd, S.E., Radkowski, M.A., Flannery, A., McLone, D.G. (1990) 'The clinical and radiological evaluation of absence of the corpus callosum.' *European Journal of Radiology*, **10**, 65–73.

Campbell, S., Pryse-Davies, J., Coltart, T.M., Seller, M., Singer, J.D. (1975) 'Ultrasound in the diagnosis of spina bifida.' *Lancet*, **1**, 1065–1068.

Cayea, P.D., Balcar, I., Alberti, O. Jr, Jones, T.B. (1984) 'Prenatal diagnosis of semilobar holoprosencephaly.' *American Journal of Roentgenology*, **142**, 401–402.

Chervenak, F.A., Berkowitz, R.L., Tortora, M., Chitkara, U., Hobbins, J.C. (1984) 'Diagnosis of ventriculomegaly before fetal viability.' *Obstetrics and Gynecology*, **64**, 652–656.

Comstock, C.H., Culop, D., Gonzalez, J., Boal, D.B. (1985) 'Agenesis of the corpus callosum in the fetus: its evolution and significance.' *Journal of Ultrasound in Medicine*, **4**, 613–616.

Davis, P.C., Hoffman, J.C., Ball, T.I., Wyly, J.B., Braun, I.F., Fry, S.M., Drvaric, D.M. (1988) 'Spinal abnormalities in pediatric patients: MR imaging findings compared with clinical, myelographic and surgical findings.' *Radiology*, **166**, 679–685.

El Gammal, T., Mark, E.K., Brooks, B.S. (1988) 'MR imaging of Chiari II malformation.' *American Journal of Roentgenology*, **150**, 163–170.

Filly, R.A. (1988) 'The "lemon" sign: a clinical perspective.' *Radiology*, **167**, 573–575.

—— Chinn, D.H., Callen, P.W. (1984) 'Alobar holoprosencephaly. Ultrasonographic prenatal diagnosis.' *Radiology*, **151**, 455–459.

Gowland, M. (1988) 'Fetal abnormalities diagnosed from early pregnancy.' *Clinical Radiology*, **39**, 106–108.

Guit, G.L., van de Bor, M., den Ouden, L., Wondergem, J.H. (1990) 'Prediction of neurodevelopmental outcome in the preterm infant: MR-staged myelination compared with cranial US.' *Radiology*, **175**, 107–109.

Harwood-Nash, D.C.F., Fitz, C.R., Resjo, M., Chung, S. (1978) 'Congenital spinal and cord lesions in children and computed tomographic metrizamide myelography.' *Neuroradiology*, **16**, 69–70.

Heinz, E.R., Rosenbaum, A.E., Scarff, T.B., Reigel, D.H., Drayer, B.P. (1979) 'Tethered spinal cord following meningomyelocoele repair.' *Radiology*, **131**, 153–160.

Hill, A., Volpe, J.J. (1982) 'Decrease in pulsatile flow in the anterior cerebral arteries in infantile hydrocephalus.' *Pediatrics*, **69**, 4–7.

Hirsch, J.H., Cyr, D., Eberhardt, H., Zunkel, D. (1983) 'Ultrasonographic diagnosis of an aneurysm of the vein of Galen in utero by Duplex scanning.' *Journal of Ultrasound in Medicine*, **2**, 231–233.

—— Pierre Kahn, A., Reiner, D., Sainte-Rose, C., Hoppe-Hirsche, E. (1984) 'The Dandy-Walker malformation: a review of 40 cases.' *Journal of Neurosurgery*, **61**, 515–522.

Hoffman-Tretin, J.C., Horoupian, D.S., Koenigsberg, M., Schnur, M.J., Llena, J.F. (1986) 'Lobar holoprosencephaly with hydrocephalus: antenatal demonstration and differential diagnosis.' *Journal of Ultrasound in Medicine*, **5**, 691–697.

Holt, P.J. (1989) 'Posthemorrhagic hydrocephalus.' *Journal of Child Neurology*, **4**, (Suppl.), S23–S31.

Hope, P.L., Costello, A.M. de L., Cady, E.B., Delpy, D.T., Tofts, P.S., Chu, A., Hamilton, P.A., Reynolds, E.O., Wilkie, D.R. (1984) 'Cerebral energy metabolism studied with NMR spectroscopy in normal and birth asphyxiated infants.' *Lancet*, **2**, 336–339.

Jaspan, T., Worthington, B.S., Holland, I.M. (1988) 'A comparative study of magnetic resonance imaging and computed tomography-assisted myelography in spinal dysraphism.' *British Journal of Radiology*, **61**, 445–453.

Johnson, M.A., Pennock, J.M., Bydder, G.M., Steiner, R.E., Thomas, D.J., Haywood, R., Bryant, D.K.T., Payne, J.A., Levene, M.I., Whitelaw, A., Dubowitz, L.M.S., Dubowitz, V. (1983) 'Clinical NMR imaging of the brain of children: normal and neurologic disease.' *American Journal of Neuroradiology*, **4**, 1013–1026.

Manelfe, C., Rochiccioli, P. (1979) 'CT of septo-optic dysplasia.' *American Journal of Roentgenology*, **133**, 1157–1160.

Manning, F., Harrison, M., Rodeck, C. and members of the International Fetal Medicine and Surgical Society (1986) 'Catheter shunts for fetal hydronephrosis and hydrocephalus.' *New England Journal of Medicine*, **315**, 336–340.

Mansfield, P., Stehling, M.K., Ordidge, R.J., Coxon, R., Chapman, B., Blamire, A., Gibbs, P., Johnson, I.R., Symonds, E.M., Worthington, B.S., Coupland, R.E. (1990) 'Echo planar imaging of the human fetus in utero at 0.5T.' *British Journal of Radiology*, **63**, 833–841.

Mark, A.S., Feinberg, D.A., Brant-Zawadski, M.N. (1987) 'Changes in size and magnetic resonance signal intensity of the cerebral CSF spaces during the cardiac cycle, as studied by gated, high resolution MRI.' *Investigative Radiology*, **22**, 290–297.

Martin, A.J., Drake, J.M., Lemaire, C., Henkelman, R.M. (1989) 'Cerebrospinal fluid shunts: flow measurements with MR imaging.' *Radiology*, **173**, 243–247.

102

Naidich, T.P., McClone, D.G., Mutluer, S. (1983) 'A new understanding of dorsal dysraphism with lipoma (lipomyeloschisis): radiographic evaluation and surgical correction.' *American Journal of Roentgenology*, **140**, 1065–1078.

—— Fernbach, S.K., McLone, D.G., Shkolnik, A. (1984) 'Sonography of the caudal spine and back: congenital anomalies in children.' *American Journal of Roentgenology*, **142**, 1229–1242.

Nicolaides, K.H., Gabbe, S.G., Campbell, S., Guidetti, R. (1986) 'Ultrasound screening for spina bifida: cranial and cerebellar signs.' *Lancet*, **2**, 72–74.

—— Campbell, J. (1989) 'Neural tube abnormalities.' *In* Hobbins, J.C., Benacerraf, B.R. (Eds) *Clinics in Diagnostic Ultrasound, No. 25: Diagnosis and Therapy of Fetal Anomalies.* London: Churchill Livingstone. pp. 55–65.

Nicolini, U., Ferrazzi, E., Massa, E., Minonzio, M., Pardi, G. (1983) 'Prenatal diagnosis of cranial masses by ultrasound: report of five cases.' *Journal of Clinical Ultrasound*, **11**, 170–174.

Nokes, S.R., Murtagh, F.R., Jones, J.D. III, Downing, M., Arrington, J.A., Turetsky, D., Silbiger, M.L. (1987) 'Childhood scoliosis: MR imaging.' *Radiology*, **164**, 791–797.

Nyberg, D.A., Mack, L.A., Hirsch, J., Mahoney, B.S. (1988) 'Abnormalities of fetal cranial contour in sonographic detection of spina bifida: evaluation of the "lemon" sign.' *Radiology*, **167**, 387–392.

Pearce, J.M., Little, D., Campbell, S. (1985) 'The diagnosis of abnormalities of the fetal central nervous system.' *In* Sanders, R.C., James, A.E. (Eds) *The Principles and Practice of Ultrasound in Obstetrics and Gynecology.* New York: Appleton-Century-Crofts. pp. 243–256.

Pilu, G., De Palma, L., Romero, R., Bovicelli, L., Hobbins, J.C. (1986) 'The fetal subarachnoid cisterns: an ultrasound study with report of a case of congenital communicating hydrocephalus.' *Journal of Ultrasound in Medicine*, **5**, 365–372.

Raghavan, N., Barkovich, A.J., Edwards, M., Norman, D. (1989) 'MR imaging in the tethered spinal cord syndrome.' *American Journal of Neuroradiology*, **10**, 27–36.

Raghavendra, B.N., Epstein, F.J. (1985) 'Sonography of the spine and spinal cord.' *Radiologic Clinics of North America*, **23**, 91–105.

Roberts, C.J., Evans, K.T., Hibbard, B.M., Laurence, K.M., Roberts, E.E., Robertson, I.B. (1983) 'Diagnostic effectiveness of ultrasound in detection of neural tube defects: the South Wales experience of 2509 scans (1977–1982) in high-risk mothers.' *Lancet*, **2**, 1068–1069.

Robertson, W.C., Gomez, M.R. (1978) 'External hydrocephalus: early finding in congenital communicating hydrocephalus.' *Archives of Neurology*, **35**, 541–544.

Rothwell, C.I., Forbes, W.StC., Gupta, S.C. (1987) 'Computed tomographic myelography in the investigation of childhood scoliosis and spinal dysraphism.' *British Journal of Radiology*, **60**, 1197–1204.

Samuelsson, L., Bergstrom, K., Thuomas, K-A., Hemmingsson, A., Wallensten, R. (1987) 'MR imaging of syringohydromelia and Chiari malformations in myelomeningocele patients with scoliosis.' *American Journal of Neuroradiology*, **8**, 539–546.

Scheible, W., James, H.E., Leopold, G.R., Hilton, S.W. (1983) 'Occult spinal dysraphism in infants: screening with high-resolution real-time ultrasound.' *Radiology*, **146**, 743–746.

Sherman, J.L., Barkovich, A.J., Citrin, C.M. (1987) 'The MR appearance of syringomyelia: new observations.' *American Journal of Roentgenology*, **148**, 381–391.

Siebert, J.J., McCowan, T.C., Chadduck, W.M., Adametz, J.R., Glasier, D.M., Williamson, S.L., Taylor, B.J., Leithiser, R.E., McConnell, J.R., Stansell, C.A., Rodgers, A.B., Corbitt, S.L. (1989) 'Duplex pulsed Doppler US versus intracranial pressure in the neonate: clinical and experimental studies.' *Radiology*, **171**, 155–159.

Stehling, M.K., Firth, J.L., Worthington, B.S., Guilfoyle, D.N., Ordidge, R.J., Coxon, R., Blamire, A.M., Gibbs, P., Bullock, P., Mansfield, P. (1991) 'Observation of cerebrospinal fluid flow with echo-planar magnetic resonance imaging.' *British Journal of Radiology*, **64**, 89–97.

Szalay, E., Roach, J., Smith, H., Maravilla, K., Partain, C.L. (1987) 'Magnetic resonance imaging of the spinal cord in spinal dysraphism.' *Journal of Pediatric Orthopedics*, **7**, 541–545.

Williams, J.L., Faerber, E.N. (1985) 'Septooptic dysplasia (de Morsier's syndrome).' *Journal of Ultrasound in Medicine*, **4**, 265–266.

Wilson, D.A., Prince, J.R. (1989) 'MR imaging determination of the location of the normal conus medullaris throughout childhood.' *American Journal of Roentgenology*, **10**, 259–262.

Winter, R.K., McKnight, L.G., Byrne, R.A., Wright, C.H. (1989) 'Diastematomyelia: prenatal ultrasonic appearances.' *Clinical Radiology*, **40**, 291–294.

7
WALKING AIDS

David I. Rowley and Gordon Rose

Myelomeningocele presents with a wide range of paralytic deficiencies, many of which can now be dealt with by standard combinations of surgery, orthoses and physiotherapy. In complete paraplegia the position is not so clearly established, although the restoration of standing and walking has been the subject of considerable research and experience in the last 25 years.

After 1945 the approach to traumatic paraplegia was dominated by the teaching of Ludwig Guttman, who, with a combination of realism and optimism, laid down therapeutic principles which have stood the test of time. In the complete paraplegic, he believed that trying to achieve functional ambulation was a waste of valuable rehabilitation time but that the inevitable failure to achieve this would only cause depression in the patient. He advocated strongly the acceptance of the wheelchair. This view inevitably coloured attitudes to other pathologies, although Guttman later said that 'The great therapeutic value of daily standing and walking . . . should always be stressed', clearly regarding such activities as promoters of general health only (Guttman 1976). A more objective view has been provided by Mazur *et al.* (1989) who demonstrated that if children with a high-level spina bifida were encouraged to walk early, they had fewer fractures, fewer pressure sores and were more independent and even if they subsequently went into a wheelchair permanently, they had better transfer capacity than a matched control series who went straight to the wheelchair.

In the early 1960s, when there was an absolute increase in the incidence of myelomeningocele for reasons which are not yet clear, advances in paediatric surgery meant that orthopaedic clinics (in which the condition had hitherto been a rarity) experienced a progressive increase in the number of patients who presented an unprecedented challenge, with their multiple problems of hydrocephalus, urinary dysfunction and locomotor disability. Some orthopaedic and orthotic experience existed from the earlier problems of poliomyelitis epidemics, but the absence of sensation and proprioception brought new problems.

There were two orthopaedic attitudes prevailing: the piecemeal correction of deformities, and the traditional use of orthoses to stabilise paralysed joints. Only with growing experience has it become apparent: (i) that orthotic function has to be expanded to control of motion and used for the transmission of energy from working muscles to an appropriate ground reaction; and (ii) that surgery should be limited to those procedures which, in the light of possible orthotic design, could improve locomotor efficiency. Lorber (1971) studied a group of 41 patients, who had had on average nine orthopaedic operations each, and found that all had remained wheelchair-bound.

This represents a reversal of priorities, justified only by the basic principles underlying the achievement of walking, which ideally has four criteria: (i) low-energy ambulation at a reasonable speed (25 to 50 per cent of normal); (ii) independent transfer; (iii) independent 'doff and don' (assumption and removal of orthoses); and (iv) ability to surmount a step of 15cm and to walk up and down a 1:10 slope.

Although not all patients will achieve these, it is certain that a few exhausting steps with high ground friction should never be dignified as walking. While these ambitions seem reasonable in the lower lesions, such ambitions in the paraplegic patient might take us back to the pre-Guttman era. However, there is some evidence that even standing can have quite a profound physiological effect (Runcie 1979), judged by blood electrolytes. Experience certainly suggests that bowel and bladder function may improve and that the so-called spontaneous fractures may disappear with the response to longitudinal loading of the bones. The psychological benefits of adhering to the normal stage of development are often shared by the parents.

Achieving the optimum result requires a return to basic principles:
(1) an understanding of the mechanisms of normal walking and the extraction from these of the minimum factors required to achieve restoration of walking
(2) a recognition of the extent of the pathology and in particular the small number of components of ambulation which are available, and
(3) an efficient orthotic design tested for function and reliability which lends itself to commercial production. Nothing proved more disheartening for patients and staff than orthoses which were slow in appearing, often with modifications which could reduce efficiency, and which spent more time being repaired than being used.

Any form of walking, normal or otherwise, requires components of locomotion (all of which are mandatory) and components of gait (some or all of which may be used).

Components of locomotion
These consist of:
(1) stabilisation of the multisegment skeleton both intrinsically (to prevent collapse of one segment on the other) and extrinsically (to prevent the intrinsically stabilised structure from falling over by keeping the centre of mass within the support area)
(2) the achievement of propulsion by transmission of available muscular energy through various forms, potential, kinetic and inertial to a ground reaction. Any orthosis must be as rigid as possible mechanically if energy is not to be wasted flexing the device. Similarly joints and any cables or gearbox should move as freely as possible

105

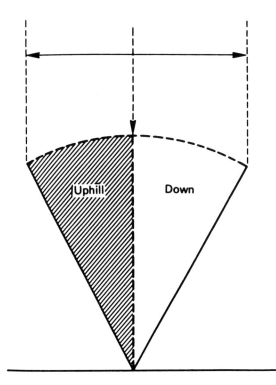

Fig. 7.1. With a straight leg during stance phase the 'uphill' segment requires an injection of energy which will be returned substantially in the 'downhill' segment.

Uphill   Down

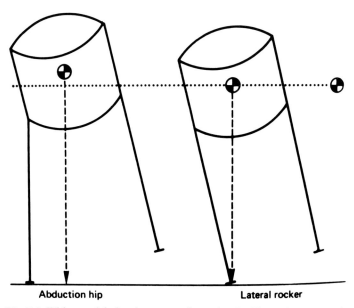

Abduction hip   Lateral rocker

Fig. 7.2. With a straight leg the centre of mass is raised less using a ground rocker compared with a hip abduction hinge and requires less energy, therefore with the added advantage of better rigidity.

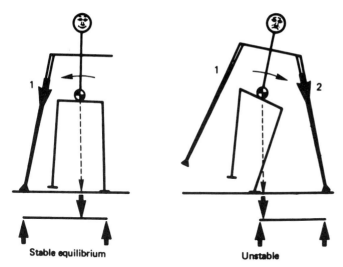

Stable equilibrium   **Unstable**

Fig. 7.3. *Left:* the geometry of the optimum abduction stance in relationship to the position of the body centre of mass. With pressure down one crutch ground clearance is obtained, and potential energy is stored which will return the foot to the ground at the end of the step with an inertial spill over to assist rocking onto the other foot. *Right:* one crutch is used as before but because the leg segment adducts the other must then be used to stop the patient falling and to return the swing leg to the ground, *i.e.* an unsafe, high-energy broken rhythm form of gait.

(3) control mechanisms. In the normal these are highly complex but in the paraplegic orthoses are small in number and therefore each must work optimally. They are again dependent on rigidity.

Components of gait

These consist of:

(1) leg pendulum. If the body is inclined forwards and one foot raised from the ground, the leg swings forward under the influence of gravity if the hinge is unconstrained, with no energy cost. If the legs are interconnected, either by cables or gearbox, the extension of one hip flexes the other using energy transmitted from the arms

(2) leg vaulting. This requires an injection of energy for the uphill phase, but the downhill phase is powered by the descent of the centre of body mass by gravity (Fig. 7.1)

(3) horizontal rotation occurring normally at the hips, which is precluded in an orthosis extending above the hips and must occur either at the footwear/floor level (high energy cost) or in swivel footplates, and

(4) lateral rocker to achieve foot clearance, which occurs at the footwear/floor level. With rigid legs, this is more efficient than imitating normal hip abduction (Fig. 7.2). Where such rigidity does not exist there is inevitably an unnecessary energy cost due to the friction of inadequate foot clearance and/or double crutch usage (Fig. 7.3).

Historically the empirical approach to the problem of walking restoration in these patients was the use of the so-called 'full-set' which stabilised the knees, had crude hip articulations, was highly flexible and required time and assistance for its assumption. In the light of present understanding of the mechanical principles, it is not surprising that it was highly disappointing and soon abandoned.

Speilrein, an engineer, first elucidated the scientific principles of swivel walking when presented with an amelic patient. He used lateral rocking at floor level and horizontal rotation at bearings in a footplate with a self-return mechanism and a side-to-side curvature with a precise radius putting the oscillation centre above the centre of body mass which, if moved forward by the patient when one footplate was raised, would cause a rotation forward under the influence of gravity without further energy expenditure by the patient. His findings were first published in an Australian engineering journal (Speilrein 1963), and only became available in general medical literature some eight years later (Speilrein 1971). The design was modified in Canada (Motloch and Elliot 1966, Woolridge 1969) when the curved footplates were replaced by flat ones with a dihedral (sloping upwards like aeroplane wings) which increased the speed of movement and crucially allowed the patient to vary this, which had been denied by the rather inflexible pattern imposed by Speilrein's design. Recognition of desirability of the patient controlling the device, rather than the device controlling the patient, has proved to be an important factor in acceptance. Strictly speaking the result was a prosthesis, and transforming this into an orthosis had its own design challenges. The presence of lower limbs limited the space for bearings and the complete exoskeleton necessary for intrinsic stabilisation meant that the patient could no longer move the centre of mass forward. The geometry of the orthosis had to ensure that this was forward of the bearing axis, and a simple device was provided to check this (Rose and Henshaw 1972).

Research into swivel walker orthoses in the late 1960s occurred in two major centres, one in England, at Shrewsbury (Edbrooke 1970, DHSS 1973) (a department funded by the government and charitable contributions which was later to be expanded into the Orthotic Research and Locomotor Assessment Unit, ORLAU, at the Robert Jones and Agnes Hunt Orthopaedic Hospital, Oswestry), and the other in Canada at the Ontario Crippled Children's Centre, Toronto. Rather surprisingly, in dealing with myelomeningocele patients the Canadians abandoned the footplates in favour of the Parapodium (Motloch 1971), with a single footplate holding both feet with a rather high friction as this rotated on the floor surface and with articulations at knee and hip for sitting, two features which increased wear and rate of breakdown. In England the swivel feature was retained, and the engineering was designed to improve rigidity and robustness and to allow rapid and independent doff and don, thus eliminating the need for articulations (Fig. 7.4) (Stallard *et al.* 1978). Despite the value of this device, and particularly its unique suitability from the age of one upwards, it was becoming apparent that some form of acceptable reciprocal walking was desirable particularly for the older patients

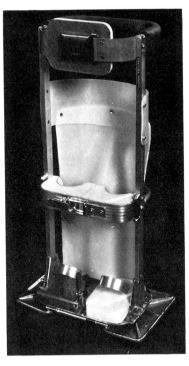

Fig. 7.4. *Left:* modern swivel walker for independent doff and don.

Fig. 7.5. *Below left:* too much hip flexion allows the centre of body mass to be behind the support leg, the patient tends to fall backwards and no ground reaction of the crutch is possible. *Below right:* centre of mass ahead of the stance leg enables satisfactory function of arm muscles to pull the patient forward during the 'uphill' phase of walking.

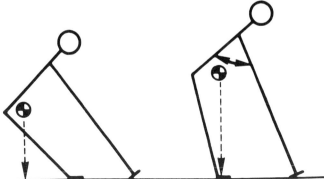

(five and upwards). A study of this problem resulted in the identification of the principles and practice of a 'hip guidance orthosis' (HGO) (Rose 1979), later to be commercially renamed the Parawalker (Fig. 7.5). This study re-emphasised the need for rigidity, a difficult engineering problem in conjunction with the need to rock from side to side to achieve alternate foot clearance (Fig. 7.6). The hip articulations must be freely moving but precisely limited in flexion range if walking is to be possible (Fig. 7.3), but they must have a release for sitting. With the development of this device a rational and not empirical choice could be made for each patient (Rose 1980), and the factors required for each of these orthoses could be identified.

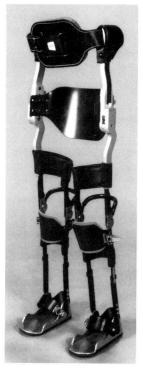

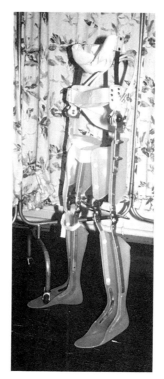

Fig. 7.6. The Parawalker.   **Fig. 7.7.** The RGO.

Outline approach to 'walking aids'

Attempts at reciprocal walking in the seriously paralysed are well established. The concept of transferring action from one leg to the other, either by a gearbox (Woolridge 1969) or by cables (Scrutton 1971), originated in the 1960s. They did not emerge from the research stage possibly because of the inevitable patterning of gait, but the addition of moulded plastic leg pieces has achieved some popularity as the 'reciprocating gait orthosis' (RGO) (Fig. 7.7).

No single device has all the virtues, and assessment must take account of patient preference and individual priorities. However, to avoid delay and disappointment it is the responsibility of the prescriber to make an informed choice.

Theoretical considerations

SWIVEL WALKER

The components of locomotion are:

(1) stabilisation: intrinsic (full exoskeleton) and extrinsic (large footplates)
(2) propulsion: footplate bearings related to the centre of body mass combined with rigid structure and inertial energy from body and arm sway, and

110

(3) control: intrinsic (footplate axis, sensory/non-sensory interface), and extrinsic (footplate noise)

The components of gait are:

(4) rotation at footplates, and

(5) rocker at footplate dihedral.

The *advantages* include the low energy requirement (see below), and the fact that it can be used from 12 months of age, therefore matching normal development. It leaves the hands free, and its modern design provides independent transfer and doff and don (Fig. 7.4). With crutches, a swing through is possible. It can be used with associated hemiplegia, spinal orthoses, where there is considerable deformity and up to c6 level. It is also commercially available with high reliability and wear characteristics, and in school and other situations it takes up much less room than a wheelchair.

The *disadvantages* are that it is relatively slow, with a maximum 25 per cent average speed; it can be used without crutches only for level floor walking; and its movement has only one element of normal gait, which reduces dynamic cosmesis, as does the clicking noise (although this is a valuable extrinsic feedback control).

FORMS OF RECIPROCAL WALKERS

For totally paralysed legs (and it can be debated whether this form of orthosis is required for lower-lesion levels) the components of locomotion are:

(1) stabilisation: intrinsic (crutches with hip articulated knee-ankle-foot-orthoses) and extrinsic (crutches plus a specified hip range limited by articulation stops or cables)

(2) propulsion: swing (gravity or cable transfer), uphill stance (arm/trunk muscles acting through crutches plus some enhancement from inertial overspill of energy from the downhill phase), and downhill stance (gravity/body mass); and

(3) control: sensory/non-sensory interface with hip-flexion limitation (Fig. 7.5).

The components of gait are:

(1) leg pendulum

(2) leg vaulting, and

(3) lateral rocker at footwear/floor level

The *advantages* include its low energy cost; its speed (up to 50 per cent normal); and its ability to surmount 15cm step and a slope up or down of one in 10, on all surfaces (external roads and fields). It has a good dynamic cosmesis. Independent transfer and doff and don can be achieved by its design features, and it is commercially available for children and adults.

Its *disadvantages* are that it is unsuitable for patients with associated hemiplegia or marked spinal deformity; also patients need to be four or five years of age, and need crutches or rollator (depending on the orthosis used).

Assessment of results of usage

Assessment demands a high level of discipline on the part of the research team if like is to be compared with like. Data must include precise recording of the level of paralysis, joint position sense if any (the occasional presence of this can account for surprisingly good performance), and joint contracture.

The most important test of the effectiveness of an orthosis is the overall performance. It is helpful to use a modified Hoffer *et al.* (1973) classification, which divides disabled people into four categories:

(1) community ambulators, who are able to walk indoors and outdoors, who use wheelchairs only for long trips, with independent transfer and doff and don
(2) household ambulators, as above but walking limited to indoors
(3) non-functional ambulators, using indoor walking therapeutically, and
(4) non-ambulators, who are restricted to a wheelchair.

Energy cost, which may be monitored by speed related to energy consumption, is most conveniently measured by rise in heart rate relative to walking speed: the so-called physiological cost index (PCI) (MacGregor 1981). In the normal subject this varies from 0.2 to 0.7 and is independent of age (Butler *et al.* 1984). The principal value of this test is in comparisons of performance, such as the evaluation of the improvements produced by design changes in orthoses. For example, the average PCI with conventional orthoses at 9.7 dropped to 5.5 with the use of ORLAU orthoses in 1979, and currently to 3.3 in 17 post-traumatic adults.

Experience shows that independent doff and don ranks higher with the patient than concealment of the orthosis except on special occasions. Patients will have differing attitudes towards apparatus design, the style of walking, and additional walking aids required (crutches or rollator). The patient must be able to accept the constraints and advantages of the orthosis and particularly to have total control of it, compared with the constraints imposed by a joined legs system.

Costs include not just the initial outlay (for the device and training); they must also take account of growth adjustment and reliability. And when structural overload occurs (as will happen sooner or later with all devices) the design must fail in a safe manner.

There is no doubt that many individuals have derived great psychological and social benefits from them (Sankarankutty *et al.* 1979, Rose *et al.* 1983), together with important practical advantages which certainly include reduction in fractures and improved transfer ability (Mazur *et al.* 1986). The experience of over 15 years has confirmed that they are here to stay even in their present form. There is good cause to be optimistic about current research projects, especially functional electrical stimulation (FES).

Effective maintained locomotion is not the only benefit to be gained by the use of these devices, but the ideal objective is to achieve categories (1) or (2) of Hoffer *et al.*'s (1973) criteria (above). Using these categories, the Parawalker (Stallard *et al.* 1991) can be compared with the old orthodox braces used in similar cases by Asher and Olsen (1983). The new orthoses have improved performance by at least one category, and only 8 per cent of patients remained chairbound compared with 52 per cent reported by Hoffer *et al.* (1973), although only 17 per cent in his series

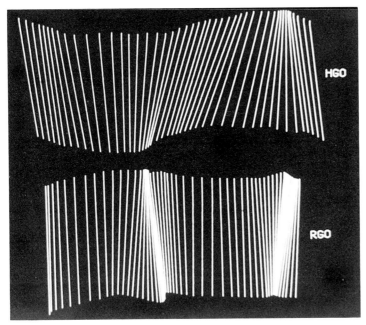

Fig. 7.8. Comparative (stick) diagrams of the HGO and RGO. Note the smooth progression of the Parawalker, which reduces energy consumption.

were thoracic lesions compared with 51 per cent at ORLAU.

The use of PCI and gas exchange is to set present standards and monitor improvements in energy expenditure. Cerny *et al.* (1980) and Williams (1983) demonstrated that in terms of energy cost the wheelchair was by far the most effective device, despite the problems of moving on varying levels and its inability to provide useful scope for reaching.

The swivel walker was given an optimistic outlook by Zakia *et al.* (1978), who suggested that the device had reasonably low energy expenditure, although more recent work by Ogilvie *et al.* (1988) has challenged this. Results are all relative. The figures given later for PCI seem to give some support to this challenge, but the increase in these values is not a linear one. Of course, ambulation in orthoses cannot nearly match the superb efficiency of normal gait, and exchange studies suggest that the energy cost for ambulation with this level of disability is some five to six times normal.

Predictably, the HGO is more efficient than the RGO because of the lack of frictional resistance that has to be overcome in the latter device. The recent Salford study (Ogilvie *et al.* 1988) and a similar piece of work from the Nuffield centre in Oxford (Whittle and Cochrane 1989) confirmed this. The Oxford study also highlighted the HGO's smooth line of forward progression, compared to the RGO, with a commensurate improvement in energy return from the downhill component of the orthosis gait cycle (Nene and Patrick 1989).

113

These studies, using different measures of energy cost, find that the level of energy required is remarkably high and in all cases is akin to a normal person moving about at a brisk trot but without the associated productivity of distance. In these circumstances the differences between RGO and HGO are less significant and overridden by the general high levels of energy consumption recorded (Fig. 7.8).

The Oxford and Salford surveys both showed that nearly all subjects felt tremendous psychological benefits from using walking aids. They felt physically better and noted a general improvement in their sense of purpose. This is not to be minimised and requires further evaluation. In individual cases (according to anecdotal evidence) there were remarkable improvements in lifestyle. We must therefore accept that many patients will gain from their use, and the decision of what to use and when will remain a matter of judgement on the part of both the user and the therapist.

One novel approach taken in Salford has been to design the swivel walker so that it may be donned by folding the device around the patient—the so-called 'front-loading' technique. The wheelchair seat can then be raised hydraulically so that the patient and the walker come upright simultaneously and the device is then locked out and used. The process can be reversed to reseat the patient. This appears to make maximum use of the wheelchair to cover larger distances efficiently, with the swivel walker being used when reaching is required. Unfortunately the excessive price of the package means that the numbers of patients deriving such a benefit will be quite small.

The way forward
In all mechanical devices the energy required for locomotion must come from the remaining muscles under voluntary control used in the most efficient way. Theoretically a further potential source can be tapped by electrical stimulation of muscles which have been removed by the lesion from this control: the hybrid mechanical FES.

In traumatic paraplegics the neuromuscular system is intact until the moment of injury, after which the two components are dissociated, although the muscles themselves are intrinsically normal. In the congenital paraplegic the picture is more complex, and it is doubtful whether there is useful muscle at all. Alternatives for the traumatic paraplegic may therefore include a system of stimulating the uncoordinated muscles with electrical signals controlled by a microcomputer. It would be an oversimplification to suggest the same for myelomeningocele: alternative energy sources in such cases must be extrinsic to the body, and some sort of hydraulic controller may be sought. A combination of both sources is possible, particularly in the acquired paraplegic.

FES is not new (Kralj and Bajd 1989), and it has many problems both in relation to the stimulation of the muscles themselves and perhaps more formidably in the control of muscle activity. Functionally stimulated muscle is especially prone to fatigue because current techniques are very crude in recruiting only a small number of muscle fibres in an all-or-none activity, whereas the natural situation is for a more modulated response with different fibres being recruited in turn, so maintaining an overall net activity. In terms of control it is often forgotten that paraplegics are also sensorily destitute: even if power can be restored, normal sensory feedback (and so intrinsic modulation) is still absent.

Many of the problems outlined will have solutions in the future and the inherent problems of FES will be reduced by implantable electrodes and more careful manipulation of the electrical signal. The long-term aim is to achieve useful control of stimulation.

At the moment most progress is being made with the open loop feedback system. The subject makes a conscious decision to instigate an electrically stimulated muscle contraction by means of a switch which produces an all-or-none twitch in the muscle. This produces an effect that the patient monitors using vision and sound along with sensation and proprioception from more proximal intact sensory apparatus. The patient has to concentrate so hard to coordinate activity that usually s/he can do nothing else.

Ideally a closed loop control system is required, where the locomotor system has both motor output and sensory input from remote devices which report on position and load. This reduces the need for a higher sensory overriding system, and so less conscious effort is devoted to ambulation. This is a formidable problem and requires a lot from both elements of the control loop.

Many muscles are required to produce useful walking or even standing, and to react properly each muscle requires its action to be modulated via appropriate sensors placed strategically on each motivated body segment. This results in a serious logistical problem.

One solution would be to combine the energetically advantageous properties of FES with the relative simplicity of orthoses. In very simple terms, orthoses are capable of supporting the body against gravity within the constraints of an equilibrium and FES may provide the means of maintaining that state of equilibrium or moving the orthotically clad body from one state of equilibrium to another during ambulation. Also, by having the body surrounded by an orthosis, the number of ways in which the body can be allowed to move can be restricted, and angle and load can be monitored easily through readily available sensors. The ankle may be fixed in an ankle-foot orthosis, for instance, obviating the need to stimulate calf or foot muscles; the knee will be restricted by a unipivotal hinge to one angular motion and subjected to one turning moment. Such a system would have only two degrees of freedom and so the control problem would be far more easily handled.

Such hybrid systems are under active consideration in a number of centres (Andrews 1986, Solomonow *et al.* 1989). For example, theoretically adding to the HGO stimulation of hip abductors could assist the raising of one foot from the ground by improving the overall stiffness of the device. HGO stimulation of the hip extensors would reduce energy demand for the uphill phase, and a quadriceps assist would help significantly in getting up from the sitting position.

In limited practice the theory has been confirmed. One immediate result of the first two has been a reduction of fatigue and discomfort in the arms after prolonged usage. However the costs, in terms of time and material resources, demand that tangible benefits must accrue if these devices are to be provided from already scant resources within disability services.

In patients with lower lumbar lesions, for instance, standing may be maintained using an ankle-foot orthosis and functional stimulation of the quadriceps to maintain knee extension. Andrews *et al.* (1989) described their orthosis as maintaining the centre of gravity of the body in front of the knee; any change in body position, resulting in the axis falling behind the knee, results in a quadriceps twitch to extend the knee and restore equilibrium. Sensation may be provided through a heel and toe sensor, or by placing a transducer behind the orthosis which monitors pressure between it and the patella.

Already we can see the introduction of conditions into this control system. All we have is a very simple set of rules which states 'if something happens' then 'do this'. We must develop this sort of conditional control system into a hierarchy of conditions which may be both positive and negative (Andrews *et al.* 1989). As more elements are added to such a system, the more ranks there will be in the hierarchy. In order to keep within practical boundaries, expert computer techniques (akin to artificial intelligence) will be required even in a hybrid system.

The addition of mechanical drivers (such as hydraulics) as a supplement to or substitute for muscle activity has also been considered (Tomovic *et al.* 1972). Much of the energy expended in walking in orthoses is concerned with lifting the centre of gravity of the body upwards so that the foot of the non-weight-bearing limb clears the ground. This is normally achieved in part by flexing the knee and dorsiflexing the foot. The possibility of doing either or both of these procedures mechanically would reduce the complexity of the muscular control and leave that element for other activities. The problem is that such patients would feel that they were being driven, which may be very uncomfortable if not frightening. Again the solution will require careful consideration to the control system, to anticipate movements and provide a fail-safe device being operated in the event of a fall or other accident. The boundaries between orthotics, prosthetics and indeed robotics will become less and less distinct.

Conclusion

At the heart of the problem is a collection of essential biomechanical conditions which must be fulfilled to overcome the problems of gravity and friction. Our understanding of the problem may not have improved greatly, but new solutions have come from often unrelated technologies. The fields of microelectronics and computing must now be explored, in search of an elegant solution for the paraplegic. The art is to combine what is technically possible with what is clinically and ethically reasonable.

REFERENCES

Andrews, B.J., Bajd, T. (1984) 'Hybrid orthoses for paraplegics.' *Proceedings of the International Symposium on External Control of Human Extremities, Dubrovnik.* pp. 55–59.

—— Barnett, R.W., Phillips, G.F., Kirkwood, C.A., Donaldson, N., Rushton, D.N., Perkins, T.A. (1989) 'Rule based control of a hybrid FES orthosis for assisting paraplegic locomotion.' *Automedica*, **11**, 175–199.

Asher, M., Olsen, J. (1983) 'Factors affecting the ambulatory status of patients with spina bifida cystica.' *Journal of Bone and Joint Surgery*, **65A**, 350–356.

Butler, P., Englebrecht, M., Major, R.E., Tait, J.H., Stallard, J., Patrick, J.H. (1984) 'Physiological cost index of walking for normal children and its use as an indicator of physical handicap.' *Developmental Medicine and Child Neurology*, **26**, 607–612.

Cerny, K., Walters, R., Hislop, H., Perry, J. (1980) 'Walking and wheelchair energetics in persons with paraplegia.' *Physical Therapy*, **60**, 1133–1139.

DHSS (1973) *Shrewsbury Walking Appliance. Notes for Guidance.* Ref: Sal 73 10, Blackpool.

Edbrooke, H. (1970) 'Clicking splint.' *Physiotherapy*, **56**, 148–153.

Guttman, L. (1976) *Spinal Cord Injuries: Comprehensive Management and Research. 2nd Edn.* Oxford: Blackwell.

Hoffer, M., Felwell, E., Perry, J., Bonnett, C. (1973) 'Functional ambulation in patients with myelomeningocoele.' *Journal of Bone and Joint Surgery*, **55A**, 137–148.

Kralj, A., Bajd, T. (1989) *Functional Electrical Stimulation: Standing and Walking after Spinal Cord Injury.* Boca Raton: CRS Press.

Lorber, J. (1971) 'The results of treatment of myelomeningocoele.' *Developmental Medicine and Child Neurology*, **13**, 279–303.

MacGregor, J. (1981) 'Evaluation of patient performance using long term ambulatory monitoring technique in domestic environment.' *Physiotherapy*, **67**, 30–38.

Mazur, J., Menelaus, M.B., Dickens, D.R.V., Doig, W.G. (1986). 'Efficacy of surgical management of scoliosis in myelomeningocele: correction of deformity and alteration of functional status.' *Journal of Pediatric Orthopaedics*, **6**, 568–575.

—— Shurtleff, D., Menelaus, M.B. (1989) 'Orthopaedic management of spina bifida. Early walking compared with early use of a wheelchair.' *Journal of Bone and Joint Surgery*, **71A**, 56–61.

Motloch, W.M. (1971) 'The parapodium: an orthopaedic device for neuromuscular disorders.' *Artificial Limbs*, **15**, 36–47.

—— Elliot, J. (1966) 'Fitting and training children with swivel walkers'. *Artificial Limbs*, **10**, 27–38.

—— Major, R.E., Butler, P.B. (1991) 'The orthotic ambulation performance of paraplegic myelomeningocoele children using the ORLAU parawalker treatment system.' *Clinical Rehabilitation*, **5**, 23–26.

Nene, A.V., Patrick, J.H. (1989) 'Energy cost of paraplegic locomotion with ORLAU parawalker.' *Paraplegia*, **27**, 5–18.

Ogilvie, C., Messenger, N., Bowker, P. (1988) 'Orthotic compensation for non-functioning hip extensors.' *Zeitschrift für Kinderchirurgie*, **43** (Suppl. II), 33–35.

Rose, G.K. (1979) 'The principles and practice of hip guidance articulations.' *Prosthetics and Orthotics International*, **3**, 37–43.

—— Henshaw, J.T. (1972) 'A swivel walker for paraplegics: medical and technical considerations.' *Journal of Biomedical Engineering*, **7**, 420–425.

—— Stallard, J., Sankarankutty, M. (1983) 'A clinical review of the orthotic treatment of myelomeningocele patients.' *Journal of Bone and Joint Surgery*, **68B**, 242–246.

Runcie, J. (1979) *Personal Communication.*

Sankarankutty, M., Rose, G.K., Stallard, J. (1979) 'The effect of orthotic treatment on spina bifida patients.' *Spina Bifida Therapy*, **1**, 187–196.

Scrutton, D. (1971) 'A reciprocating brace with polyplanar hip hinges used on spina bifida children.' *Physiotherapy*, **57**, 61–66.

Solomonow, M.R., Baratta, R., Shoji, D., D'Ambrosia, N., Rightar, W., Walker, R., Beandette, R. (1989). 'FES powered reciprocating gait orthosis for paraplegic locomotion.' *Proceedings of the 3rd Vienna International Workshop on Electrical Stimulation.* p. 81.

Speilrein, R.E. (1963) 'An engineering approach to ambulation without the use of external power sources, of severely handicapped individuals.' *Journal of Institute of Engineers, Australia*, **35**, 321–326.

—— (1971) 'Australian contribution to the ambulation of legless individuals.' *Medical Journal of Australia*, **2**, 152–161.

Stallard, J., Rose, G.K., Farmer, I.R. (1978) 'The ORLAU swivel walker.' *Prosthetics and Orthotics International*, **2**, 35–42.

Tomovic, R., Vukobratovic, M., Vodovnik, L. (1972) 'Hybrid actuators for orthotic systems: hybrid assistive systems.' *Proceedings of the 4th International Symposium on Control of Human Extremities, Dubrovnik*. pp. 73–79, ETAN Belgrade.

Whittle, M.W., Cochrane, G.M. (1989) 'A comparative evaluation of the hip guidance orthosis (HGO) and reciprocating gait orthosis (RGO).' Health Equipment Information, DHSS Procurement Dept Room 423, 14 Russell Square, London WC1B 5EP.

Woolridge, C. (1969) 'Bracing of children with paraplegia resulting from spina bifida and cerebral palsy.' University of Virginia: Committee on Prosthetics Research and Development Report.

Zakia, Z.A., Griffiths, J.C., Heywood, O.B. (1978). 'Ambulatory monitoring of heart rate in spina bifida children in swivel walkers.' *Proceedings of the 2nd International Symposium on Ambulatory Monitoring*. Middlesex: Academic Press. pp. 239–246.

8
RECENT CONCEPTS IN PHYSIOTHERAPY

Carole Sobkowiak

The amount of physiotherapy which disabled children receive is a cause of concern for most parents, and can lead them to search for more and more treatment in their desperate desire to see their child walking. Whether their perception of physiotherapy is accurate or not, there are those who will continue to search. This may culminate in the pilgrimage effect.

The combined advances in bioengineering and orthopaedic management, such as the development of the hip guidance orthosis (Ogilvie *et al.* 1988), have enhanced the locomotor prospects for children with spina bifida and hydrocephalus. This has greatly simplified the physiotherapist's task, but what remains difficult is the training of high-quality motor skills leading towards a life of independence for the young person concerned. Residual problems are seen in young adults who, after years of physiotherapy, still require checklists or verbal prompting from an adult in order to cope with everyday activities. In these situations, the question arises whether this is due to a lack of appropriate training or the presence of an inherent factor. It is very important therefore that physiotherapists should be seen as teachers of movement rather than just 'givers' of exercises.

One solution has been to try to integrate motor activities into the educational system whether it be mainstream, special schooling or a mixture of both, ranging from nursery education up until school-leaving age. Physiotherapy can be incorporated into classroom activities (see p. 124).

The principles of paediatric physiotherapy are as follows:
1. Treatment of the child is the education of the family.
2. Early intervention begins soon after birth.
3. Therapy is achieved through play activities.
4. Partnerships are formed with parents, extended family, carers, teachers and other professionals so that programmes are continued at home and in school.
5. Physiotherapy should become part of everyday life.

Early counselling
Informing the parents of their child's disability is never easy and will produce intense grief reactions in the parents and the extended family. The timing of the introduction of the physiotherapist must be carefully considered. It is crucial for the physiotherapist to see the parents together in order to listen to their expectations. Early involvement of a specialist social worker or health visitor may be valuable not only to the family but also to the physiotherapist by providing a reflection of the

family's understanding of the situation. In this way an attempt can be made to allay misconceptions about physiotherapy and to build the foundation for a trusting relationship with parents so that anxieties may be shared.

At the beginning much time is spent establishing such a relationship as well as obtaining an accurate assessment of the child. During early assessment it is impossible to predict the outcome with accuracy. It is important to explain these facts to the parents at the outset, and to indicate that the initial frequency of visits will diminish as they learn to take over some of the treatment. Unless adequately prepared, some parents may feel let down and understandably begin to search for new solutions. Reassurances can be given of long-term support and access to a telephone lifeline. It is advisable to arrange blocks of treatment sessions in order to achieve a particular goal. This will help to prevent the long-term dreary pitfall of weekly therapy, with its monotony and lack of direction.

It is taken for granted in society that all babies and young children will play and develop; indeed it is impossible to stop a healthy child from developing in a normal environment. It is not until a disabled baby is born that a family's perceptions of child development come under scrutiny. It is especially difficult for parents of a firstborn, who have had no previous experience of child-rearing. Frequently to be heard is the question 'What should s/he be doing?' An in-depth knowledge of normal child development is essential so that individual physiotherapy programmes can be planned. These are taught through play, since this is how children learn, and the pleasurable responses of babies will encourage parents to persevere. The individual programmes are eventually linked to the preschool educational system, when children move from solitary play into group activities.

Parents may find it difficult to handle and play with their children when they are so distressed. To share the burden, other members of the family and respite carers can be shown the basic techniques of handling and positioning during the day and at night. Video recordings of treatment programmes can be made for use in the home, nursery and school, so that physiotherapy is built into everyday activities.

Physiotherapy has been linked traditionally to the orthopaedic management of children with spina bifida. There is still an important role for this, and attention should be given to the care of joint ranges, early weight-bearing to promote bone growth, prevention of acetabular dysplasia, postoperative rehabilitation and the strengthening of muscle groups, especially the trunk and shoulder girdle prior to ambulation. By working as a member of a team with the paediatrician, orthopaedic surgeon and orthotist, the physiotherapist will play an important part in the assessment of orthoses and walking aids. It is extremely desirable to have the benefit of advances in bioengineering and the use of gait analysis facilities. If these are not available locally, it is worth sending children with complex problems to a gait analysis laboratory where computer-assisted analysis will enable the fine tuning of orthoses and aids. If there is doubt about such a referral, a video recording of the child's gait sent in advance will usually confirm the necessity for a visit. Repeated visits to hospital, loss of school time and frustration levels for the family can be minimised in the long term. It is only relatively recently that there have been major advances in ambulation with low energy expenditure (Rose 1979, Ogilvie *et al.* 1988).

The other problems surrounding the condition are related to the hydrocephalus and morphological changes such as syringomyelia or the Arnold-Chiari malformation. There are children who have hydrocephalus without spina bifida, including that due to intraventricular bleeding, infections and malignancies. These children will have varying degrees of disability and may present with signs and symptoms similar to those children with neurological disorders who are unskilled and have learning difficulties, *e.g.* children who were of low birthweight (Dunn *et al.* 1986) or who are described as clumsy (Gubbay 1975).

Patterns of myelination
The recent use of magnetic resonance imaging (MRI) has shown the pattern of myelination in the normal child. At two months of age myelin is present only in the middle cerebellar peduncles, but by eight months it has extended into the internal capsule, corpus callosum and the central white matter (Harbord *et al.* 1990). In an earlier study, Gadsdon *et al.* (1979) showed that myelin formation in the white matter of the corpus callosum was reduced in the presence of hydrocephalus and can be restored with the relief of hydrocephalus. It will be interesting to see if this can be confirmed by MRI. Further investigations of myelination patterns extending into the hydrocephalic group would be of great value.

Myelination progresses in a cephalocaudal direction with ventral roots myelinating before dorsal ones (Sutherland *et al.* 1988). This means that the motor nerves will mature before the sensory ones, and the lumbar dorsal roots are the last to myelinate (Rafalowska 1979).

Children with hydrocephalus often take longer to acquire balancing skills and there is a likelihood of a similar situation in those with spina bifida and hydrocephalus, except that it will be masked by the paralysis.

The different rates of phasic muscle development should be taken into account during tendon transfer, especially at the distal end of the limb. Similarly the distal development of hand praxis and fine motor skills may be delayed (Wallace 1973; Minns *et al.* 1977; Mazur *et al.* 1986, 1988; Jacobs *et al.* 1988).

Early therapeutic intervention includes stimulation of visual awareness and of the vestibular system. 'The semicircular canals signal the angular velocity of the head, and stabilise it by evoking postural reflexes that also activate appropriate antigravity trunk/limb muscles. The vestibulospinal tract is the path through which extensor antigravity muscles are adjusted in relationship to the position of the head' (Brooks 1986).

Certain stimulus positions have been described (Katona 1988), in particular the 'sitting in air' position, when the baby is held by the thighs and lifted into a sitting position. Initially the spine is flexed and the head falls forward. Eventually the head is lifted and the baby will look round and visually fixate on an object while there is elevation of the upper extremities. The vestibulospinal and reticulospinal pathways come into action, the receptors in the neck are stimulated and so is the vestibular receptor system.

Sensory integration techniques can be used with young babies to give varied labyrinthine and optical stimulation (Ayres 1972). The techniques involve body orientation in space, vibration and rolling to provide tactile and proprioceptive training.

Parents are often afraid to handle and move their babies in case they cause damage to the lesions on the back or to the valve, especially when they take their child home following hospitalisation. Early advice about the best way to hold and carry their baby will help to reassure parents. Caution is given regarding the risk of fracture when paralysis is present in the lower limbs. Play programmes can be performed while the baby is being nursed on an adult's knee, or using different tactile surfaces such as underinflated beach balls, lilo beds and swings, or indeed any suitable piece of household furniture, so that therapy can be carried out unobtrusively in the home rather than introducing too much specialised equipment which may seem out of place.

The discrimination of multisensory information can be observed when the child is moved from one position to another and on different surfaces which will permit the development of righting reactions and postural control.

The sequencing of movement up the motor hierarchy from one position to another is complex. For example, to get from the sitting position onto all fours, prior to crawling, requires not only the will to move but also the ability to initiate such a movement, followed by trunk rotation, inclining the eyes and head through different planes, crossing one arm over the midline to contact a new surface accompanied by a series of muscle contractions to achieve another stable posture in a different position. The continued sequencing of movement for verticalisation is equally complex as more distal components become involved. Ayres (1979) said that this early stimulation enables the brain to plan the kind of messages to send to the muscles, and the sequence in which to send them.

White (1984) wrote: 'As the infant matures and childhood experiences broaden, he develops more abstract concepts. The early vestibular, proprioceptive and tactile play will enable the child to develop the form and space perception that is the foundation for complex manipulative skills and for later abstract concepts such as number and letter recognition'.

The lack of motivation in children with spina bifida and/or hydrocephalus is a common feature which is still poorly understood. A child may be given a command and be completely unable to execute the motor movement without further verbal prompting. It may also be necessary to break the task down into very small stages.

During early treatment, there is emphasis on the development of spatial awareness and sequencing of movement as motor activities are learned through spatial memories (Sutherland 1988). During and after this period, it is crucial to develop good quality gross motor activities as these precede the development of fine motor skills which are required for precise and detailed hand praxis. Gross motor activities (e.g. rolling, creeping and crawling) will progress towards the high-quality skills involving the distal joints (jumping, standing on one leg and hopping). There are some children, especially in the hydrocephalic group, who will develop a certain degree of gross motor agility with time but who are slower to acquire the competence of fine motor hand skills.

Development of upper-limb skills
With maturation comes the development of large arm movements, starting proximally at the shoulder girdle and progressing distally with the later emergence of hand skills and discrete finger movements.

It used to be postulated that lack of experience was responsible for poor upper-limb function in children with spina bifida, especially in those with high lesions who had to use their arms for support. However, similar neurological signs can be found in the upper limbs of children with hydrocephalus only, and those with other aetiologies mentioned previously, who may have less obvious neurological impairment.

There are common features in the elicited neurological signs, including finger agnosia, graphaesthesia, astereognosis for shape and texture, difficulty with individual finger sequencing, right/left confusion and cerebellar signs such as dysdiadochokinesia, dysmetric finger/nose test, hand-patting and finger-tapping responses which manifest as poor co-ordination. The presence of mirror movements and associated movements can also indicate minor neurological impairment (Touwen and Prechtl 1970, Denkla 1978). Mirror movements of the hands can persist. One hand may copy the manipulative pattern of the hand performing the task, thus making it difficult for one hand to work in isolation or for both hands to perform separate skills simultaneously. Conversely there may be an inhibitory effect when one hand is attempting a complex skill such as writing or unscrewing a lid, and the other is holding down the paper or holding the jar.

The persistence of associated movements in the upper limbs can also contribute towards decreased function. They are exacerbated by increased effort and stressful situations. In ambulant children it is possible to measure them by using the Fog test (Fog and Fog 1963, Connolly and Stratton 1968). Walking on heels, toes and outer or inner borders of the feet will produce synkinetic overflow movements in the arms and the hands (Wolff *et al.* 1983, 1985).

In clinical practice, strong links have been found between the neurological examination of the upper limbs and the results of psychometric testing carried out by the educational psychologist. Poor motor sequencing can affect handwriting, for example, and difficulty with right/left orientation and astereognosis for shape can relate to deficits in mathematical concepts. These links form a baseline for the measurement of neurological progress, as well as enabling programmes to be devised jointly by the educational psychologist and the physiotherapist.

It has been shown that the measurement of associated movements may act as a marker of developmental state, independent of chronological age (Wolff *et al.* 1985).

The case for intervention into adult life is strengthened by the fact that the neurological signs and associated signs may still be present in the teenager and even young adult with spina bifida and/or hydrocephalus. Wolff *et al.* (1985) described the relationship betwen neuromotor status and psychological investigations. Their findings suggest that motor signs may give clues about the development of motor coordination and language competence.

Education-based approaches

Conductive Education (CE) was pioneered at the Petö Institute, an educational establishment under the auspices of the Hungarian Ministry of Education. CE is not claimed to be a treatment (Hári and Tillemans 1984), but a system whereby children are given opportunities to facilitate learning. The Institute is a training centre for the conductors, who work hard to motivate the children and help them find enjoyable ways round their problems. Conductors strive to achieve maximum independence and will try to avoid holding the child unless failure is imminent (Hári and Tillemans 1984). In contrast to individual therapy, CE uses group work for its methods of teaching and utilises the benefits of collective activity. Tasks can also be built up in small stages towards a common goal with the use of speech, chanting, inner language and rhythm to reinforce the learning process.

A crucial distinction is that in Hungary a child cannot attend a normal school or a school for the physically disabled unless s/he is able to walk. There is therefore a great emphasis on walking. Those children not attending school receive six hours home tuition per week or are cared for in other state institutions.

The Petö Institute has a philosophy of managing with the minimum use of aids and appliances. It is not known what happens to the joints in the long term, however, and whether further deformities may develop. It is hoped that longitudinal studies will eventually become available (Sobkowiak 1990).

Integrated learning programmes have been devised in the United States to help parents and children learn self-care skills, and for teachers to present academic material effectively (Lollar 1990).

In Britain the integration of motor activities into the school curriculum is desirable in order to combine the strengths of the health and education services. The physiotherapist remains a generic specialist offering help and advice within the education framework.

A model has been pioneered in a school for children with severe learning difficulties which necessitates the breaking down of tasks into small stages. This method also lends itself well to children with spina bifida and/or hydrocephalus. It can be applied in other educational establishments, including mainstream schools, and a consistent method can therefore apply throughout the educational system.

In order for physiotherapy to become integrated into the school activities and to monitor progress, a number of methods are used:

TABLE 8.I

TABLE 8.I

Factors observed during gross motor screening

Time taken to process information
Quality of movement
Sequencing of movement
Equilibrial reactions
Awareness of others
Body image
Spatial concepts including right/left orientation
Auditory and visual memory

TABLE 8.II

Factors observed during hand function testing

Muscle tone
Motor profile
Sensory profile
Neurological signs
Hand praxis to include writing and drawing

1. There is an annual gross motor screening of each child which is done jointly by the physiotherapist and teacher (see Table 8.I). This takes approximately one hour and is separate from detailed assessments which the physiotherapist may be carrying out at other times. A developmental proforma has been designed, ranging from rolling up to higher agility skills. It is coded qualitatively and quantitatively, and is sensitive to whether the child performs better with an auditory command or whether visual reinforcement is required. For children with severe learning difficulties there is a code for the use of gesture such as Makaton (Walker 1985) or Link (Smith 1985).

2. The Derbyshire Language Scheme (Knowles and Masidlover 1982) is used during the gross motor screening with young children and those with learning difficulties. The scheme is concerned with language rather than speech and is developmentally based: arranged in levels according to the developmental sequence of normal children's language. The scale extends from a two-word level, at 18 months, to a 10-word level or more at 48 months as utterances become longer and more complex. The use of the scheme will focus upon the correct level of comprehension for each child, and thereby determine the appropriate verbal instructions to be given during the motor screening.

3. Detailed hand-function assessment, compiled by the author from a previous study (Minns *et al.* 1977), will enable the items shown in Table 8.II to be identified.

Results of screening and use of data

So far we have only computer data for the gross motor screening which is processed in our medical physics department. This is represented by a bar line, easily seen by teachers, parents and children. The movement is scored on a scale of 0 to 3 (no attempt to good attempt). The verbal instructions are scored according to whether gesture (G) is required (such as the use of Makaton or Link for a child with severe learning difficulties), whether a visual (V) demonstration is needed or ultimately whether the child can perform the activity with just an auditory (A) command. The proforma and data show not only the level at which the child is currently functioning but also the progress over the years. Conversely it can alert the physiotherapist to areas of underperformance or even deterioration. The data form part of the school and medical records, and families may have a copy so that information can travel with the child or young adult.

In future we hope to develop a movement score and to obtain further correlation between gross motor activities, hand function and language development.

Teachers can use the data to determine the exact level at which a child is functioning, and to compare different managements in the infant.

Overlap between physiotherapy and teaching methods
It is easy to go from a physiotherapy-based approach towards a teaching situation for preschool children, as the two professions overlap. Many early aims of physiotherapy (visual tracking, fixation and awareness, vocal responsiveness, spatial relationships, tactile sensation, gross motor activities and symbolic play) will dovetail into the early sensory training outlined in the national curriculum. These aims would tie in with the teaching of language, early science and pre-reading skills, *e.g.* visual perception, mathematical concepts including number classification, sequencing of body action, and appreciation of money and time. It would be very desirable if these aims could be incorporated into every preschool timetable, maintaining regular assessment.

As the child progresses from the early sensory curriculum towards the first level of the national curriculum, it is possible to incorporate activities into subjects such as physical education, movement and music, hand skills groups, writing, more advanced mathematics, drama and extended sensory work in science subjects.

The use of gross motor activities as an adjunct to learning is vital, especially at the stage of teaching prepositions. A child can be told to crawl *under* the table, sit *in* the tunnel or jump *on* the mat.* Visual and auditory memory can be reinforced in this way by extending the length of commands and using different pieces of apparatus. Mathematical concepts can be taught through gross motor activities (*e.g.* rolling, crawling or walking round a circle, square or triangle). In order to enhance the learning process, counting and measuring time, distance and speed, as well as right/left orientation, can be included in these activities.

Spatial orientation
Putting young children into wheelchairs used to be frowned upon, for fear of

---

*'In', 'on' and 'under', for instance, are at the two-word level on the Derbyshire Language Scheme, and 'front' and 'back' are at the seven-word level.

obesity and prevention of walking. Given a well motivated family and a good diet in school, then we would positively encourage the use of such equipment for severely disabled children who are slow-moving (with aids or independently) so that they can join in activities with their peers. This should not detract from positive attempts at ambulation. Disillusionment may set in during the teenage years, when encouragement should be given to return to a walking programme when the family are ready. There are many fun go-karts, power driven 'comets' and turbo chairs and specially adapted bicycles on the market, as well as a variety of sports wheelchairs. Self esteem and keeping up with the others are important; indeed some children become the envy of their peers with modern high-tec equipment. The principle here is no different from using one's car for a quick dash to the shops or for an outing. Early identification of landmarks and problem solving may contribute towards orienteering and driving ability in young adult life (Simms 1987).

Joint programmes worked out by the teacher, educational psychologist and therapist are useful when observing children in different settings: during outings or visits to other schools for mainstream integration. This is equally important for pupils who already attend mainstream school. Wherever the placement may be, difficulties can be encountered when the child or young person is moving from the place in which the skill has been learned into the new environment. This highlights the need for further intervention in order to consolidate the task. The real test for pupils with spina bifida and/or hydrocephalus is to be able to perform at the same level in a wide variety of circumstances.

Varied opportunities can be sought through leisure activities, *e.g.* the Outward Bound scheme, canoeing, sailing, abseiling and sporting competitions. It has often been said that these children do not manifest a competitive spirit and it is difficult to know if this is due to lack of opportunity. Many of the activities described can be achieved from a wheelchair. The young people concerned should be encouraged to help with the organisation of events from an early age so that they do not become used to being passengers in society. Apart from their perceptual and learning difficulties (Holgate 1985), the children may have a poorly identified sense of the future. Encouragement for future planning should be included in training programmes.

Well documented physiotherapy assessments, accompanied by computerised results, make a valuable interdisciplinary contribution towards realistic expectations and achievements for the young person. They provide a sound platform from which to plan the progression of the young person's passage into further education or placement in a sheltered work environment, and highlight the relevance of continued education in these developing areas well into adult life.

Summary

Physiotherapy has an important role to play in the early intervention and teaching of motor patterns, using a task analysis approach together with the use of language to internalise spatial concepts. While the acquisition of walking is a high priority, it should not be the only goal.

Physiotherapy should be integrated into the home environment and the school timetable where possible, so that the child does not have to be withdrawn from the classroom for 'exercises'. It is hoped that this will help to alleviate family stress and concern about how often their child receives physiotherapy, and therefore enhance the philosophy that therapy is a way of life.

REFERENCES

Ayres, A.J. (1972) *Sensory Integration and Learning Disorders*. Los Angeles: Western Psychological Services. pp. 11–12, 114–115.
—— (1979) *Sensory Integration and the Child*. Los Angeles: Western Psychological Services. pp. 181–185.
Brooks, V.B. (1986) *The Neural Basis of Motor Control*. Oxford: Oxford University Press. p. 25.
Code, C. (1987) *Language, Aphasia, and the Right Hemisphere*. Chichester: John Wiley.
Connolly, K., Stratton, P. (1968) 'Developmental changes in associated movements.' *Developmental Medicine and Child Neurology*, **10**, 49–56.
Denkla, M.B. (1978) 'Minimal brain dysfunction.' *In* Call, J., Mirsky, A.F. (Eds) *Education and the Brain*. Chicago: University of Chicago Press.
Dunn, H.G., Ho, H.H., Crichton, J.U., Robertson, A.-M., McBurney, A.K., Grunau, R.V.E., Penfold, P.S., Schulzer, M. (1986) 'Evolution of minimal brain dysfunctions to the age of 12 to 15 years.' *In* Dunn, H.G. (Ed.) *Sequelae of Low Birthweight: The Vancouver Study. Clinics in Developmental Medicine, Nos 95/96*. London: S.I.M.P. with Blackwell Scientific; Philadelphia: J.B. Lippincott. pp. 249–272.
Fog, E., Fog, M. (1963) 'Cerebral inhibition examined by associated movements.' *In* Bax, M., Mac Keith, R. (Eds) *Minimal Cerebral Dysfunction. Clinics in Developmental Medicine, No. 10*. London: S.I.M.P. with Heinemann; Philadelphia: J.B. Lippincott. pp. 52–56.
Gadsdon, D.R., Variend, S., Emery, J.L. (1979) 'Myelination of the corpus callosum. II: the effect of relief of hydrocephalus upon the processes of myelination.' *Zeitschrift für Kinderchirurgie*, **28**, 314–321.
Gubbay, S.S. (1975) *'The Clumsy Child: A Study of Developmental Apraxic and Agnostic Ataxia.'* Philadelphia: W.B. Saunders.
Harbord, M.G., Finn, J.P., Hall-Craggs, M.A., Robb, S.A., Kendall, B.E., Boyd, S.G. (1990) 'Myelination patterns on magnetic resonance of children with developmental delay.' *Developmental Medicine and Child Neurology*, **32**, 295–303.
Hári, M., Tillemans, T. (1984) 'Conductive education.' *In* Scrutton, D. (Ed.) *Management of the Motor Disorders of Children with Cerebral Palsy. Clinics in Developmental Medicine, No. 90*. London: S.I.M.P. with Blackwell Scientific; Philadelphia: J.B. Lippincott. pp. 19–35.
Holgate, L. (1985) 'Young people with spina bifida and/or hydrocephalus—learning and development.' Peterborough: Association for Spina Bifida and Hydrocephalus.
Jacobs, R.A., Wolfe, G., Ramuson, M. (1988) 'Upper extremity dysfunction in children with myelomeningocele.' *Zeitschrift für Kinderchirurgie*, **43**, 19–21.
Katona, F. (1988) 'Developmental clinical neurology and neurohabilitation in the secondary prevention of pre- and perinatal injuries of the brain.' *In* Vietze, P.M. (Ed.) *Early Indentification of Infants with Developmental Disabilities*. Orlando, FL: Grune & Stratton. p. 129.
Knowles, W., Masidlover, M. (1982) *Derbyshire Language Scheme*. Derbyshire County Council.
Lollar, D. J. (1990) 'Learning patterns among spina bifida children.' *Zeitschrift für Kinderchirurgie*, **45**, 39.
Mazur, J.M., Menelaus, M.B., Hudson, I., Stillwell, A. (1986) 'Hand function in patients with spina bifida cystica.' *Journal of Pediatric Orthopedics*, **6**, 442–447.
—— Aylward, G.P., Colliver, J., Stacey, J., Menelaus, M. (1988) 'Impaired mental capabilities and

hand function in myelomeningocele patients.' *Zeitschrift für Kinderchirurgie*, **43**, 24–27.

Minns, R.A., Sobkowiak, C.A., Skardoutsou, A., Dick, K., Elton, R.A., Brown, J.K., Forfar, J.O. (1977) 'Upper limb function in spina bifida.' *Zeitschrift für Kinderchirurgie*, **22**, 493–506.

Ogilvie, C., Messenger, N., Bowker, P., Rowley, D.I. (1988) 'Orthotic compensation for non-functioning hip extensors.' *Zeitschrift für Kinderchirurgie*, **43**, 33–35.

Rafalowska, J. (1979) 'Some problems of development and ageing of the nervous system. II: Myelination of spinal roots in the second half of life and in early infancy.' *Neuropatalogia Polska*, **3**, 407–420.

Rose, G.K. (1979) 'The principles and practice of hip guidance articulations.' *Prosthetics and Orthotics International*, **3**, 37.

Simms, B. (1987) 'The route learning ability of young people with spina bifida and hydrocephalus and their able-bodied peers.' *Zeitschrift für Kinderchirurgie*, **42**, 53–56.

Smith, C. (1985) *Communication Link.* Middlesbrough, Cleveland: Beverley School for the Deaf.

Sobkowiak, C.A. (1990) 'Conductive education.' *Link*, **127**, 6–7.

Sutherland, D.H., Olshen, R.A., Biden, E.N., Wyatt, M.P. (1988) *The Development of Mature Walking. Clinics in Developmental Medicine, Nos 104/105.* London: Mac Keith Press with Blackwell Scientific; Philadelphia: J.B. Lippincott.

Touwen, B.C.L., Prechtl, H.F.R. (1970) *The Neurological Examination of the Child with Minor Nervous Dysfunction. Clinics in Developmental Medicine, No. 38.* London: S.I.M.P. with Heinemann; Philadelphia: J.B. Lippincott.

Walker, M. (1985) *Revised Makaton Vocabulary, 4th Edn.* Camberley, Surrey: Makaton Vocabulary Development Project.

Wallace, S. (1973) 'The effect of upper limb function on mobility of children with myelomeningocele.' *Developmental Medicine and Child Neurology*, **15**, 84–91.

White, R. (1984) 'Sensory integrative therapy for the cerebral-palsied child.' *In* Scrutton, D. (Ed.) *Management of the Motor Disorders of Children with Cerebral Palsy. Clinics in Developmental Medicine, No. 90.* London: S.I.M.P. with Blackwell Scientific; Philadelphia: J.B. Lippincott. pp. 86–95.

Wolff, P.H., Gunnoe, C.E., Cohen, C. (1983) 'Associated movements as a measure of developmental age.' *Developmental Medicine and Child Neurology*, **25**, 417–429.

—— —— —— (1985) 'Neuromotor maturation and psychological performance: a developmental study.' *Developmental Medicine and Child Neurology*, **27**, 344–354.

129

9
SURGERY OF THE VERTEBRAL COLUMN

John V. Banta

Scoliosis

Incidence

Congenital scoliosis and kyphosis were first described by Marsh *et al.* (1885). However, only two cases of curvature of the spine were included in the detailed analysis of 245 cases of myelomeningocele reported to the Clinical Society of London. The early report of Barden *et al.* (1975), indicating an 11 per cent incidence of scoliosis among adults, was an underestimate partly due to subsequent improvement in perinatal care and medical advances which have led to the survival of more children with neural tube defects with higher levels of paralysis. The relationship between spinal deformity and the level of the dysraphic defect was first noted by Barson (1970), who described a 27 per cent incidence of kyphosis in an analysis of 601 newborns. The incidence of scoliosis is directly related to the neurosegmental level (Shurtleff *et al.* 1976, Piggott 1980, Becker and Banta 1986) as well as to the level of the last intact laminar arch (Piggott 1980). The differentiation between developmental or paralytic curvature and curves of congenital origin was noted by Raycroft and Curtis (1972). Earlier reports suggested that scoliosis was unlikely to become a clinical problem if curvature was not present by the age of nine years (Raycroft and Curtis 1972, Piggott 1980). More recent studies, however, indicate that clinically significant paralytic spinal deformity, with curves in excess of 20°, does occur beyond the first decade of life (Fig. 9.1) (Becker and Banta 1986), and in older children the deformity may be related to unrecognised cord pathology (Samuelsson *et al.* 1987).

In a study of 100 children with myelomeningocele (Becker and Banta 1986), scoliosis (defined as a curve in excess of 20°) was analysed according to the correlation of incidence with motor level and age (Fig. 9.2). Although the overall incidence of scoliosis was 42 per cent, it rose to over 90 per cent in individuals with thoracic level motor function, and a 70 per cent incidence was noted in children with asymmetric motor levels and with spasticity.

The relationship of hip dislocation to the presence of scoliosis has been controversial. An earlier study (Raycroft and Curtis 1972) suggested that unilateral hip dislocation could be an infrapelvic cause of scoliosis; recent clinical reports, however, relate curve direction to pelvic obliquity but not to hip dislocation (Samuelsson and Eklöf 1988). The status of the range of motion of the hip is important regardless of whether or not the hip is dislocated. Asymmetric hip-flexion contractures can contribute to the rate of progression of an already established curve in the lower thoracic or lumbar spine.

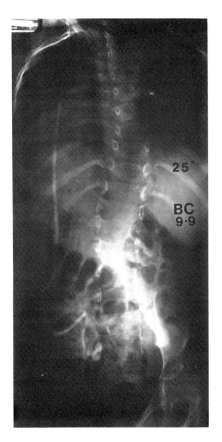
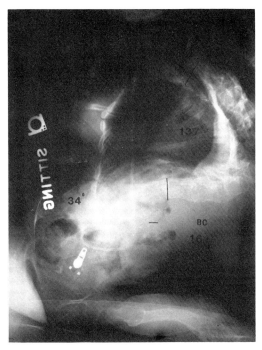
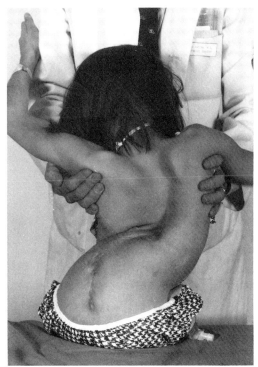

Fig. 9.1. *Above:* x-ray of child (aged 9 yrs 9 mths) with a 25° thoracolumbar curve. The child was lost to follow-up until she returned at age 16 with a 137° scoliosis which was inoperable due to severe pulmonary disease (*above right and bottom right*).

131

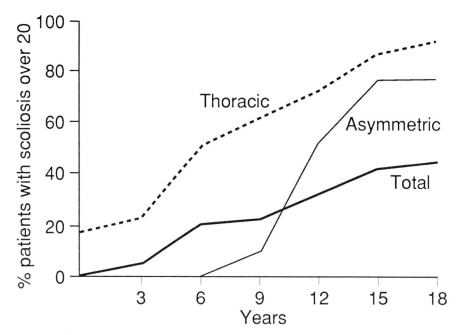

Fig. 9.2. Line graph showing correlation of curve progression with motor level and age.

The neurological lesion in myelomeningocele is not always static. Slow progressive deterioration in motor function has been recognised clinically, although the cause was not readily apparent until the emergence of newer imaging techniques. Hall *et al.* (1979) first noted the relationship between scoliosis and hydrocephalus in children with shunt obstruction. Following shunt revision in seven of 11 children, improvement occurred for up to 20 months in curves less than 55°. Syringohydromyelia and Chiari malformations are common in children with spinal dysraphism but the relationship to developmental scoliosis is not clearly defined (Samuelsson *et al.* 1987).

The incidence of congenital scoliosis ranges from 15 to 38 per cent (Piggott 1980, Samuelsson and Eklöf 1988). Congenital curves are classified as resulting from either a failure of formation or a failure of segmentation of the vertebral elements, both of which are recognisable at birth and frequently demonstrate rapid progression (Fig. 9.3) (Winter 1983). There is also some evidence of an aetiological relationship between multiple vertebral anomalies and neural tube defects (Wynne-Davies 1977, Lendon *et al.* 1981). Early surgical treatment is indicated since conservative orthotic management is unsuccessful. Duckworth *et al.* (1968) coined the term 'hemimyelocele' for an unusual congenital anomaly characterised by unilateral paralysis, the presence of a hemivertebra, and progressive scoliosis. The seriousness of this condition is apparent in a report of 10 patients who all had severe scoliosis and limb length inequality, and six of whom had renal anomalies (Maguire *et al.* 1982).

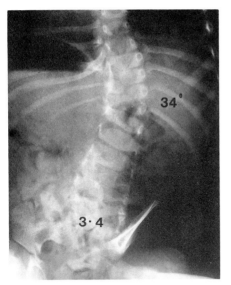

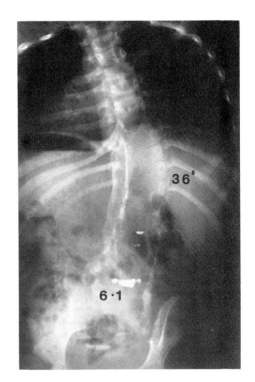

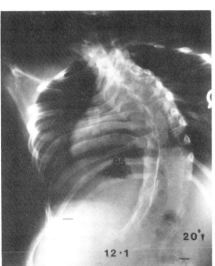

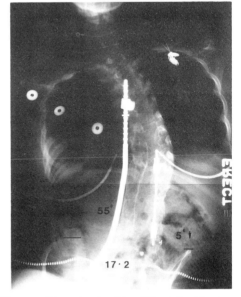

Fig. 9.3. *Top left:* x-ray of a girl with hemimyelo-meningocele with a congenital scoliosis secondary to a hemivertebra and contralateral unsegmented bar at the thoracolumbar junction measuring 34° at age 3 yrs 4 mths. *Top right:* following an *in situ* fusion to arrest the deformity, a solid fusion was obtained with the curve measuring 36°. *Bottom left:* without a brace during growth, the curve progressed from 36° to 95° at age 12 yrs 1 mth with a 20° pelvic obliquity. *Bottom right:* the curve was corrected to 55° at age 13 by a two-stage spinal osteotomy and fusion with Harrington implants; pelvic obliquity was corrected to 5° with preservation of the left side-L4 motor function allowing independent self transfers.

133

Treatment

The treatment goal of scoliosis in spinal dysraphism is to preserve body symmetry and to allow the child an erect sitting posture over a level pelvis without spinal decompensation. Equally important is the preservation of anatomic spinal contours in the sagittal plane, and hip mobility to enable ambulation or to facilitate independent standing transfers in patients with functional (antigravity grade three) motor levels above the third lumbar neurosegmental level. Most children with developmental curves can be managed conservatively until puberty with a total contact thoracolumbosacral orthosis (TLSO). This orthosis can be fabricated from lightweight polypropylene, either from standard modules for lesser degrees of deformity or by custom moulding for children with more severe deformity (Griffiths and Taylor 1980).

Orthotic treatment in neuromuscular scoliosis is palliative and not curative, as the desired therapeutic benefit is to delay surgery to allow the child to obtain near-normal skeletal height in the sitting position. For this reason, it is frequently advisable to leave the child out of the orthosis at night to maintain skin tolerance over potential pressure areas (Banta *et al.* 1990).

Orthoses are indicated when deformity in the erect position results in spinal decompensation that interferes with sitting balance. This applies to ambulatory children with thoracic levels of paraplegia or to children who have a trunk imbalance or pelvic obliquity interfering with clearance of the swing-phase limb. A recent advance in orthotic design, the Reciprocal Gait Orthosis (Durr-Fillauer, Chattanooga, Tennessee) and the Parawalker Orthotic System from the Orthotic and Research Locomotion Analysis Unit (ORLAU, Oswestry, United Kingdom), allow children with thoracic and upper lumbar neurosegmental levels to apply a custom-moulded trunk, hip-knee-ankle-foot orthosis over a total contact spinal orthosis and remain upright with household walking skills.

Surgery is recommended for neuromuscular scoliosis when the deformity exceeds 45° (Allen and Ferguson 1979). At this magnitude of deformity, the surgery is technically easier and the resulting curve correction is greater. Most important of all, the pelvic obliquity associated with paralytic lumbar and thoracolumbar curves can be corrected to provide a level pelvis. If the pelvic obliquity is left uncorrected, the long-term risk of pressure sores of the pelvis is greatly increased. Using a pressure device with pressure-resistant transducers, Drummond *et al.* (1985) demonstrated that pressure sores were commonly associated with a 30 per cent increase of weight borne by one ischial tuberosity or with a 55 per cent shift of total bodyweight to the ischia and sacrococcygeal areas.

The decision for surgery is best determined by analysis of the rigid structural deformity as measured on supine bending films. Before adolescence, a child with a thoracolumbar curve measuring 75° erect can be safely managed with an orthosis to allow for further growth as long as the curve measures less than 50° on supine side-bending x-rays. Supine traction films are of more value in the preoperative planning phase for the analysis of trunk balance and pelvic obliquity. This traction film allows the surgeon to analyse the effect of residual hip-flexion contracture on lumbar lordoscoliosis and to determine the degree of compensatory upper thoracic curve that would be desirable to restore spinal compensation over a level pelvis.

The decision for surgery is based not only on an appraisal of curve magnitude but also on an estimate of the remaining growth and general health of the child. Anthropomorphic studies confirm that trunk height at maturity is indirectly proportional to the level of paralysis (Duval-Beaupère *et al.* 1987), so that individuals with thoracic levels of paraplegia commonly demonstrate a reduction in trunk height and shortened lower extremities. As a consequence, such children with high levels of paralysis present unique problems in the determination of ideal bodyweight because preoperative nutritional assessment is critical when performing staged anterior and posterior spinal arthrodesis.) Accurate measurement of ideal bodyweight can be calculated by determining the percentile of weight for stature based on arm-span measurements (Jaivin *et al.* 1991).

The optimum age for surgery is 10 to 12 years (Menelaus 1976). At puberty, the average child has attained 80 per cent of adult sitting height and by this time more adequate bone stock is available and body size allows the application of most spinal implants. With increasing spinal deformity there is often a corresponding increase in pelvic obliquity which becomes a major impediment to ambulation (Kahanovitz and Duncan 1981). The effect of spinal fusion on walking potential is controversial. Mazur *et al.* (1986), in a review of 49 children treated between 10 and 12 years of age, suggested that a decline in functional performance accompanied spinal arthrodesis. All of their patients, however, were immobilised in plaster body casts for six months postoperatively. Most children who decline in walking activity do so by the onset of their second decade as energy demands for gait increase relative to body mass. For the child with antigravity hamstring function (fourth lumbar neurosegmental level), arthrodesis of the spine with correction of pelvic obliquity and any residual hip contractures followed by rapid mobilisation with a bivalved custom-moulded spinal orthosis should not result in a loss of walking potential.

An impairment in vital capacity is noted in patients with thoracic curves exceeding 60°. As curves progress beyond 70°, there is often a progressive decline in functional vital capacity, functional expiratory volume and functional reserve capacity. In children with thoracolumbar paralytic curves, a lack of trunk stability results in increased pressure of the intra-abdominal viscera on the diaphragm. Pulmonary function studies in a small number of children undergoing combined anterior and posterior fusion have indicated an improvement in peak flow, maximum voluntary ventilation and functional reserve capacity, all of which suggest an improvement in thoracic mechanics (Banta and Park 1983). Preoperative pulmonary function studies are essential since anterior surgical approaches to the spine frequently require exposure of the lower thoracic and lumbar spine through a transthoracic retroperitoneal approach. Such patients frequently require ventilator support during the immediate postoperative period.

TABLE 9.I
Surgical results of treatment for scoliosis in patients with myelomeningocele

	Patients (N)	Non-unions N (%)	Infections N (%)	Deaths N (%)
Sriram *et al.* 1972	33	14 (42.4)	7 (21.2)	0
Osebold *et al.* 1982	40	9 (22.5)	16 (40)	2 (5)
McMaster 1987	23	9 (39.1)	2 (8.6)	1 (4.3)

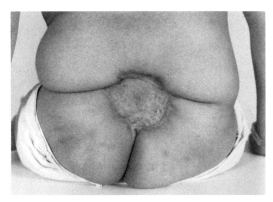 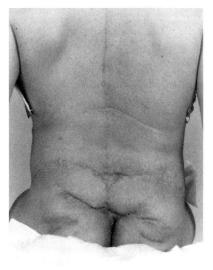

Fig. 9.4. *Left:* 14-year-old girl who presented with a 65° right thoracolumbar scoliosis. The defect had been closed with a split thickness skin graft applied directly to the dura. *Right:* following a first-stage bilateral Y-V plasty, repair of the skin defect, and brace treatment for a year to allow maturation of the soft tissue repair, a two-stage fusion and instrumentation was performed without complication.

The evolution of surgical technique to achieve correction of dysraphic spinal deformity without unacceptable rates of pseudoarthrosis has been long and characterised by high complication rates (Table 9.I). Sriram *et al.* (1972) reported seven major wound infections in a study of 33 patients when surgery was performed in the presence of an unrepaired sac. While some authors recommend using an inverted Y incision in which dissection is on either side of the midline along each osteochondral ridge (Allen and Ferguson 1979, Osebold 1982), I prefer a direct midline approach to avoid occasional wound healing problems at the apex of the three limbs of the Y incision. Skin having a questionable appearance or irregular residual scar from a sac allowed to heal by epithelialisation of the sac should be excised and covered with a rotational flap and allowed to mature prior to definitive spinal surgery (Fig. 9.4).

Unacceptably high pseudoarthrosis rates are common when single-stage posterior arthrodesis of the dysraphic spine is attempted (Osebold 1982, Mazur *et al.* 1986, Ward *et al.* 1989). The magnitude of this problem was demonstrated by Osebold *et al.* (1982), who noted a 42 per cent pseudoarthrosis rate with

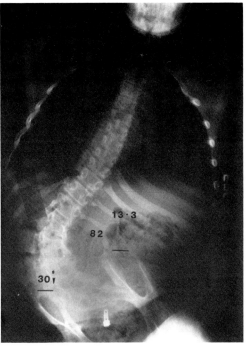

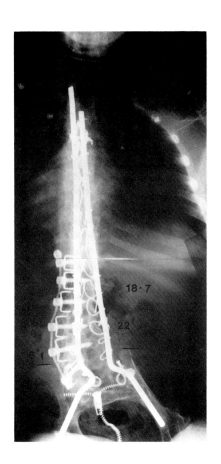

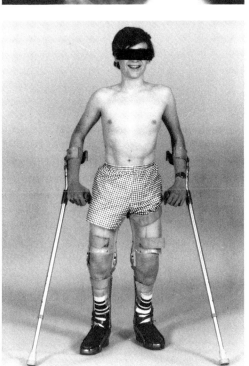

Fig. 9.5. *Top left:* x-ray of a 13-year-old ambulatory male with an 82° scoliosis and a 30° pelvic obliquity. *Top right:* scoliosis was corrected to 22° and the pelvic obliquity reduced to 8° by combined anterior and posterior arthrodesis using anterior Dwyer instrumentation and posterior Luque segmental fixation to the pelvis with the Galveston technique. *Left:* patient remained ambulatory with hip-knee-ankle orthoses and forearm crutches.

conventional posterior techniques which was reduced to only 23 per cent when combined anterior and posterior fusion techniques were used. The first-stage anterior arthrodesis accomplishes two important goals. First, removal of the anterior longitudinal ligament, the annulus, and the intervertebral disc, increases the mobility of the spine and allows greater correction of the scoliosis and equally important, the pelvic obliquity. Second, anterior arthrodesis provides a large area of bone for a solid fusion in the lumbar region where the dysraphic vertebrae provide minimal posterior bone (Fig. 9.5).

Anterior instrumentation, popularised by Dwyer *et al.* (1969) and Zielke and Pellin (1976), provides excellent correction and stabilisation of the spine and is helpful when using Harrington distraction rods at the time of the posterior fusion (Dickens 1979). McMaster (1987) reported correction of up to 50 per cent with anterior fusion with Dwyer implants and an additional 20 per cent of correction with a second-stage fusion with Harrington rods; the pseudoarthrosis rate was less than 6 per cent. The incidence of perioperative complications associated with the Dwyer implant has been low (McMaster and Silber 1975) with only one reported case of retroperitoneal fibrosis affecting renal function. With the refinement of the segmental spinal fixation technique which was developed by Luque and Cardoso (1977), and with the use of the Galveston pelvic fixation technique (Allen and Ferguson 1979), rigid posterior fixation has in most instances obviated the need for anterior instrumentation in the correction of scoliosis in patients with myelomeningocele (Ferguson and Allen 1983, Banta 1990).

The development of the Texas-Scottish-Rite Hospital Spinal Implant System (Danek Medical, Memphis, Tennessee) allows the surgeon to combine the mechanically more rigid Galveston pelvic fixation with two appropriately con-toured rods with a cross linkage to a pair of rods contoured to correct both coronal- and sagittal-plane deformities of the thoracic and lumbar spine. By means of this unique combination, derotation corrective force can be applied to the spine and selective distraction and compression forces can be exerted on the pelvis to correct pelvic obliquity (Fig. 9.6).

Further refinement in segmental fixation techniques led to the Cotrel-Dubousset (Cotrel *et al.* 1988, Denis 1988) and the Texas-Scottish-Rite systems in which multiple pedicle and laminar hooks are applied to each rod, allowing simultaneous compression and distraction and derotation forces to be applied to the spine. Unfortunately the intraoperative time is often increased and the

Fig. 9.6. (*Opposite page.*) *Top:* preoperative anteroposterior and lateral x-rays of a 14-year-old girl with a 76° scoliosis, tethered cord, 65° bilateral hip-flexion contractures, and a subarachnoid cyst at the cervicothoracic junction. She presented with back pain, increasing scoliosis, and progressive loss of walking ability. Hip contractures were released by intertrochanteric extension osteotomy. *Bottom:* following anterior interbody fusion from T9 to S1, the second-stage posterior arthrodesis was performed using the Galveston technique, Texas-Scottish-Rite cross-link system, and Cotrel-Dubousset segmental fixation, reducing the scoliosis to 12° and the pelvic obliquity to 5°. Untethering the conus and decompression of the subarachnoid cyst relieved her pain.

138

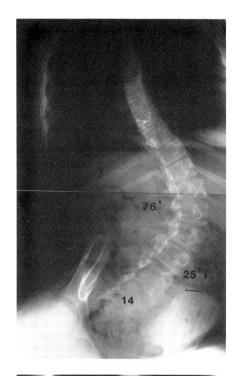
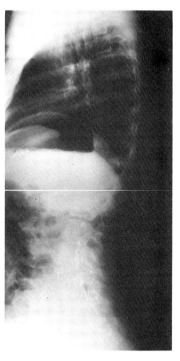
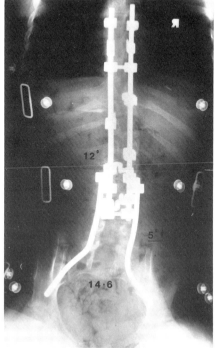
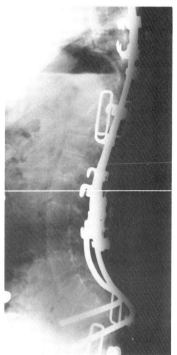

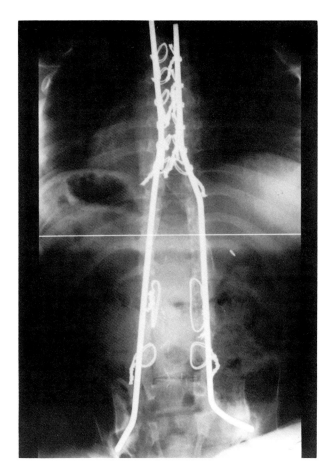

Fig. 9.7. Luque-Galveston technique with pedicular wiring as fixation spanning a dysraphic spine from T8 to the sacrum.

concentrated forces applied to the often osteopenic vertebral elements can result in loss of fixation. This loss of purchase is particularly evident when sacral and iliosacral screws are used for pelvic fixation for children with neuromuscular scoliosis (Johnston *et al.* 1987*a*). Allen and Ferguson (1979) described circumferential wiring of the pedicles in the dysraphic lumbar spine. With this technique, the author has successfully spanned as many as eight vertebral levels without nonunion (Fig. 9.7). Segmental fixation with sublaminar wires with Luque rods remains a valuable surgical technique especially in patients with immature or osteopenic spines. Luque rods cross-linked with the Texas-Scottish-Rite cross-link system afford improved rigidity to the spinal construct to resist torque and bending moments (Johnston *et al.* 1987*b*).

Operative technique
Meticulous preoperative planning is essential to achieve solid arthrodesis with minimal complications. Evaluation and management of the patient's nutritional

status, pulmonary and renal function, will help to avoid skin breakdown, ventilator dependency and urinary tract infection. Sterilisation of the urinary tract is attained as needed with appropriate antibiotics started preoperatively, followed by perioperative prophylactic antibiotics which are routinely given for 72 hours following surgery. The neurological status of the child must be critically examined. A computerised axial tomographic (CAT) scan should be performed to confirm the anatomic position and the function of any shunt system. Magnetic resonance imaging (MRI) of the brainstem is now commonly employed to ascertain whether a Chiari malformation or cord syrinx may be contributing to the scoliosis. Suspected shunt malfunction should be repaired prior to correction of the spinal deformity, whether it be a scoliosis or kyphosis. Theoretically, a correction of a large curve could exert axial traction on the spinal cord and brainstem although the dentate ligaments should dissipate the traction force over a few vertebral levels. Occult lesions such as diastematomyelia should be identified preoperatively and the surgeon should be prepared to remove them, if necessary, at the time of the posterior fusion. I have encountered two instances in which, in the presence of a known diastematomyelia in children with thoracic paraplegia, a first-stage anterior arthrodesis and partial correction of a thoracolumbar scoliosis resulted in lower-extremity pain which was subsequently relieved by resection of the bone spur at the second-stage fusion.

The question of cord tether and cord syrinx will be addressed below (p. 154), but the surgeon must realise the importance of upper motor neuron lesions in spinal dysraphism. Children exhibiting progressive motor loss and spasticity of the lower extremities can be effectively managed with selective anterior rhizotomy, a procedure which is best performed at the second-stage posterior approach when the dural sac is exposed. In practice, many patients exhibit extensive scarring of the conus medullaris and terminal cord; in these cases, distal cordectomy can be performed (McLaughlin *et al.* 1986).

Many children present with lordoscoliosis with the lordosis resulting from fixed hip contractures. In these children, the hip deformity is best corrected either by soft tissue release alone or in combination with a posterior directed wedge extension osteotomy in the intertrochanteric region of the femur. This results in a more accessible approach to the anterior aspect of the lumbar spine and also reduces the stress exerted across the pelvis on the maturing fusion mass. Care must be taken to calculate the appropriate osteotomy angle so that the child retains a functional arc of 90° of motion to sit with and to assure that there will be equal weight distribution on the thighs and pelvis as well as provision for sufficient extension of the hips to allow for self transfers or ambulation. Spinal surgery using rigid internal fixation can be performed once the soft tissues have healed. The convex side of the curve is exposed through a conventional anterior approach through a thoracoabdominal incision centred over the rib adjacent to the uppermost vertebra in the proposed fusion. The excised rib is used as a graft for the intervertebral disc spaces. The incision should extend to the pubic tubercle to allow access to the disc space between the fifth lumbar and first sacral vertebrae; this disc space is included in the fusion in instances in which the fusion is extended to the pelvis to reduce the likelihood of lumbosacral pseudoarthrosis. To promote a solid arthrodesis, meticulous removal of all disc material at the lateral margins of the convexity of the curve is important; this allows complete derotation of the thoracolumbar spine as well as maximum curve correction and close approximation of the subchondral vertebral endplate. Occasionally, because of severe acute angular deformity at the thoracolumbar junction, a wedge resection osteotomy of the vertebral body is indicated, in order to allow for maximum correction of deformity by performing a one- or two-stage osteotomy of the spine. When a two-stage osteotomy is planned, haemostasis following the anterior resection can usually be effected by the use of bone wax supplemented with thrombin-soaked pledgets of gelfoam or the application of Surgicel (Johnson & Johnson Patient Care, New Brunswick, New Jersey) or Avitene (Alcon, Puerto Rico) to the exposed bone surfaces. Maximum haemostasis, however, is usually achieved at the time of closure with repair of the anterior longitudinal ligament which should be preserved by careful subperiosteal dissection during the approach to the intervertebral discs. All disc spaces should be packed with autogenous rib graft supplemented with homologous bone graft. Anterior instrumentation is no longer used by most surgeons but the Dwyer apparatus is still useful in the correction of severe lordotic deformities when it is inserted in the mid-sagittal plane.

The second-stage posterior arthrodesis is normally scheduled seven to 10 days after the anterior fusion. Both stages can be performed at the same time, thereby avoiding a second anaesthetic; however, the complexity of the deformity and the combined operative time generally dictates the two-stage procedure. The posterior approach is performed in stages. First the dysraphic spinal region is exposed, dissecting distally from the last intact laminar arch, preferably through a midline incision, then dissecting laterally beneath the splayed lumbar muscles in a subperiosteal fashion to the level of the transverse processes. The pelvis is then prepared for the internal fixation of choice. Rhizotomy or untethering of the cord can be accomplished at this stage and the exposure of the normal proximal spine is then completed. With a staged exposure, blood loss can be more easily controlled and the entire spine remains exposed for a brief period for fusion and instrumentation.

Unfortunately, with the introduction of segmental fixation techniques, an anterior arthrodesis was thought by some to be unnecessary and this resulted in a higher rate of pseudoarthrosis. Rods $3/16$-inch in diameter provide excellent fixation for young children who weigh less than 30kg but these rods are not capable of withstanding the repetitive stress concentrated at the thoracolumbar and lumbo-sacral junction, the most common sites of pseudoarthrosis. Therefore $1/4$-inch Luque rods or the 7mm Cotrel-Dubousset rods are preferred. A solid arthrodesis is essential to success and a thorough decortication of all exposed bone and an abundant amount of bone graft is crucial to a successful fusion. With strict attention to the intraoperative details and the precautions described above, a pseudoarthrosis rate of under 6 per cent can be anticipated (Mayfield 1981, McMaster 1987, Banta 1990).

It is questionable whether the fusion should always extend to the pelvis. It can be argued that for the exceptional instance, where there is no pelvic obliquity and the lower end of the curve ends at or above the fifth lumbar vertebra, the fusion need not extend to the pelvis; however the lower end of the implant will frequently end at a dysraphic vertebra with inadequate bone to provide adequate fixation. While pedicle screw fixation is possible, there are no published clinical end-result studies of this technique. The fusion area in curves of neuromuscular aetiology should extend from the upper thoracic spine to the pelvis. Because the bone is frequently osteopenic in the non-ambulatory patient, protection of the healing fusion mass with a bivalved polypropylene total contact spinal orthosis is considered an important part of the postoperative management of these children (Broom *et al.* 1989). For this reason, patients should be protected during the first six months following surgery with a bivalved total contact spinal orthosis. Once the orthosis is delivered and the family is instructed in its proper use, the patient is discharged and appropriate radiographs to monitor the rate of fusion are obtained at four-monthly intervals.

Two postoperative complications, though uncommon, may compromise the final result. Residual pelvic obliquity with resultant breakdown of the soft tissue over the prominent ischial tuberosity must be avoided, since most if not all patients will remain seated for extended periods. Lindseth (1978) described a bilateral posterior iliac osteotomy whereby up to 14° of pelvic obliquity can be corrected. The use of a gel cushion seat insert (Akros by Lumex, Bayshore, New York) or an inflated Roho seat cushion (Roho, Belleville, Illinois) in the patient's wheelchair has proven invaluable in preventing skin breakdown over the ischia in children with minor degrees of pelvic obliquity. Residual stiffness of the hip may also compromise an otherwise successful fusion; the radical Girdlestone resection arthroplasty (Castle and Schneider 1978) has helped some patients with totally ankylosed hips to regain an erect sitting posture.

Kyphosis

In children with myelomeningocele, the incidence of kyphosis has been reported to range from 10 or 12 per cent (Hoppenfield 1967, Cotta *et al.* 1971) to as high as 27 per cent (Barson 1970). The kyphotic deformity is most common in the lumbar spine, with the dysraphism often extending from the lower thoracic spine to the sacrum. The higher incidence of kyphosis reported by Barson (1970) is partially explained by the 91 cases of anencephaly included in his study of 601 dysraphic spines. Many affected infants have associated defects including a high level of paraplegia and other congenital defects as noted by Lorber (1972). The extent of the vertebral defect is best appreciated in the lateral radiograph which shows a loss or reversal of the normal lumbar lordosis. The vertebral body is characteristically rounded and the anterior vertebral notch thought to represent the residual intersegmental artery is usually absent (Naik 1972). Defects of formation may result in an apical wedge vertebra directed posteriorly. In this case, the magnitude of the deformity increases rapidly at an average of 8° per year (Banta and Hamada 1976). Defects of segmentation are less common and result in anterior unsegmented bars or kyphoscoliosis. As noted by Hoppenfeld (1967) in a study of 12 necroscopy specimens, the pedicles rotate laterally with the accompanying hypoplastic facets assuming a coronal orientation. The rudimentary laminae at the apex are rotated 180° and at the apex of the deformity are nearly parallel to the subjacent vertebral body.

The pelvis is characteristically hypoplastic with the iliac wings assuming a more sagittal orientation separated by a dysraphic sacrum. When a severe angular kyphotic deformity is present, the lower thoracic spine rapidly assumes a compensatory lordotic contour. The quadratus lumborum and erector spinae muscle groups are displaced laterally and the deformed spine is at risk for progressive collapse by the unopposed action of the psoas muscles and the crura of the diaphragm (Sharrard and Drennan 1972).

As cited by Bunch *et al.* (1977), Euler developed mathematical analyses to quantitate the critical load necessary to cause a column to buckle. With only one end of a column fixed, the weight-bearing ability of a column is reduced by a factor of 16; as the length of the column increases, the load necessary to create deformation of the column rapidly diminishes. Hence kyphotic spinal deformity is not only progressive with growth, but will also recur following surgical treatment unless complete correction is obtained.

Typically, the great vessels span the kyphosis in children born with congenital kyphosis in contradistinction to children with acquired kyphotic deformity when the retroperitoneal structures are progressively drawn back into the prevertebral concavity. Arteriographic studies have shown that the aortic bifurcation is lower than usual, arising between the fourth lumbar vertebra and the sacral brim. The aorta is reduced in calibre, and abnormal segmentation of the lumbar arteries is common (Watt and Park 1978). The kidneys assume an abnormal axis due to the spinal collapse, and the alteration of the renal axis as seen on intravenous pyelograms may be misinterpreted as an apparent horseshoe kidney (Fernbach and Davis 1986).

Surgical treatment
The surgical correction of kyphosis by spinal osteotomy was first performed by Sharrard in 1966, and the early results of apical vertebrectomy with preservation of the dural contents and roots were reported by him in 1968. The neural elements were preserved in the hope that neurological recovery would occur in patients in whom faradic stimulation showed muscle contraction. Clinical experience has shown that much, if not all, of the lower-extremity movement noted in such children is reflexive and is rapidly lost; now the atretic cord is resected, with care

144

TABLE 9.II
Surgical results of treatment for kyphosis in patients with myelomeningocele

	Patients (N)	Deaths N (%)	Pseudoarthrosis N (%)	Loss of correction N (%)
Sharrard and Drennan 1972	13	3 (23.0)	2 (15.3)	15 (at 1 yr)
Lowe and Menelaus 1978	11	2 (18.1)	2 (18.1)	30
Lindseth and Stelzer 1979	12 (Group III)	0	1 (8.3)	24
Heydemann and Gillespie 1985	12	0	1 (8.3)	8

taken to oversew the dura at the level of the normally functioning spinal cord. Care must be taken to ensure that the distal cord remains free with open communication of the central canal to the subdural space to avoid acute elevation of intracranial pressure, which can be fatal (Winston *et al.* 1977).

Sharrard and Drannan (1972) described a technique of osteotomy and excision of the cephalad limb of the kyphosis in older children. Total correction of the deformity and spinal fixation, however, remained a problem: of 18 cases undergoing surgery at an average age of seven years a 33° improvement in deformity was achieved, but an average of 15° of recurrent deformity was evident in the first two years after surgery. There were two instances of pseudoarthrosis and three deaths. The surgical correction of this deformity is a formidable challenge to the surgeon and many fixation devices have been recommended, including staples and crossed pins (Sharrard and Drennan 1972), Kirschner wires (Lowe and Menelaus 1978), Harrington rods (Leatherman and Dickson 1978), ankle orthosis (AO) plates (Hellinger 1981), anterior plates with shackles (Hall and Poitras 1977), and Dwyer cables and screws (McMaster 1988). Segmental fixation with Luque rods currently affords the best stabilisation for the older child undergoing kyphectomy with apical vertebral resection and arthrodesis.

Lindseth and Stelzer (1979) compared three techniques of vertebral excision for kyphosis: apical wedge resection, apical vertebral body resection plus excision of one or more adjacent vertebrae, and resection of the proximal lordotic segment including a partial resection of the apical vertebra. By resecting the lordotic segment in combination with a short fusion, 12 children achieved growth with only a 24 per cent loss of correction; this compares favourably with results reported in other series (Table 9.II).

The dilemma that confronts the surgeon in attempting to achieve total correction is the fine line between fusing a minimum number of segments to allow for spinal growth and making the fusion long enough to avoid loss of correction with further growth. The so-called 'Luque Trolley' technique of segmental spinal instrumentation, without arthrodesis to allow for growth of the immature spine, has recently been used in a few selected patients with variable results (Fig. 9.8). This is an intriguing concept in the young child requiring lumbar kyphectomy and fusion plus support of the thoracic spine to allow further growth. Zembo *et al.* (1990)

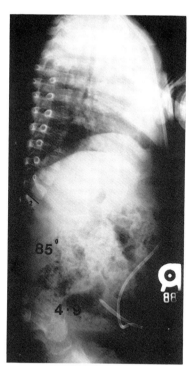

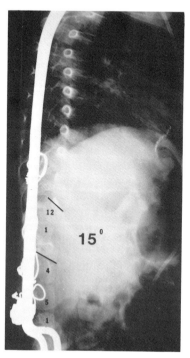

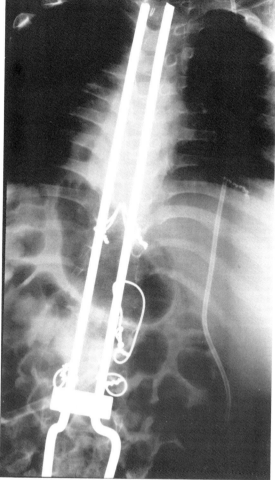

Fig. 9.8. *Left:* lateral x-ray of a child aged 4.9 years with an 85° mid-lumbar kyphosis and compromised skin over the apex of the kyphosis. *Below left and right:* postoperative x-rays following resection of the distal spinal cord, decancellation of the second lumbar and resection of the third lumbar vertebra. Arthrodesis was limited to the lumbar region and sublaminar Merselene tapes were used to secure the Luque rods to the thoracic spine without arthrodesis to allow for longitudinal growth.

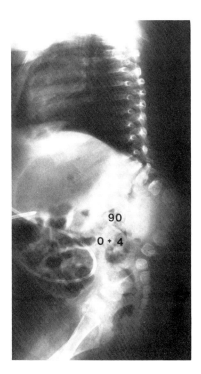

Fig. 9.9. Lateral x-rays of (*top*) four-month-old child with a 90° mid-lumbar kyphosis, corrected to 34° (*bottom left*) by an apical kyphectomy and (*bottom right*) maintained for three years with a custom spinal orthosis with recurrent deformity of 15°. Extension of the fusion will be required at puberty.

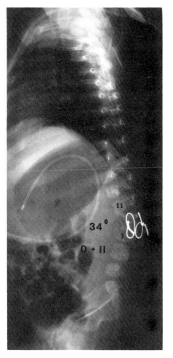

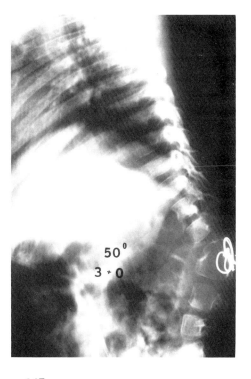

147

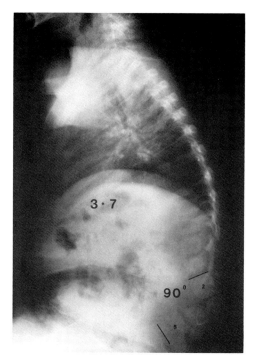
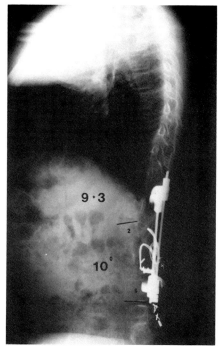

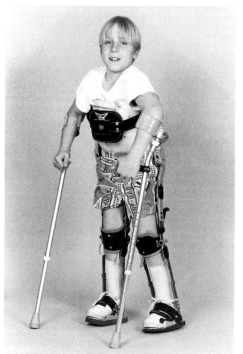

Fig. 9.10. *Above left:* lateral x-ray of a three-year-old with a congenital kyphosis from L2 to L5. *Above right:* a posterior kyphectomy and limited posterior fusion provided correction to 11° which has been maintained for six years. *Left:* patient has a spinal orthosis and is walking in the community with a Parawalker, but he may require extension of the fusion at skeletal maturity.

148

reported success in four cases with myelodysplasia with an average growth of 1cm per year for three years. Mardjetko *et al.* (1990), however, reported failure in nine cases of young children with unspecified spinal deformity. Alternatively, neonatal apical kyphectomy and fusion performed at the time of closure with preservation of remaining lumbar vertebrae, followed by use of an external spinal orthosis, allows the child to attain increased sitting height prior to extending the fusion from the upper thoracic spine to the pelvis (Fig. 9.9). A recent report of this technique (Crawford 1990) suggests that correction can be maintained for up to four years.

The optimum age for surgery in the postnatal period is not well defined. Sharrard and Drennan (1972) noted that children who survived to age three continued to thrive; in two other reported series (Hall and Poitras 1977, Lindseth and Stelzer 1979), the earliest age at which surgery was undertaken was between three and four years (Fig. 9.10). Technically the procedure is easier in the older child with greater bone size (Channon and Jenkins 1981); with growth, however, the compensatory lower thoracic lordosis presents obstacles to correction and fixation as well as progressive impairment of pulmonary function.

The decision for kyphectomy with vertebral resection and arthrodesis in the older child must be made by the parents on the basis of proper information, since the reported morbidity is significant and there is a real risk of death (Table 9.II). The same preoperative guidelines described in the scoliosis section apply here, with the additional caveat that specific attention must be given to the patient's nutritional status. With the advent of improved spinal implants, there is always a risk of infection and late skin breakdown because of inadequate soft-tissue coverage of prominent hardware. The incidence of skin breakdown in patients with thoracic level paralysis and the cost of care in patients with such lesions is greater than previously recognised (Harris and Banta 1990).

Two-stage anterior and posterior arthrodesis of the spine for congenital kyphosis has a very limited role. For rigid congenital curves, the two-stage anterior strut graft with interbody fusion in combination with a conventional posterior arthrodesis (Brown 1978) is indicated only as a salvage procedure when additional anterior fusion and strut graft is required to stabilise recurrent deformity following pseudoarthrosis or in cases of wound infection when the posterior fixation must be removed. On the other hand, in children with progressive collapsing paralytic or developmental kyphosis, the deformity can be safely corrected with less morbidity by a two-stage procedure. In this case, the optimal candidate for a two-stage procedure must demonstrate a 50 per cent correction of the deformity on a hyperextension radiograph without evidence of rigid angulation of the apical vertebra (Fig. 9.11).

Operative technique
The newborn child with congenital kyphosis frequently presents problems for the neurosurgeon attempting adequate wound closure following repair of the neural defect. Resection of the dysplastic neural elements with resection of the apical

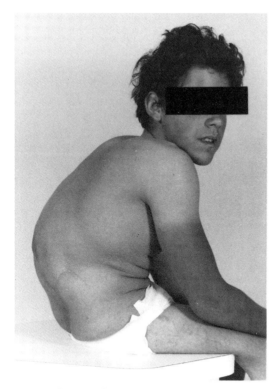
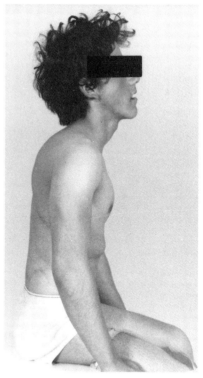

Fig. 9.11. Preoperative and postoperative photographs illustrating correction of paralytic kyphosis by a two-stage anterior fusion and posterior fusion using ¼-inch rods and the Luque-Galveston technique.

vertebrae and posterior elements allows soft-tissue mobilisation and closure. Decancellation of the vertebral bodies allows them to be progressively flattened and pushed forward into a horizontal plane and maintained with a posterior longitudinal suture acting as a tension band (Lindseth 1990). This recently recommended technique holds promise because theoretically it allows for some further spinal growth from the undisturbed vertebral endplates.

Relaxing chevron-shaped flank incisions to mobilise soft tissue to the posterior midline (Sharrard 1968) is to be avoided since the resulting scars can interfere with subsequent definitive spinal fusion by restricting adequate mobilisation of soft tissue necessary for wound closure over the spinal implant.

The surgical technique for kyphectomy with vertebral resection and arthrodesis uses a vertical midline incision, preferably following the incisional scar of previous repair, although straight midline incisions have been reported without subsequent skin problems (Heydemann and Gillespie 1987). The scarred dura and atrophic neural elements at the apex of the kyphosis are incised transversely and dissection is carried proximally to the level of the functional cord which corresponds approximately to the level of the last intact laminar arch. Resection of the most caudal intact laminar arch facilitates the exposure of the normal dura at the site of the proximal repair of the dural sac. Great care must be taken to perform meticulous coagulation with electric cautery of the segmental vessels at the level of each foramen. Use of bone wax is helpful in controlling brisk venous bleeding which is occasionally encountered from the vertebral bodies. Distal dissection of the scarred dura and posterior longitudinal ligament is necessary to expose the intervertebral discs for subsequent fusion. The sacral segment of the cord and dura need not be resected routinely as the vascular supply in this region is abundant and further excessive blood loss can be avoided. Careful anterior dissection around the apical vertebral body allows the anterior longitudinal ligament and soft tissue to be safely retracted. The bone of the resected proximal limb of the kyphos is used as bone graft and a large amount of graft is placed anterior to the site of the vertebrectomy (Fig. 9.12).

Segmental instrumentation with $^3/_{16}$-inch Luque rods and the Galveston technique for pelvic anchoring of the implant is my preferred method of fixation. The size of the transverse bar of the ilium can be accurately determined preoperatively with a CAT scan to determine if the intramedullary space of the ilium at that level will accommodate the fixation. An alternative method of fixation, with a step cut contoured rod introduced into the sacrum through the first sacral foramen, can be used if the iliac bone stock is inadequate (Fackler et al. 1990).

Following osteotomy, the deformity is reduced to restore a flat spinal contour and segmental wires are tightened around the rods and intact lamina in the lower thoracic spine. Additional wires are passed around the intact pedicles adjacent to the osteotomy site and are tightened to create a posterior tension band at the level of the osteotomy. Resection of the previously exposed intervertebral discs is easily accomplished; packing the resultant cavities with bone graft completes the lumbar fusion. The remaining exposed cortical bone is decorticated and the operation is completed by making a two-layer closure over a retained suction drainage.

Potential intraoperative complications incude acute elevation of the intra-cranial pressure secondary to inadvertent constriction of the transected end of the spinal cord (Winston et al. 1977), excessive haemorrhage, intraoperative air embolism (Banta 1990), and acute hypotension at the time of correction of the kyphosis as the segmental instrumentation is being secured. The latter problem is probably related to relative distraction of the vena cava as the spinal column is relatively elongated, resulting in decreased venous return. This emphasises that sufficient bone must be resected to shorten the spinal column to allow complete correction of the deformity withut undue tension on the retroperitoneal structures. Immobilisation with a bivalved total contact TLSO is necessary to protect the spinal construct as the fusion matures (Banta 1990).

Using Luque segmental fixation, Heydemann and Gillespie (1987) reported correction in 12 children with the mean kyphosis decreasing from 124° to 33°. McMaster (1988) reported on 10 children in whom a mean correction from 131° to

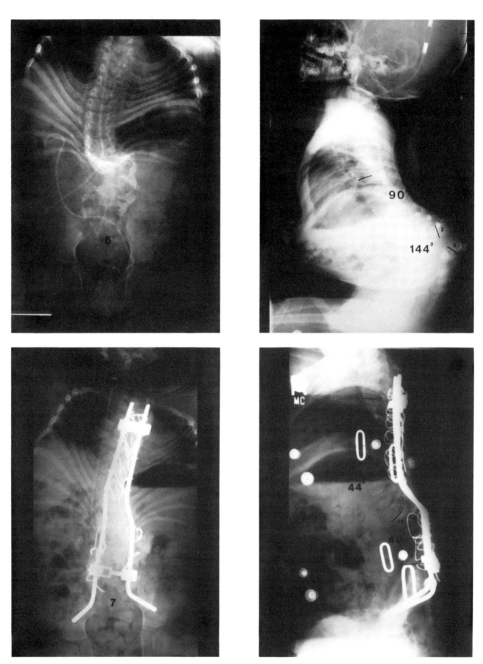

Fig. 9.12. *Top:* preoperative anteroposterior and lateral x-rays of a six-year-old male with a 144° kyphosis and a 90° lower thoracic lordosis with an 80° scoliosis at the thoracolumbar junction. *Bottom left:* postoperative x-ray showing correction of coronal deformity with a compensated spine. *Bottom right:* postoperative lateral x-ray demonstrates correction of the kyphosis to 40° by cordectomy and apical vertebral resection from T12 to L3. The thoracic hyperlordosis has been corrected to 44°.

152

44° was obtained using Dwyer cables and compression plates; however, there were four cases of instrument failure. Using this technique in 16 children, Banta (1990) obtained an average correction of 69 per cent with the mean deformity of 113° being reduced to 35°.

The occurrence of pseudoarthrosis following posterior vertebrectomy and osteotomy and fusion is usually a result of inadequate bone graft anterior to the osteotomy site or an incomplete interbody fusion from the initial posterior approach. In these instances, salvage can be obtained by means of an anterior approach with disc excision, interbody grafting, and placement of an anterior strut graft of tibial autograft. The tibia is preferable to the fibula for grafting because the latter is extremely atrophic in patients with midthoracic paraplegia. Resection of the anterior two thirds of the tibial diaphysis with careful repair of the periosteal sleeve usually results in adequate regeneration of the donor site at the tibial diaphysis. The tibial graft is mortised into the anterolateral aspect of the vertebral bodies at either end of the concave deformity and additional bone is packed into the remaining void between the strut and the vertebral bodies.

The unresolved question concerning the treatment of kyphosis in myelo-meningocele is that of appropriate patient selection. Many affected children present with a high level of paralysis, mental retardation and a marginal nutritional status. In these high-risk patients, the development of improved surgical techniques and spinal implants places the surgeon in the unenviable position of having to recommend to the parents a surgical decision that will have a major impact on the child's future life. These operations should be performed in hospitals where an experienced surgical team has a full complement of technical support personnel and adequate medical facilities to care for the problems which can occur with reconstructive spinal surgery of this magnitude.

The ultimate decision rests with the surgeon. And in the words of Eckstein and Vora (1972): 'This type of operation is only performed in exceptional circumstances and . . . one's endeavor to keep a patient alive may be somewhat limited by sound judgement'.

Future developments

Improvement in the care of the child with myelomeningocele will ultimately depend upon a better understanding of the neurological lesion. The presence of an upper motor neuron lesion in up to 50 per cent of patients (Stark and Baker 1967, Stark and Drummond 1973) is well recognised but sometimes overlooked in a busy clinical service where reconstructive surgical procedures are being proposed for recurrent lower-limb deformities. The natural history of scoliosis in myelodysplasia is well documented in studies of older children (Piggott 1980, Becker and Banta 1986) that were conducted before the availability of today's imaging techniques. The clinical significance of brainstem compression by the Chiari malformation, syrinx formation, and scarring and nerve root adherence at the site of repair and their relationship to scoliosis requires collaborative long-term clinical study by neurosurgeons and orthopaedic surgeons (Rothwell *et al.* 1987). MRI has been invaluable in the identification of a low-lying conus and in identifying cord tethers. The specificity, however, is less in differentiating a thickened filum and intradural scar in conjunction with a repaired myelomeningocele (Moufarrij *et al.* 1989). To 'detether' a spinal cord is not an innocuous procedure, as further neurological loss can occur (Schmidt and Yngve 1988). Park *et al.* (1985) reported improvement in eight of 12 patients undergoing obex plugging procedures for adolescents with progressive spasticity motor weakness and scoliosis. There was a reduction in spasticity with increased upper-extremity motor strength but no improvement in the magnitude of the scoliosis. Curves measuring less than 30° may show improvement following detethering, at least in the short term, but large curves do not. These results, however, are preliminary and patients undergoing such procedures must be monitored closely until they reach skeletal maturity (Dias and Hughes 1989).

There has been much controversy about the possible cause-and-effect relationship between hip dislocation and scoliosis. The indications for surgery of the hip and spine are now becoming clearer through collaborative end-result study and consensus conferences (Beaty and Canale 1990). Increased recognition of the incidence and natural history of scoliosis in patients with myelomeningocele will allow physicians and parents to plan the major procedures their children will require as they attain skeletal maturity.

REFERENCES

Allen, B.L., Jr., Ferguson, R.L. (1979) 'The operative treatment of myelomeningocele spinal deformity.' *Orthopedic Clinics of North America*, **10**, 845–862.
Banta, J.V. (1990) 'Combined anterior and posterior fusion for spinal deformity in myelomeningocele.' *Spine*, **15**, 946–952.
—— Hamada, J.S. (1976) 'Natural history of the kyphotic deformity in myelomeningocele.' (Abstract.) *Journal of Bone and Joint Surgery*, **58A**, 279.
—— Park, S.M. (1983) 'Improvement in pulmonary function in patients having combined anterior and posterior spine fusion for myelomeningocele scoliosis.' *Spine*, **8**, 765–770.
—— Lin, R., Peterson, M., Dagenais, T. (1990) 'Team approach in the care of the child with myelomeningocele.' *Journal of Prosthetics and Orthotics*, **15**, 263–273.
Barden, G.A., Meyer, L.C., Stelling, F.H. (1975) 'Myelodysplastics—fate of those followed for twenty years or more.' *Journal of Bone and Joint Surgery*, **57A**, 643–647.
Barson, A.J. (1970) 'Spina bifida: the significance of the level and extent of the defect to the morphogenesis.' *Developmental Medicine and Child Neurology*, **12**, 129–144.
Beaty, J.H., Canale, S.T. (1990) 'Current concepts review. Orthopaedic aspects of myelomeningocele.' *Journal of Bone and Joint Surgery*, **72A**, 626–630.
Becker, G.J., Banta, J.V. (1986) 'The natural history of scoliosis in myelomeningocele.' *Orthopaedic Transactions*, **10**, 18.
Broom, M.J., Banta, J.V., Renshaw, T.S. (1989) 'Spinal fusion augmented by Luque-rod segmental instrumentation for neuromuscular scoliosis.' *Journal of Bone and Joint Surgery*, **71A**, 32–44.
Brown, H.P. (1978) 'Management of spinal deformity in myelomeningocele.' *Orthopedic Clinics of North America*, **9**, 391–402.
Bunch, W.H., Smith, D., Hakala, M. (1977) 'Kyphosis in the paralytic spine.' *Clinical Orthopaedics and Related Research*, **128**, 107–112.

Castle, M.E., Schneider, C. (1978) 'Proximal femoral resection-interposition arthroplasty.' *Journal of Bone and Joint Surgery*, **60A**, 1051–1054.

Channon, G.M., Jenkins, D.H.R. (1981) 'Aggressive surgical treatment of secondary spinal deformity in spina bifida children. Is it worthwhile?' *Zeitschrift für Kinderchirurgie*, **34**, 394–398.

Cotrel, Y., Dubousset, J., Guillaumat, M. (1988) 'New universal instrumentation in spinal surgery.' *Clinical Orthopaedics and Related Research*, **227**, 10–23.

Cotta, V.H., Parsch, K., Schulitz, K.P. (1971) 'Die Behandlung der Lumbalkyphose bei Spina Bifida Cystica.' *Zeitschrift für Orthopädie und ihre Grenzgebiete*, **108**, 567–574.

Crawford, A.H. (1990) 'Effects of neonatal kyphectomy on preventing development of deformity in myelomeningoceles.' *57th Annual Meeting of the American Academy of Orthopaedic Surgeons, Paper No. 268*. New Orleans, Louisiana, February 10, 1990.

Denis, F. (1988) 'Cotrel-Dubousset instrumentation in the treatment of idiopathic scoliosis.' *Orthopedic Clinics of North America*, **19**, 291–311.

Dias, L., Hughes, W.A. (1989) 'Scoliosis in myelomeningocele: the role of tethered cord and hydromyelia.' *Annual meeting of the Pediatric Orthopaedic Society of North America, Paper No. 76*. Hilton Head, South Carolina, May 17–May 20, 1989.

Dickens, D.R.V. (1979) 'The surgery of scoliosis and spina bifida.' (Abstract.) *Journal of Bone and Joint Surgery*, **61B**, 386.

Drummond, D., Breed, A.L., Narechania, R. (1985) 'Relationship of spine deformity and pelvic obliquity on sitting pressure distributions and decubitus ulceration.' *Journal of Pediatric Orthopaedics*, **5**, 396–402.

Duckworth, T., Sharrard, W.J., Lister, J. (1968) 'Hemimyelocele.' *Developmental Medicine and Child Neurology*, **10** (Suppl. 16), 69–75.

Duval-Beaupère, G., Kaci, M., Lougovoy, J., Caponi, M.F., Touzeau, C. (1987) 'Growth of trunk and legs of children with myelomeningocele.' *Developmental Medicine and Child Neurology*, **29**, 225–231.

Dwyer, A.F., Newton, N.C., Sherwood, A. (1969) 'An anterior approach to scoliosis. A preliminary report.' *Clinical Orthopaedics and Related Research*, **62**, 192–202.

Eckstein, N.B., Vora, R.M. (1972) 'Spinal osteotomy for severe kyphosis in children with myelomeningocele.' *Journal of Bone and Joint Surgery*, **54B**, 328–333.

Fackler, C.D., Warner, W.C., Woude, L.V. (1990) 'A comparison of two instrumentation techniques in the treatment of lumbar kyphosis in myelodysplasia.' *57th Annual Meeting of the American Academy of Orthopaedic Surgeons, Paper No. 269*. New Orleans, Louisiana, February 10, 1990.

Ferguson, R.L., Allen, B.L., Jr. (1983) 'Staged correction of neuromuscular scoliosis.' *Journal of Pediatric Orthopaedics*, **3**, 555–562.

Fernbach, S.K., Davis, T.M. (1986) 'The abnormal renal axis in children with spina bifida and gibbus deformity—the pseudohorseshoe kidney.' *Journal of Urology*, **136**, 1258–1260.

Griffiths, J.C., Taylor, A.G. (1980) 'The production of spinal jackets for children with spina bifida.' *Journal of Medical Engineering and Technology*, **4**, 10–23.

Hall, J.E., Poitras, B. (1977) 'The management of kyphosis in patients with myelomeningocele.' *Clinical Orthopaedics and Related Research*, **128**, 33–40.

Hall, P., Lindseth, R., Campbell, R., Kalsbeck, J.E., Desousa, A. (1979) 'Scoliosis and hydrocephalus in myelocele patients. The effects of ventricular shunting.' *Journal of Neurosurgery*, **50**, 174–178.

Harris, M.B., Banta, J.V. (1990) 'Cost of skin care in the myelomeningocele population.' *Journal of Pediatric Orthopaedics*, **10**, 355–361.

Hellinger, J. (1981) 'Die Resektionskolumnotomie bei der myelodysplastischen Lumbalkyphose.' *Pädiatrie und Grenzgebiete*, **20**, 313–322.

Heydemann, J.S., Gillespie, R. (1987) 'Management of myelomeningocele kyphosis in the older child by kyphectomy and segmental spinal instrumentation.' *Spine*, **12**, 37–41.

Hoppenfeld, S. (1967) 'Congenital kyphosis in myelomeningocele.' *Journal of Bone and Joint Surgery*, **49B**, 276–280.

Jaivin, J.S., Banta, J.V., Milanese, A., Hight, D.W., Alexander, F. (1991) 'Perioperative J-tube feeding in reconstructive spinal surgery.' *Developmental Medicine and Child Neurology*, **33**, 225–231.

Johnston, C.E., II, Ashman, R.B., Corin, J.D. (1987*a*) 'Mechanical effects of crosslinking rods in Cotrel-Dubousset instrumentation.' (Abstract.) *Orthopaedic Transactions*, **11**, 96–97.

155

—— —— Sherman, M.C., Eberle, C.F., Herndon, W.A., Sullivan, J.A., King, A.G.S., Burke, S.W. (1987b) 'Mechanical consequences of rod contouring and residual scoliosis in sublaminar segmental instrumentation.' *Journal of Orthopaedic Research*, **5**, 206–216.

Kahanovitz, N., Duncan, J.W. (1981) 'The role of scoliosis and pelvic obliquity on functional disability in myelomeningocele.' *Spine*, **6**, 494–497.

Leatherman, K.D., Dickson, R.A. (1978) 'Congenital kyphosis in myelomeningocele. Vertebral body resection and posterior spine fusion.' *Spine*, **3**, 222–226.

Lendon, R.G., Lendon, M., Wynne-Davies, R. (1981) 'Congenital vertebral anomalies and the possible aetiological relationship with spina bifida.' *Zeitschrift für Kinderchirurgie*, **34**, 390–395.

Lindseth, R.E. (1978) 'Posterior iliac osteotomy for fixed pelvic obliquity.' *Journal of Bone and Joint Surgery*, **60A**, 17–22.

—— Stelzer, L., Jr. (1979) 'Vertebral excision for kyphosis in children with myelomeningocele.' *Journal of Bone and Joint Surgery*, **61A**, 699–704.

—— (1990) *Personal Communication*.

Lorber, J. (1972) 'Spina bifida cystica. Results of treatment of 270 consecutive cases with criteria for selection for the future.' *Archives of Disease in Childhood*, **47**, 854–873.

Lowe, G.P., Menelaus, M.B. (1978) 'The surgical management of kyphosis in older children with myelomeningocle.' *Journal of Bone and Joint Surgery*, **60B**, 40–45.

Luque, E.R., Cardoso, A. (1977) 'Segmental correction of scoliosis with rigid internal fixation.' *Orthopaedic Transactions*, **1**, 136–137.

Maguire, C.D., Winter, R.B., Mayfield, J.K., Erickson, D.L. (1982) 'Hemimyelodysplasia: a report of 10 cases.' *Journal of Pediatric Orthopaedics*, **2**, 9–14.

Mardjetko, S.M., Hammerberg, K.W., Lubicky, J.P. (1990) 'The Luque trolley revisited: review of nine cases requiring revision.' *Paper presented at the 25th Annual Meeting of the Scoliosis Research Society*. Honolulu, September 1990.

Marsh, N., Gould, A.P., Clutton, H.H., Parker, R.W. (1885) 'Report of a committee of the society nominated Nov. 10, 1882, to investigate spina bifida and its treatment by the injection of Dr Morton's iodoglycerine solution.' *Transactions of the Clinical Society of London*, **18**, 339–434.

Mayfield, J.K. (1981) 'Severe spine deformity in myelodysplasia and sacral agenesis. An aggressive surgical approach.' *Spine*, **6**, 498–509.

Mazur, J., Menelaus, M.B., Dickens, D.R.V., Doig, W.G. (1986) 'Efficacy of surgical management for scoliosis in myelomeningocele: correction of deformity and alteration of functional status.' *Journal of Pediatric Orthopaedics*, **6**, 568–575.

McLaughlin, T.P., Banta, J.V., Gahm, N.H., Raycroft, J.F. (1986) 'Intraspinal rhizotomy and distal cordectomy in patients with meylomeningocele.' *Journal of Bone and Joint Surgery*, **68A**, 88–94.

McMaster, M.J. (1987) 'Anterior and posterior instrumentation and fusion of thoracolumbar scoliosis due to myelomeningocele.' *Journal of Bone and Joint Surgery*, **69B**, 20–25.

—— (1988) 'The long-term results of kyphectomy and spinal stabilization in children with myelomeningocele.' *Spine*, **13**, 417–424.

McMaster, W.C., Silber, I. (1975) 'An urological complication of Dwyer instrumentation. Case report.' *Journal of Bone and Joint Surgery*, **57A**, 710–711.

Menelaus, M.B. (1976) 'Orthopaedic management of children with myelomeningocele: a plea for realistic goals.' *Developmental Medicine and Child Neurology*, **18** (Suppl. 37), 3–11.

Moufarrij, N.A., Palmer, J.M., Hahn, J.F., Weinstein, M.A. (1989) 'Correlation between magnetic resonance imaging and surgical findings in the tethered spinal cord.' *Neurosurgery*, **25**, 341–346.

Naik, D.R. (1972) 'A sign of spina bifida cystica on lateral radiographs of the spine.' *Clinical Radiology*, **23**, 193–195.

Osebold, W.R., Mayfield, J.K., Winter, R.B., Moe, J.H. (1982) 'Surgical treatment of paralytic scoliosis associated with myelomeningocle.' *Journal of Bone and Joint Surgery*, **64A**, 841–856.

Park, T.S., Cail, W.S., Maggio, W.M., Mitchell, D.C. (1985) 'Progressive spasticity and scoliosis in children with myelomeningocele. Radiological investigation and surgical treatment.' *Journal of Neurosurgery*, **62**, 367–375.

Piggott, H. (1980) 'The natural history of scoliosis in myelodysplasia.' *Journal of Bone and Joint Surgery*, **62B**, 54–58.

Raycroft, J.F., Curtis, B.H. (1972) 'Spinal curvature in myelomeningocele: natural history and etiology.' *American Academy of Orthopaedic Surgeons Symposium on Myelomeningocele*. Saint

Louis: C.V. Mosby. pp. 186–201.

Rothwell, C.I., Forbes, W. St C., Gupta, S.C. (1987) 'Computed tomographic myelography in the investigation of childhood scoliosis and spinal dysraphism.' *British Journal of Radiology*, **60**, 1197–1204.

Samuelsson, L., Bergström, K., Thoumas, K-A., Hemmingsson, A., Wallensten, R. (1987) 'MR imaging of syringohydromelia and Chiari malformations in meyolemingocele patients with scoliosis.' *American Journal of Neuroradiology*, **8**, 539–546.

—— Eklöf, O. (1988) 'Scoliosis in myelomeningocele.' *Acta Orthopaedica Scandinavica*, **59**, 122–127.

Schmidt, F., Yngve, D. (1988) 'Tethered cord release, risks and benefits.' (Abstract.) *Orthopaedic Transactions*, **12**, 571.

Sharrard, W.J.W. (1968) 'Spinal osteotomy for congenital kyphosis in myelomeningocele.' *Journal of Bone and Joint Surgery*, **50B**, 466–471.

—— Drennan, J.C. (1972) 'Osteotomy—excision of the spine for lumbar kyphosis in older children with myelomeningocele.' *Journal of Bone and Joint Surgery*, **54B**, 50–60.

Shurtleff, D.B., Goiney, R., Gordon, L.H., Livermore, N. (1976) 'Myelodysplasia: the natural history of kyphosis and scoliosis: a preliminary report.' *Developmental Medicine and Child Neurology* (Suppl. 37), 126–133.

Sriram, K., Bobechko, W.P., Hall, J.E. (1972) 'Surgical management of spinal deformities in spina bifida.' *Journal of Bone and Joint Surgery*, **54B**, 666–676.

Stark, G.D., Baker, G.C.W. (1967) 'The neurological involvement of the lower limbs in myelomeningocele.' *Developmental Medicine and Child Neurology*, **9**, 732–744.

—— Drummond, M. (1973) 'Results of selective early operation in myelomeningocele.' *Archives of Disease in Childhood*, **48**, 676–683.

Ward, W.T., Wenger, D.R., Roach, J.W. (1989) 'Surgical correction of myelomeningocele scoliosis: a critical appraisal of various spinal instrumentation systems.' *Journal of Pediatric Orthopaedics*, **9**, 262–268.

Watt, I., Park, W.M. (1978) 'The abdominal aorta in spina bifida cystica.' *Clinical Radiology*, **29**, 63–68.

Winston, K., Hall, J., Johnson, D., Micheli, L. (1977) 'Acute elevation of intracranial pressure following transection of non-functional spinal cord.' *Clinical Orthopaedics and Related Research*, **128**, 41–44.

Winter, R.B. (1983) *Congenital Deformities of the Spine*. New York: Thieme-Stratton.

Wynne-Davies, R. (1977) 'Scoliosis, vertebral anomalies and spina bifida.' *Birth Defects Original Article Series*, **XIII**, 75–83.

Zembo, M.M., King, A.G., Burke, S.W. (1990) 'Successful use of the Luque trolley to preserve trunk growth in children with paralytic spiral deformity.' *Paper presented at the 25th Annual Meeting of the Scoliosis Research Society*. Honolulu, September 1990.

Zielke, K., Pellin, B. (1976) 'Neue instrumente und implante zur Ergänzung des Harrington systems.' *Zeitschrift für Orthopädie und Ihre Grenzgebiete*, **114**, 534–537.

157

10
THE EFFECTS OF SPINA BIFIDA AND HYDROCEPHALUS UPON LEARNING AND BEHAVIOUR

Brian Tew

The psychological study of children with spina bifida and hydrocephalus has a shorter history than that of many other childhood disabilities. It is only 30 years since Doran and Guthkelch (1961) first reported the results of intelligence tests given to a series of spina bifida children.

Since then the problems presented by children with neural tube defects (NTDs) have been studied mainly by educational and clinical psychologists, but also by teachers and doctors and very recently by neuropsychologists. Doctors and teachers have also used psychological tests. Information from these different sources has established a solid body of knowledge, although controversy still exists in a number of areas. One of the reasons for the conflicting findings is that the treatment of the child with myelomeningocele and hydrocephalus is always evolving, so that findings obtained under a particular regimen may have only a modest relationship with the findings from present practice.

The following review highlights several areas where psychologists have made a distinctive contribution to the understanding of spina bifida and hydrocephalus.

Changes in surgical policy and its effect upon intelligence
Measuring the intelligence of spina bifida children can provide information about likely academic potential and thus appropriate schooling. A more detailed analysis of scores, along with other psychometric data, often indicates particular cognitive impairment requiring remediation or strengs which can be built upon in a treatment programme. Knowledge of the extent of intellectual retardation was implicit in establishing a selective treatment policy, even though the results of psychological assessment tend to come some years after changes in management when there is a wider repertoire of behaviour to assess.

In Britain the treatment of spina bifida children falls into three fairly distinct phases, with some evidence of variation in intellectual outcome. The first phase of 'conservative care' ended in the early 1960s. Relatively few children received immediate surgery, and those who survived mostly escaped hydrocephalus. This was the case in the South Wales studies of Laurence and Tew (1967, 1971), which recorded a survival rate of less than 10 per cent up to the children's 11th birthday. The overall IQ of the 36 cases of myelomeningocele was in the low average range of

158

ability, 89 (SD 17), but with a spread of scores of around 100 IQ points.

The decade from about 1963 saw the adoption of unselective surgical treatment virtually all over Britain, leading to a huge increase in survival rates. A comparison of children treated under the 'conservative' and 'aggressive' regimens revealed a significant decline (p<0.01) in the IQs of children with myelomeningocele, and a significant increase in the extent of their physical disability (p<0.02) (Laurence 1974). The mean IQ of children with myelomeningocele was found to be 77 (SD 22), indicating that a substantial proportion of children had learning difficulties requiring special educational provision.

The current trend of selective surgery resulted largely from Lorber's (1971) review of the consequences of aggressive treatment policies. Studies from several centres (Guiney and MacCarthy 1981, Lorber and Salfield 1981, Sklayne 1982) show that the proportion of severely physically disabled children has decreased with the current policy: fewer were confined to wheelchairs or had epilepsy and more were reliably continent, but a substantial minority still had significant disability. The South Wales study (Tew *et al.* 1985; Tew 1988, 1989*a,b*) was a total population survey which dealt with the psychological consequences of a benevolent but selective treatment policy. It included 18 children who had been denied immediate care because of adverse physical criteria, but who were treated later when their survival was obvious, and 59 who had had prompt treatment. Those treated early had a full-scale IQ of 88 (SD 21.5): only 1 point different from the conservatively treated sample (Laurence and Tew 1971) described earlier, but 8 IQ points higher than the average of the unselectively treated sample born in the 1960s. The difference between IQs was not significant. The mean IQ of spina bifida children given active treatment remains about 1SD below the population mean.

Children denied immediate care had a significantly lower (p<0.02) full-scale IQ of 72 (SD 22) than those promptly treated. The scores of those denied immediate care show that a postponement of treatment does not necessarily have a disastrous effect upon intelligence. Three had IQs above 100 and two attended ordinary school, suggesting that neonatal characteristics do not always correlate well with some aspects of later development. On the other hand, unforeseen complications can invalidate initial optimism, and three promptly treated children had IQs of 30 due to later intracranial infection.

Verbal-performance differences in intelligence
Since the 1950s, studies of children with brain injury have emphasised that cognitive abilities may be differentially impaired, with visuoperceptual, spatial and motor skills being more affected than verbal abilities (Strauss and Lehtinen 1947). Many psychologists have looked for similar difficulties on the Wechsler scales, which are particularly suitable for such an analysis, even though Rutter *et al.* (1970) argued that verbal-performance discrepancies are of little use in diagnosing brain damage.

One of the first studies to report significant differences between verbal and

159

performance quotients among spina bifida and hydrocephalic children was by Badell-Ribera *et al.* (1966), who considered this to be a 'characteristic sign of brain damage', because there were no marked differences between quotients in those with spina bifida only. Lonton's study (1977) showed that verbal ability was between 13 and 20 points greater than performance intelligence, regardless of the site of the lesion. A particularly unusual finding was that performance IQ was 22 points lower among children with meningocele who rarely experience brain involvement. The second study by Lonton (1979) found that ventricular dilatation had a very significant effect ($p < 0.001$) on performance intelligence only. In France, Billard *et al.* (1986) found that the majority of their series had verbal scores greater than performance scores, with a mean difference of 14 points.

Other studies provide weaker evidence that performance IQ is particularly affected. The Greater London Council (GLC) study (Halliwell *et al.* 1980) recorded a mean difference of just 7 points in favour of verbal IQ ($p < 0.05$), exactly the same difference found by Mazur *et al.* (1988). Superior performance IQs were sometimes reported when IQ scores were grouped according to the frequency of shunt revision—the need for which may suggest raised intracranial pressure and/or intracranial infection. A few small studies have reported higher performance IQs among a number of their subjects (Scherzer and Gardiner 1971, Herren *et al.* 1972).

The likelihood of differences between verbal and performance IQ occurring in a 'normal' population has been calculated by Field (1960) and Sattler (1982). For example, 10 per cent of the population will have differences of 23 points or more. Wills *et al.* (1990) compared Wechsler IQ scores among children with myelomeningocele against the theoretical frequencies in a normal population, and found that a difference of more than 12 points was twice as great among the spina bifida sample, providing some evidence of differential cognitive impairment.

Reliability of intelligence test scores
Barring further insults to the central nervous system, IQ scores show an unusually high reliability over time. A correlation of $+0.82$ between scores at 18 months and five years of age was reported on a shunted series by Fishman and Palkes (1974) even when different tests were used. Serial assessment of an unselectively treated series using the WPPSI scale at 5, the WISC at 10 and the WISC-R at 16 showed intercorrelations of between $+0.88$ and $+0.93$ on the separate scales. Over the 11 years of study, the 16-year-olds were only about 5 points lower than their five-year-old score. Most of the changes could be accounted for by losses in IQ of more than 1SD among children with valve complications and/or intracranial infection (Tew and Laurence 1983).

Sex differences in intelligence
Spina bifida is more common among females (Doran and Guthkelch 1961). Some studies have identified them as having more severe physical disabilities (Tew and Laurence 1972, Halliwell *et al.* 1980) and as more likely to be shunted (Hunt 1981).

The South Wales study (Tew and Laurence 1982) was alone in finding that girls had significantly lower (p<0.001) IQs than boys. A study of nearly 1400 children predominantly with myelomeningocele (Lonton 1985) showed no differences between the sexes in terms of IQ, reading, degree of physical disability or incontinence.

Site of the spinal lesion

Psychologists have used different approaches to assess the severity of physical disability and its association with intelligence, for example using categories of disability (Halliwell *et al.* 1980), the upper sensory level of the spinal lesion (Badell-Ribera *et al.* 1966), or the number of vertebral segments occupied by the lesion (Lonton 1977).

There is general agreement that IQ scores are inversely related to the site of the lesion. For example, children with sacral lesions had a mean IQ of 100 but those with thoracolumbar-sacral lesions had a mean IQ of 75 (Lonton 1977). A similar distribution of scores occurred in the study by Halliwell *et al.* (1980), where children with no disability had a full-scale IQ of 99 (compared to a mean of 112 for the controls) while those defined as very severely physically disabled had a mean IQ of 75. Among 'aggressively' treated children with lesions below L3, 82 per cent were of normal intelligence with an IQ greater than 80 (Hunt 1990).

As there is a clear association between shunted hydrocephalus and the site of the lesion, however, it is likely that variations in IQ could be affected by shunting as well as by paraplegia. One attempt to separate out these variables was made by Badell-Ribera *et al.* (1966) who showed that hydrocephalics had lower IQ scores than non-hydrocephalics when classified according to the severity of their disability, but a more precise indication of the relative effects of hydrocephalus and overall physical disability would have been possible if multivariate statistical analysis had been used.

Labour and vaginal delivery may be associated with pressure on exposed nerve roots resulting in additional loss of neural function (Stark and Drummond 1970), and in view of the studies quoted above, intelligence could be affected. Luthy *et al.* (1991) tested this hypothesis by comparing outcomes among three groups of children, all with uncomplicated myelomeningocele, who were (i) delivered by caesarean section prior to labour (N 47), (ii) delivered by caesarean section after a period of labour (N 35) or (iii) delivered vaginally (N 78).

Children delivered after labour were twice as likely to have severe paralysis as those delivered by elective section. Additionally the elective caesarean section group had a level of paralysis about three segments below the anatomical level of the lesion. At 24 months all were assessed on the Bayley Scales (excluding the Psychomotor parts). The elective section group had a mean score of 94 (SD 15), compared to 85 (SD 22) for the two groups experiencing labour. Although this difference is not significant, the results are in line with the finding that as the lesion descends the spine, IQ improves. A follow-up of this series would be of interest.

The effects of hydrocephalus

During the 1970s there was a shift away from analyses based upon disease categories to ones which recognised the crucial effect of hydrocephalus, and especially shunting, upon cognitive functioning. Shunt insertion is undertaken when demonstrable clinical signs of ventricular dilatation are observed by which time there has been some insult to cognitive function, perhaps largely irreversible. Shunting may prevent further intellectual deterioration or death taking place, but it does not restore normal neuropsychological function (Prigatano *et al.* 1983). Consequently a dichotomy of shunted and non-shunted cases was widely adopted by psychologists. Children who had shunts tended to have significantly lower IQs and poorer scores on all psychometric tests than children who had escaped this complication, although there was some overlap between the scores of the two groups (Spain 1974, Tew and Laurence 1975).

There may be a third group of children, known as 'arrested' hydrocephalics, who show early evidence of raised intracranial pressure which is not sufficiently serious to warrant surgery before their hydrocephalus seems to stop increasing spontaneously. Assessment reveals IQ scores midway between those with spina bifida only and those with shunts inserted. Their losses in intelligence are probably due to their transient ventricular dilatation (Tew and Laurence 1975, Halliwell *et al.* 1980). 'Normal-pressure' hydrocephalus, alleged to be present among many children, seems to have been reported in only a dozen cases (Milhorat and Hammock 1972, Hammock *et al.* 1976). Typically there is a progressive disparity between psychomotor development and normal maturation, suggesting insidious ventriculomegaly. Increases in IQ of 15 to 20 points were reported after shunting. Such a claim clearly demands corroboration, but significant gains in neuropsychological functioning have been documented among aged adults (Stambrook *et al.* 1988).

Further evidence that the shunted/non-shunted dichotomy may be an oversimplification is highlighted by the effects of intracranial infection upon cognitive function. Selker *et al.* (1973) observed that 'major infection remains the most profound cause of poor future performance with no appreciable evidence of being able to regain lost ground'. Confirmation of this viewpoint came from McClone *et al.* (1982) and Mapstone *et al.* (1984). McClone *et al.* reviewed 167 children with myelomeningocele. Thirty-nine who were not shunted had a mean IQ of 102 (SD 18), while 86 who had shunts but were free from infection had a non-significantly lower IQ of 95 (SD 19); but 42 who had shunts and were experiencing complications such as ventriculitis had a significantly lower mean IQ of 73 (SD 26). Although no clear relationship could be demonstrated between the severity and duration of infection and cognitive function, they concluded that 'mental retardation associated with myelomeningocele is not an associated trait but rather an acquired deficit related to the onset of ventriculitis and meningitis'.

There are important implications if this is the case. First, better control of intracranial infection seems to be the most obvious way of preserving intellectual function and is meeting with increasing success. In Lorber's (1971) series, 18 per cent of the sample developed ventriculitis in the newborn period, but only 2.5 per cent did so in the Chicago study (McClone *et al.* 1982). Second, as we have discussed elsewhere, the prediction of outcome from characteristics assessable at birth (Laurence *et al.* 1976, Lonton 1982) can be confounded by events such as intracranial infection. Third, studies of outcome should explicitly describe and analyse separately those with intracranial infection, rather than include them among shunt-treated children as was the case in earlier work.

Hydrocephalus is so varied a state, even within apparently homogeneous groups (Welch 1980), that the presumed cause of the hydrocephalus should be described for some conditions. Porencephalic cysts and the Dandy-Walker syndrome, for instance, are associated with extremely low levels of intelligence (Raimondi and Soare 1974), and including them into broader categories of hydrocephalus will distort their overall distribution of ability.

A 'new' category of hydrocephalic children has recently been seen in special baby-care units as a result of increasingly skilled management of very low-birthweight babies, who are especially vulnerable to intracranial haemorrhage interrupting the free circulation of CSF. Their outcome is extremely variable, with 30 per cent having no disability or just a mild variation from normal functioning (Etches *et al.* 1989) but up to 40 per cent having an increased liability to learning difficulties, though they seem to escape more severe physical disability (Stellman and Bannister 1982, 1985) and need detailed assessment prior to, and during, the early years of schooling.

Epilepsy
A major complication of hydrocephalus is epilepsy. Previously occurring in 30 to 40 per cent of all hydrocephalics (Hosking 1974, Lorber *et al.* 1978), better antibiotic cover and reduction in the more severe disability under a selective treatment policy have currently reduced the prevalence of epilepsy to less than 10 per cent (Evans *et al.* 1985), but this is still an appreciably greater incidence than found among the normal population.

Children with neuroepileptic disorder of varying aetiology are likely to have some impairment of intellectual and motor function (Rutter *et al.* 1970), and to be more liable to psychiatric disorder. Hydrocephalic children are no exception: Dennis *et al.* (1981) confirmed that children who had seizures had a significantly lower overall IQ, largely due to poorer non-verbal functioning. However, as they confined their study to those with IQs above 70, they excluded those who had more extensive cerebral pathology who might have had different patterns of intelligence test scores more frequently associated with low intelligence and epilepsy (Hunt 1990).

Ocular defects
Children with spina bifida, especially those with hydrocephalus as an additional

complication, are particularly liable to squints. More than 50 per cent of shunted children are so affected (Stanworth 1969, Clements and Kaushal 1970), but even those with spina bifida only are more prone to have squints than the general population (Stanworth 1969). Studies of cerebral-palsied children and others with squints suggested that they may have difficulties especially with visuoperceptual and motor functioning (Abercrombie *et al.* 1964, Wedell 1973) and there is no reason to suppose that children with NTD differ greatly.

Tew and Laurence (1978*a*) examined the relationship between learning ability and ocular defects (mainly squints and nystagmus, but not impaired acuity), and found that those with squints had significantly lower scores on a wide range of tests than non-squinting children. But as those with squints often had shunts and high back lesions, the existence of these complications almost certainly confounded their observations.

Reductions in non-verbal IQ, considered to be due to impairments of the visual cortex among hydrocephalics, was reported by Dennis *et al.* (1981). However, other work by Prigatano *et al.* (1983) and Zeiner *et al.* (1985), also on hydrocephalics, indicated that impaired ocular motility is associated with reduction in both verbal and non-verbal functions and complex visuospatial problem solving. These investigators are unusual in having undertaken longitudinal neuropsychological assessment, but the results of their tests appeared inconclusive, some remaining constant over a two-year interval, some improving and some deteriorating. Perhaps the rather confusing picture may be partly due to a lack of sensitivity of the tests used.

Visuoperceptual difficulties
Many studies have described spina bifida-hydrocephalic children as having affected visuospatial functioning, but the assessment of such abilities invariably depends upon pencil and paper tests. So children with low scores on tests such as the Frostig or Bender-Gestalt, which purport to measure perceptual ability, may do so because of motor dysfunction rather than actual spatial impairment. One experiment, which required children to make perceptual matches without a corresponding motor act, concluded that visuoperceptual functioning was significantly poorer among hydrocephalics (Miller and Sethi 1971) than controls: but as the latter were not matched for IQ, the validity of their findings is uncertain. Further investigation of perceptual functioning using video display units and computers would be an interesting development.

Hand function
Although impairment of cognitive function among children with NTD was recognised early, the same cannot be said about upper-limb function. In fact, recognition of children's difficulties was probably set back by such statements as 'all have good hands and arms, their outlook appears brighter than that of many children with other types of physical handicap' (Henderson 1968). With the

Department of Education and Science (1969) making statements like 'the upper extremities and upper trunk develop normally and this will help the child to achieve mobility in daily living activities', it is likely that school medical examinations were confined to below the waist.

It is now abundantly clear that neurological and psychological assessment reveals impairment of coordination and manipulation sufficient to affect school performance and eventual employability. Wallace (1973) examined 225 consecutive unselected children with myelomeningocele and found that 69 per cent had significant abnormal upper-limb function associated with a variety of cerebral abnormalities. Shunting did not reduce the frequency of upper-limb abnormality: in fact 'it was present significantly more often'. No obvious relationship existed between the site of the spinal lesion and abnormal hand and arm function, indicating that all children, but especially those with hydrocephalus, should be screened early in life.

Minns *et al.* (1977) agreed with her findings, but suggested that children with meningocele may also have subtle impairment. Overall they found a significant relationship (p<0.01) between functional abnormality on skills such as buttoning, catching a ball and using a screwdriver, and more clinically assessed activities, such as stereognosis, diadochokinesia and shunted hydrocephalus. They recommended practical functional assessment by therapists, because 'on occasions, neither the neurologist nor psychologist is going to be able to predict the child with manipulative problems, for intelligence correlates better with neurological abnormality than functional difficulties'.

A further study of upper-limb function by Turner (1986) confirmed that there was no association between the level of lesion and fine motor difficulties. However, there were several methodological difficulties in this study: a range of 14 years between youngest and oldest in the sample, rather arbitrary modification of standard-ised tests and changes in the scoring systems. Moreover, this study would have benefitted from multivariate statistical analysis which would permit an analysis of the relative contributions of particular variables known to affect hand function.

Mazur *et al.* (1988) made a detailed study of the interrelationships between hand function, hydrocephalus and other intracranial complications, site of lesion and intelligence. Like Jacobs *et al.* (1988), they showed that children with higher spinal lesions had the most severely affected hand function. The Mazur study indicated that even children with well controlled hydrocephalus can have abnormal hand function, because neurological abnormality had a more profound effect upon hand function than on intelligence. The mean hand function time on the Jebsen-Taylor test was between 2 and 4sD below the mean, whereas their IQ scores were no more than 1sD below. Children with low intelligence (IQ <80) were found to have particular difficulty using their hands, as did those with high lesions and those who had more than three shunt revisions. Since all three variables overlap greatly, there is a need for more sophisticated statistical analysis.

An obvious expression of impaired hand function is poor handwriting and drawing ability, first noted by Sella *et al.* (1966). The first detailed assessment of handwriting was by Anderson (1975), who found that about 60 per cent of spina bifida hydrocephalic children were significantly slower writers than their controls, and that the presentation of their work was poorer. Her findings have been fully corroborated by Pearson *et al.* (1988) and Ziviani *et al.* (1990), the former study observing that better writing was related to intelligence and ordinary school attendance. Useful guidelines for improving handwriting have been presented by Cambridge and Anderson (1979), but a properly controlled trial to improve writing skills has yet to be undertaken.

An important and previously neglected aspect of upper-limb function is muscle strength. Manual muscle testing revealed that below-normal strength was common among children with myelomeningocele, but significantly poorer again among hydrocephalics (Hamilton and Shah 1984). Some children had 'patchy' muscle weakness, involving both intrinsic and extrinsic muscles, liable to affect a variety of gross and fine forearm and hand movements, and especially writing.

A small but useful study by Brunt (1984) examined apraxia, defined as an inability to imitate correctly non-habitual gestures and tasks of bilateral motor coordination either initiated by verbal command or direct imitation. Brunt (1984) suggested that the areas of the cortex likely to be responsible for movement sequencing may be affected by hydrocephalus, because such children's actions were often jerky, suggesting ineffective transitions from one phase of a movement to the next.

Impaired upper-limb function is due to multiple causes, notably the Arnold-Chiari malformation and associated cerebellar dysfunction, but contributory factors may include the severity of physical disability (especially paraplegia and progressive spinal deformity), low intelligence and visuoperceptual impairment, and restricted experience among the more severely disabled in the early years of life. Some improvements may result from the introduction of Portage-type learning programmes into the child's home, although an early intervention programme hoping to improve motor abilities (Rosenbaum *et al.* 1975) yielded rather disappointing results.

Left-handedness
It is still unclear why left-handedness should be more common among spina bifida-hydrocephalic children, with reported prevalence rates of 22 per cent (Lonton 1976), 29 per cent (Turner 1986), 32 per cent (Minns *et al.* 1977), and more than 40 per cent in a special school population (Field 1970). In the general population less than 10 per cent are left-handed. Lonton (1976) suggested that elevated rates of left-handedness occur among several different disabilities in childhood, but hardly of the magnitude found among children with NTD.

In the South Wales study (Tew 1989*b*), 12.5 per cent of pupils in ordinary schools wrote with their left hand, compared with 17 per cent in special schools. The reduction in left-handedness among these children, in comparison with the above estimates, may be in line with other evidence of a slight improvement of other disabilities associated with selective treatment policies (Evans *et al.* 1985).

Cocktail party syndrome

The term 'cocktail party syndrome' (CPS) was first coined by Hadenius *et al.* (1962) to describe the verbal behaviour of *some* arrested hydrocephalics 'who were mentally retarded but educable with a peculiar contrast between a good ability to learn words and talk and not knowing what they talk about. They love to chatter but think illogically'. Others added personality traits to the syndrome, describing such children as 'facile, uninhibited and cheeky' (Ingram and Naughton 1962).

It is thought that their language develops normally with appropriate syntax (Spain 1974), and their speech often includes 'impressive' words not part of the usual repertoire of children of their age. Their speech is clearly articulated, with inflections and stresses resembling adult utterances (Schwartz 1974), and full of clichés and automatic phrases. Often they have a highly selective memory for relatively trivial events. All of this leads those in contact with them, and especially their parents, to overestimate their accomplishments. When parents of children with CPS were asked to estimate their child's intelligence, their guesses were 20 to 40 IQ points above their actual scores (Tew *et al.* 1974). These parents are apt to reject the psychologist's findings regarding their child's abilities and also to be critical of teachers for not realising what they perceive to be their child's true potential. On the other hand, parents of children with normal language were often very accurate in their judgements of ability.

CPS is not a feature of all spina bifida children's language but seems to be associated in varying degrees with hydrocephalus, though not all hydrocephalics show this syndrome, for reasons not yet understood. It seems more likely to occur among children with paraplegia and low intelligence, and sometimes in children with spina bifida only, perhaps with spontaneous arrested hydrocephalus. The presence of CPS is symptomatic of low intelligence at the age of 10 (Tew 1979). Studies which report no difference between the language of hydrocephalics and normal children often consist of spina bifida children with at least average IQ (Byrne *et al.* 1990).

Estimates of prevalence vary between 28 per cent (Stough *et al.* 1988), 30 per cent (Hurley *et al.* 1990) and 40 per cent (Spain 1974). As this syndrome is reported to decline over time, the age composition of the samples under investigation is clearly important, as is their intelligence. Although children with CPS are often loquacious, they do not score highly on tests of expressive and receptive language function: in fact they score significantly below spina bifida children with normal language, who in turn have poorer language skills than normal controls (Tew 1979).

Tew (1979) used five criteria to identify children with CPS: (i) fluent, well articulated speech, (ii) excessive use of social phrases in conversation, (iii) overfamiliarity of manner, (iv) introducing personal experience into the conversation in inappropriate and irrelevant contexts, and (v) perseveration of responses. Stough *et al.* (1988) rightly pointed out that these criteria lack objectivity, being dependent upon the examiner's judgement. However, they used them in a study of the language ability of seven four- to six-year-olds and seven 14- to 16-year-olds all with spina bifida and hydrocephalus. A statistical procedure known as cluster analysis identified four children with different language scores from the rest of the sample. Their teachers also chose these children but added a further two as having characteristics of CPS. Statistical analysis showed that out of the five criteria, only irrelevant language was characteristic of CPS.

Tew's (1979) criteria were also used by Hurley *et al.* (1990) in a study of 50 persons with myelomeningocele aged between 10 and 32. To be classified as having this syndrome each person had to meet four of the five criteria independently judged by two raters. Exactly half of the sample had normal functioning, but 30 per cent had CPS, and 20 per cent were described as 'dysfunctional', defined as having two or three of Tew's criteria and also as not being able to manage their life very well, measured on an 'activities of daily living' scale.

Many of their findings confirmed Tew's (1979) observations, except that some of their subjects with CPS were within the average range of intelligence. They speculated that some of Tew's subjects who had grown out of the syndrome were those they described as 'dysfunctional', though only a longitudinal study would answer this question.

Dennis *et al.* (1987) undertook a detailed and statistically sophisticated study to trace the course language development of hydrocephalics. Their sample of 75 consisted of 30 with spina bifida, but the remainder came from about seven different disease categories, some of which consisted of one or two cases only, making generalisations very difficult. Five types of language skills were assessed on tests mostly devised by Dennis and colleagues. Both index children and controls were divided into age bands, enabling comparisons to be made over time. This showed that although language skills among hydrocephalics improved with age, they did so at a slower rate than in the normal population. Children with accompanying spina bifida seemed to have greater dysfluency than those with different aetiology. Early hydrocephalus seemed to affect the ability to monitor the appropriateness of one's speech and those with shunts tended to have more problems involving seriation, such as perseveration. Dennis *et al.* (1987) argued that CPS was not a useful term to describe hydrocephalic language, because it did not explain the course of their language development.

The cause of CPS is still obscure. Taylor (1961) thought that the child's fluency had been selectively reinforced by the family, but this seems unlikely. Most favour neuropathological explanations. McNab (1965), Emery and Svitok (1968) and Brocklehurst (1976) suggested that ventricular dilatation affects the anterior commissures which develop after birth and are associated with language function. Bodley (1982) speculated that CPS reflects difficulties in self-control and self-monitoring, analogous to disturbance in executive function found among adults with frontal-lobe damage and/or limbic-lobe disturbance. Hurley *et al.* (1990) also recognised the possibility of deficits in frontal-lobe functioning, but suggested that right hemisphere dysfunction, or at least connections to that hemisphere from the occipital area, may be a likely cause. Perhaps a more authoritative explanation of this syndrome will eventually come from neuropathologists and their findings at post-mortem examination.

Due to the improvement in physical and intellectual status of children selectively treated, and better control of intracranial infection, CPS seems to be much less frequent in young children now.

Personality and behaviour problems
The Isle of Wight study (Rutter *et al.* 1970) showed that the likelihood of psychiatric disorder among children with physical disabilities involving the brain was at least four times greater than in the general population. However, the severity of physical disability did not seem to be associated with psychiatric disorder, suggesting that environmental circumstances have an important effect upon emotional well-being (Rutter 1977). A Canadian study found that children with chronic illness and associated disability had three times more risk of psychiatric disorder and were also at considerably more risk of having social adjustment problems than an unaffected population (Cadman *et al.* 1987). A child with a complicated NTD, therefore, is likely to have an increased predisposition to some form of emotional disturbance and/or social difficulty.

However, the evidence relating to behavioural adjustment among children with NTD has often been contradictory. Some of the confusion may be due to variations in the methods used to ascertain maladjustment: *e.g.* postal surveys (Murch and Cohen 1989), parental report (Breslau 1985; Lavigne *et al.* 1988; Wallander *et al.* 1988, 1989*b*), interviews with young adults (Dorner 1976, McAndrew 1979), standardised questionnaires completed by teachers (Tew and Laurence 1973, Anderson 1975) or by the child (Moilanen *et al.* 1985), and occasionally multiple sources of data (Spaulding and Morgan 1986). Psychiatric interview has been remarkably infrequent (Kolin *et al.* 1971, Connell and McConnell 1981).

Often samples have included children with more than a 10-year age spread (Kazak and Clark 1986, Wallander *et al.* 1989*a*), and have sometimes lacked essential data describing clinical, social and intellectual characteristics (Breslau 1985, Wallander *et al.* 1988). Some samples may have uncertain bias (Wallander *et al.* 1988*b*). The absence of matched controls clearly makes comparisons more difficult (Dorner 1976). Finally, international variations in service provision may influence psychological outcome.

Studies indicating higher rates of maladjustment, emotional disturbance or behaviour disorder (the terms are often used without clear definition other than a score on a particular test) span a variety of investigations. An early study of 13 children and their parents revealed a strong relationship between degree of the child's adjustment and parental coping ability (Kolin *et al.* 1971). All of the children had moderate to intense feelings of anxiety, and a quarter were depressed. The high rate of disorder led to a suggestion that routine psychiatric screening should be undertaken for all families. An Australian study (Connell and McConnell 1981) assessed 43 hydrocephalics of varying aetiology, aged between five and 12. Overall 44 per cent had some form of psychiatric disorder, principally neuroticism. Boys were more frequently and more severely affected, while those with epilepsy as an additional complication were at particular risk of having disturbance. No obvious relationship existed between either IQ or the extent of physical disability and psychiatric disorder.

Personal interviews of the parents of adolescents with spina bifida revealed that two thirds of the young people reported serious, recurrent depression in the past year (Dorner 1976). Half of the girls and a quarter of the boys felt occasionally that 'life was not worth living', and a quarter of the girls had entertained suicidal feelings. However, none of McAndrew's (1979) Australian sample had suicidal thoughts even though the majority of them had low self-esteem. A Scandinavian study of mid-adolescents (Borjeson and Lagergren 1990) found that 10 of their sample of 25 were occasionally depressed ('wanting to cry'), but of these only three had possible endogenous depression, and only one had frank psychiatric disorder.

Surveys requiring teachers to complete standardised questionnaires on behaviour in school showed that a third of children were maladjusted (mostly neurotic difficulty) and a further 13 per cent came into the lesser category of unsettled behaviour (Tew and Laurence 1973). However, there was no clear relationship between behaviour disturbance and severity of the child's disability, a finding confirmed by Wallander *et al.* (1989*a*). Using a different inventory, Anderson (1975) found that only 11 per cent had scores indicating behaviour disorder. Differences between the scales probably account for some of the differences between the proportions of the children identified as having difficulty, but a Scottish study showed that teachers of spina bifida children in ordinary schools were not always aware of the children's feelings of inferiority (O'Hagan *et al.* 1984). This must cast some doubt on the validity of questionnaire data gathered this way. In studies of the behaviour problems occurring among spina bifida children, there is agreement that neurotic difficulty is much more common than conduct disorder (Connell and McConnell 1981, Lavigne *et al.* 1988), but one study recorded very similar rates of disturbance involving internalising behaviour, externalising behaviour and social behaviour on the Child Behaviour Checklist (Wallander *et al.* 1989*a*). However, these difficulties may be relative: 182 teachers of spina bifida children rated behaviour disorder as by far the least serious difficulty they faced in the classroom (Tew 1984).

Several small-scale epidemiological studies looking at spina bifida children alongside those with other disabilities have found high rates of emotional disturbance among the former. Breslau (1985) recorded that 27 per cent of the 63 spina bifida cases were 'severely psychiatrically impaired', but as the information was obtained from the mother, the true extent of the difficulty is uncertain. In a similar study depending upon maternal report (Wallander *et al.* 1988), only 10 per cent showed evidence of behaviour problems but a fifth had difficulties with social competence. Maladjustment among the children in the spina bifida subgroup was indistinguishable from that of children with other chronic disabilities, although all showed greater disturbance than the non-disabled population.

The self-concept of children with physical disabilities continues to be of interest to psychologists. Chairbound children or those needing appliances for movement, who may also be incontinent, can have realistic anxieties about their relationship with the non-disabled and especially with the opposite sex (Hirst 1989). Self-awareness and heterosexual interest both increase during adolescence, and the self-esteem of young people with NTD may be lower than that of the able-bodied.

The GLC study (Pearson *et al.* 1985) specifically addressed this question and found no essential differences between younger and older adolescents and matched controls, but a smaller Scandinavian study came to the opposite conclusions in their study of hydrocephalics (Moilanen *et al.* 1985). Both studies underline the importance of the family in shaping positive or negative self-concepts.

Self-concept is a heterogeneous collection of feelings about various aspects of one's life. A more clearly differentiated picture of the nature of emotional difficulties came from Kazak and Clark's (1986) study of six- to 13-year-olds with myelomeningocele against apparently socially advantaged controls. The spina bifida sample had significantly poorer self-concepts (p<0.01) and experienced more anxiety (p<0.01). They were just significantly poorer in terms of behaviour, popularity and happiness (p<0.05). Somewhat surprisingly, there was no difference between index and control groups in respect of personal appearance. Poorer self-concepts among spina bifida youngsters were also found by Campbell *et al.* (1977). This study suggested that boys expressed more concern about their body image than girls, possibly because urinary diversion may be seen to be more mutilating among males.

Both the Kazak and Clark study and that by Spaulding and Morgan (1986) used the Piers-Harris self-concept scale, but the latter study found no difference between spina bifida and control groups. Although those with spina bifida generally had severe physical disability, none had severe learning difficulties (their mean IQ was 108). Spaulding and Morgan (1986) pointed out that their findings could not be 'generalised to retarded children who represent about one third of all spina bifidas'. In spite of this limitation, they argued that the psychological functioning of the chronically ill and/or disabled child did not differ significantly from that of the general population.

Efforts to improve self-concept have mainly involved counselling and social skills training. A different approach was used by Andrade *et al.* (1991) who developed a 10-week exercise programme for adolescents: a significant increase in self-concept scores and other physiological measures was reported at the end of the study.

School attainments
Studies of school attainments have consistently shown that spina bifida children

have reading standards below their actual age (Tew and Laurence 1975, Carr *et al.* 1981, Lonton 1981). The highest reading ages occur among those free from hydrocephalus (though even these tend to be inferior to the normal population), with the lowest scores among those with shunts, indicating the important limiting effect of intelligence, perceptual difficulties (Holgate 1985) and attentional disorders (Tew *et al.* 1980), all of which appear to have an interactive effect upon literacy. However, other factors outside the child influence reading standards. Pupils at special schools had significantly lower reading ages than predicted from their age and IQ, while those attending ordinary school read at an appropriate level for their intelligence (Tew and Laurence 1978*b*).

Arithmetic skills are even poorer than reading ability, again with shunted children at the greatest disadvantage. About a third of a sample were incapable of simple counting at the age of seven (Tew and Laurence 1975). Their mathematical difficulties persisted, and reassessment of this sample at 16 showed that they had very significantly lower scores than the controls ($p<0.001$). Again those with shunts fared worst. However, slightly more optimistic results were reported by Wills *et al.* (1990) in a study of children with average intelligence; they confirmed lower group and individual scores on the Wide Range Achievement Test, but not the existence of specific arithmetic disability.

Tew *et al.* (1989*b*) noted an improvement in numerical ability over a 10-year period, but only among pupils in ordinary schools: children with shunts and especially those attending special schools remained particularly weak in this subject. It remains to be seen whether this is due to temporal and/or frontal-lobe lesions, thought to be associated with dyscalculia (O'Hare *et al.* 1991) and possibly associated with hydrocephalus. It is also unknown whether poor calculating ability is a common feature among children with other kinds of physical disability. A comparative study needs to be done.

The cause of these difficulties is certainly multifactorial: it includes the above variables, and also events such as hospitalisation after the age of six, which has a significant effect upon numerical ability but not upon reading (Carr *et al.* 1981), because mathematics has to be taught systematically, while reading is one of the most common pastimes for anyone confined to bed. Children in British special schools may have up to two hours less teaching per week than their counterparts in ordinary schools (Carr *et al.* 1983), and probably receive proportionately less teaching of arithmetic. Finally, Parfitt (1979) suggested that teachers in special schools may create a self-fulfilling prophecy, because they do not expect spina bifida children to do well in mathematics.

Schooling
Given the very wide range of disabilities (mental, physical and multiple) associated with NTD, a range of schooling options is needed. There is not just a choice between ordinary schools and special schools, because there is a wide range of special educational help for children in ordinary schools.

The introduction of selective treatment, and the reduction in the more severe forms of disability, has coincided with more positive feelings towards the integration of disabled children into ordinary schools and made it easier for spina bifida children to be educated alongside their non-disabled peers. In the Sheffield area, 82 per cent of nursery and 71 per cent of primary schoolchildren born since 1975 attended an ordinary school (Lonton *et al.* 1986), but enthusiasm for integration varies throughout the country. The South Wales study found a lower proportion (51 per cent) fully integrated, while a further 10 per cent were at special units in ordinary schools (Tew 1989*b*).

Integration is not always a straightforward process: some children experience practical problems regarding access and appropriate furniture and equipment, all of which could be resolved by better funding. Lonton *et al.* (1986) identified three areas where improvements were needed in ordinary schools: (i) employing care assistants to help with toileting *etc.*, (ii) delivering physiotherapy services to the school, and (iii) providing in-service education for teachers. Half of the teachers in Sheffield and nearly four out of five in South Wales had little knowledge of the needs of spina bifida children in their school.

Integration or mainstreaming is known to have positive advantages for students. Adolescents attending ordinary schools had better social adjustment than those in special residential schools (Anderson *et al.* 1982), but the placement of a spina bifida child in a mainstream class does not necessarily imply full integration. Some children may experience 'psychological distress' from such an arrangement (Lord *et al.* 1990).

At primary-school level the main benefits of integration appear to be academic, with higher reading ages (Tew and Laurence 1978*b*, Carr *et al.* 1981) and better mathematical skills (Tew 1988, 1989*b*). Children attending ordinary schools normally follow the same curriculum as their able-bodied peers, but special schools are too small to be able to offer a wide range of subjects, which in turn affects their pupils' examination prospects. Almost four fifths of those in special schools and three quarters of children with shunts left school without any examination achievements (Tew 1986). As these children were often the most seriously physically disabled, they were ill equipped to take up any form of employment.

Employment rates for young adults with spina bifida vary between 19 and 33 per cent (Lonton *et al.* 1984, Thomas *et al.* 1989, Hunt 1990, Tew *et al.* 1990); thus some 70 to 80 per cent of adults born during the period of aggressive care in Britain are likely to be without work. It is not known whether these rates also occur in other countries. Open employment is an unrealistic expectation for many, although one study has shown that there was no clear distinction between those in and out of work except at the extremes of the distribution (Tew *et al.* 1990). A greater proportion of young adults would be able to take up work if the government willed more resources.

Conclusion
Psychologists have made important contributions in identifying both general and

specific learning difficulties among children with NTD. Two further developments now seem to be needed.

1. Although specific neuropsychological procedures have been used occasionally over the last 10 years, it is odd that precise assessment procedures such as the Luria-Nebraska or the Halstead-Reitan scales have yet to be used in carefully defined samples. As these tests purport to assess more localised cerebral function, it should be instructive to compare the results of such assessments with the findings of brain imaging procedures in order to establish the strength of the association between anatomical abnormality and particular patterns of neuropsychological scores; one area where this could be done is among children with cocktail party syndrome. Serial neuropsychological assessment could also detect progressive deterioration of function associated with raised intracranial pressure.

2. Psychologists have largely been content to measure and describe functional limitations associated with spina bifida-hydrocephalic children, without taking the next step of introducing a controlled intervention programme. Very few studies have set out to improve specific developmental difficulties. Behavioural procedures have been used to improve motivation in adolescents (Carr 1982), with younger children (Feldman *et al.* 1982, 1983) and in association with parent training procedures (Fishman and Fishman 1975). One study has used these techniques to improve fine and gross motor coordination (Rapport and Bailey 1985). Behaviour modification and biofeedback have proved successful in treating encopresis (Pappo *et al.* 1988). Intervention studies have attempted to improve handwriting (Cambridge and Anderson 1979), visuomotor perception (Gluckman and Barling 1980) and reading comprehension (Grant and Mooney 1990), but efforts to raise mathematical achievement are still awaited.

Some psychological studies are 'snapshots' in time. More meaningful results will come from longitudinal investigation. For example, high rates of misery and depression have been reported among adolescents (Dorner 1976, Anderson *et al.* 1982), but single enquiries such as these cannot establish whether such feelings are reactive and reflect realistic worries about their ability to cope with the demands of adult life, or whether they are expressions of more long-standing emotional disturbance. But the worldwide decline in the numbers of children born with NTD (see Chapter 1) will make it more difficult to generate samples sufficiently large and homogeneous to yield meaningful results, unless there is international collaboration between different centres.

REFERENCES

Abercrombie, M.L.J., Gardner, P.A., Hansen, E., Jonckheere, J., Lindon, R.L., Solomon, G., Tyson, M. (1964) 'Visual, perceptual and visuo-motor impairments in physically handicapped children.' *Perceptual Motor Skills*, **18**, 561–624.
Anderson, E.M. (1975) *Cognitive and Motor Deficits in Children with Spina Bifida and Hydrocephalus with Special Reference to Writing Difficulties*. University of London: Ph.D. thesis.
—— Clarke, L., Spain, B. (1982) *Disability in Adolescence*. London: Methuen.
Andrade, C.-K., Kramer, J., Garber, M., Longmuir, P. (1991) 'Changes in self-concept, cardiovascular

endurance and muscular strength of children with spina bifida aged 8 to 13 years in response to a 10-week physical activity programme: a pilot study.' *Child: Care, Health and Development*, **17**, 183–196.

Badell-Ribera, A., Shulman, K., Paddock, N. (1966) 'The relationship of non-progressive hydrocephalus to intellectual functioning in children with spina bifida cystica.' *Pediatrics*, **37**, 787–793.

Billard, C.T., Santini, J.J., Gillet, P., Nargeot, M., Adrien, J. (1986) 'Long term intellectual prognosis of hydrocephalus with reference to 77 children.' *Pediatric Neuroscience*, **12**, 219–225.

Bodley, A. (1982) *Intellectual Deficits in Spina Bifida Children With and Without Hydrocephalus.* University of Melbourne: M.A. thesis.

Borjeson, M.C., Lagergen, J. (1990) 'Life conditions of adolescents with myelomeningocele.' *Developmental Medicine and Child Neurology*, **32**, 698–706.

Breslau, N. (1985) 'Psychiatric disorder in children with physical disabilities.' *Journal of the American Academy of Child Psychiatry*, **42**, 87–94.

Brocklehurst, G. (Ed.) (1976) *Spina Bifida for the Clinician. Clinics in Developmental Medicine, No. 57.* London: SIMP with Heinemann Medical; Philadelphia: J.B. Lippincott.

Brunt, D. (1984) 'Apraxic tendencies in children with meningomyelocele.' *Adapted Physical Activity Quarterly.*, **1**, 61–67.

Byrne, K., Abbeduto, L., Brooks, P. (1990) 'The language of children with spina bifida and hydrocephalus: meeting task demands and mastering syntax.' *Journal of Speech and Hearing Disorders*, **55**, 118–123.

Cadman, D., Coyle, M., Szatmari, P., Offord, D. (1987) 'Chronic illness, disability and mental and physical well-being: findings of the Ontario child health study.' *Pediatrics*, **79**, 805–813.

Cambridge, J., Anderson, E.M. (1979) *The Handwriting of Spina Bifida Children. An Advisory Booklet for Teachers and Students.* London: ASBAH.

Campbell, M.M., Hayden, P.W., Davenport, S.L.H. (1977) 'Psychological adjustment of adolescents with myelodysplasia.' *Journal of Youth and Adolescence*, **4**, 397–407.

Carr, J. (1982) 'A behavioural approach to problems of motivation in the spina bifida child.' *Zeitschrift für Kinderchirurgie*, **37**, 184–186.

—— Halliwell, M.D., Pearson, A.M. (1981) 'Educational attainments of spina bifida children attending ordinary and special schools.' *Zeitschrift für Kinderchirurgie*, **34**, 364–370.

—— Pearson, A., Halliwell, M. (1983) *The GLC Spina Bifida Survey: Follow up at 11 and 12 Years.* London: GLC Research & Statistics Branch.

Clements, D.B., Kaushal, K. (1970) 'A study of the ocular complications of hydrocephalus & meningomyelocele.' *Transactions of the Opthalmological Society (UK)*, **90**, 383–390.

Connell, H.M., McConnell, T.S. (1981) 'Psychiatric sequelae in children treated operatively for hydrocephalus in infancy.' *Developmental Medicine and Child Neurology*, **23**, 505–517.

Dennis, M., Fitz, C.R., Netley, C.T., Sugar, J., Harwood-Nash, D., Hendrick, B., Hoffman, H., Humphreys, R. (1981) 'The intelligence of hydrocephalic children.' *Archives of Neurology*, **38**, 607–615.

—— Hendrick, E., Hoffman, H., Humphreys, R. (1987) 'Language of hydrocephalic children and adolescents.' *Journal of Clinical and Experimental Neuropsychology*, **2**, 593–621.

Department of Education and Science (1969) *Health of the Schoolchild, 1966–1968.* London: HMSO.

Doran, P.A., Guthkelch, A.N. (1961) 'Studies in spina bifida cystica I. General survey and re-assessment of the problem.' *Journal of Neurosurgery and Psychiatry*, **24**, 331–345.

Dorner, S. (1976) 'Adolescents with spina bifida—how they see their situation.' *Archives of Disease in Childhood*, **51**, 439–444.

Emery, J.L., Svitok, I. (1968) 'Inter-hemispherical distances in congenital hydrocephalus associated with meningomyelocele.' *Developmental Medicine and Child Neurology*, **10** (Suppl. 15), 21–29.

Etches, P., Ward, T., Bhui, P., Peters, K., Robertson, C. (1989) 'Outcome of posthemorrhagic hydrocephalus in premature infants.' *Pediatric Neurology*, **3**, 136–140.

Evans, R., Tew, B., Thomas, M., Ford, J. (1985) 'Selective surgical management of neural tube malformations.' *Archives of Disease in Childhood*, **60**, 415–419.

Feldman, W.S., Manella, K.J., Apodaca, L., Varni, J.W. (1982) 'Behavioural group parent training in spina bifida.' *Journal of Clinical Child Psychology*, **11**, 144–150.

—— Manella, K.J., Varni, J.W. (1983) 'A behavioural training programme for single mothers of physically handicapped children.' *Child: Care, Health and Development*, **9**, 157–168.

175

Field, A. (1970) 'Spina bifida: learning problems.' *Special Education*, **59**, 14–15.
Field, J.G. (1960) 'Two types of tables for use with Wechsler's Intelligence Scales.' *Journal of Clinical Psychology*, **47**, 3–7.
Fishman, M., Palkes, H.S. (1974) 'The reliability of psychometric testing in children with malformations of the central nervous system.' *Developmental Medicine and Child Neurology*, **16**, 180–185.
Fishman, C.A., Fishman, D.B. (1975) 'A group training programme in behaviour modification for mothers of children wth spina bifida.' *Child Psychiatry and Human Development*, **6**, 3–14.
Gluckman, S., Barling, J. (1980) 'Effects of a remedial programme on visual-motor perception in spina bifida children.' *Journal of Genetic Psychology*, **136**, 195–202.
Grant, D., Mooney, A. (1990) 'Teaching reading comprehension skills to spina bifida children.' *Zeitschrift für Kinderchirurgie*, **45**, 11–13.
Guiney, E. J., MacCarthy, P. (1981) 'Implications of a selective policy in the management of spina bifida.' *Journal of Pediatric Surgery*, **16**, 136–138.
Hadenius, A.M., Hagberg, B., Hyttnas-Bensch, K., Sjögren, I. (1962) 'The natural prognosis of infantile hydrocephalus.' *Acta Paediatrica Scandinavica*, **51**, 117–123.
Halliwell, M.D., Carr, J., Pearson, A. (1980) 'The intellectual and educational functioning of children with neural tube defects.' *Zeitschrift für Kinderchirurgie*, **31**, 375–381.
Hamilton, A., Shah, S. (1984) 'Physical hand function of the child with spina bifida-myelomeningocele.' *Occupational Therapy*, **May**, 147–150.
Hammock, M., Milhorat, T., Baron, I. (1976) 'Normal pressure hydrocephalus in patients with myelomeningocele.' *Developmental Mental and Child Neurology*, **18** (Suppl. 37), 55–68.
Henderson, P. (1968) 'The educational problems of myelomeningocele.' *Hospital Medicine*, **2**, 909–914.
Herren, H., Colin, D., Goddet, F., Alcchenberger, N. (1972) 'Etude du niveau de développement neural chez les paraplégiques d'age scolaire à spina-bifida.' *Revue de Neuropsychiatrie d'Infant*, **2**, 681–700.
Hirst, M. (1989) 'Patterns of impairment and disability related to social handicap in young people with cerebral palsy and spina bifida.' *Journal of Biosocial Science*, **21**, 1–12.
Holgate, L. (1985) *Young People with Spina Bifida and or Hydrocephalus: Learning and Development*. London: ASBAH.
Hosking, G.P. (1974) 'Fits in hydrocephalic children.' *Archives of Disease in Childhood*, **49**, 633–635.
Hunt, G. M. (1981) 'Spina bifida: implications for 100 children at school.' *Developmental Medicine and Child Neurology*, **23**, 160–172.
—— (1990) 'Open spina bifida: outcome for a complete cohort treated unselectively and followed into adulthood.' *Developmental Medicine and Child Neurology*, **32**, 108–118.
Hurley, A., Dorman, C., Laatsch, L., Bell, S., D'Avignon, J. (1990) 'Cognitive functioning in patients with spina bifida, hydrocephalus, and the "cocktail party" syndrome.' *Developmental Neuropsychology*, **6**, 151–172.
Ingram, T.T.S., Naughton, J.A. (1962) 'Paediatric and psychological aspects of cerebral palsy associated with hydrocephalus.' *Developmental Medicine and Child Neurology*, **4**, 287–292.
Jacobs, R.A., Wolfe, G., Rasmuson, M. (1988) 'Upper extremity dysfunction in children with myelomeningocele.' *Zeitschrift für Kinderchirurgie*, **43**, 19–21.
Kazak, A., Clark, M. (1986) 'Stress in families of children with myelomeningocele.' *Developmental Medicine and Child Neurology*, **28**, 220–228.
Kolin, I.S., Scherzer, A.L., New, B., Garfield, M. (1971) 'Studies of the school age child with meningomyelocele: social and emotional adaption.' *Journal of Paediatrics*, **78**, 1013–1019.
Lavigne, J., Nolan, D., McClone, D. (1988) 'Temperament, coping and psychological adjustment in young children with myelomeningocele.' *Journal of Pediatric Psychology*, **13**, 363–378.
Laurence, K.M. (1974) 'Effect of early surgery for spina bifida on survival and quality of life.' *Lancet*, **1**, 301–304.
—— Tew, B.J. (1967) 'Follow up of 65 survivors from the 425 cases of spina bifida born in South Wales 1956–1962.' *Developmental Medicine and Child Neurology*, **9** (Suppl. 13), 1–4.
—— —— (1971) 'Natural history of spina bifida cystica and cranium bifidum cysticum. The major central nervous system malformations in South Wales part IV.' *Archives of Disease in Childhood*, **46**, 127–138.
—— Evans, R.C., Weeks, R.D., Thomas, M.D., Frazer, A.K., Tew, B.J. (1976) 'The reliability of prediction in spina bifida.' *Developmental Medicine and Child Neurology*, **18** (Suppl. 37), 150–156.

Lonton, A.P. (1976) 'Hand preference in children with myelomeningocele and hydrocephalus.' *Developmental Medicine and Child Neurology*, **18** (Suppl. 37), 143–149.

—— (1977) 'Location of the myelomeningocele and its relationship to subsequent physical and intellectual abilities in children with myelomeningocele associated with spina bifida and hydrocephalus.' *Zeitschrift für Kinderchirurgie*, **22**, 510–519.

—— (1979) 'The relationship between intellectual skills and the computer axial tomograms of children with spina bifida and hydrocephalus.' *Zeitschrift für Kinderchirurgie*, **28**, 368–374.

—— (1981) 'The integration (mainstreaming) of spina bifida children into ordinary schools.' *Zeitschrift für Kinderchirurgie*, **34**, 356–364.

—— (1982) 'Prediction of intelligence in spina bifida neonates.' *Zeitschrift für Kinderchirurgie*, **37**, 172–174.

—— (1985) 'Gender and spina bifida—some misconceptions.' *Zeitschrift für Kinderchirurgie*, **40**, 34–36.

—— Loughlin, A.M., O'Sullivan, A.M. (1984) 'Spina bifida adults.' *Zeitschrift für Kinderchirurgie*, **39**, 110–112.

—— Cole, M.S.J., Mercer, J. (1986) 'The integration of spina bifida children—are their needs being met?' *Zeitschrift für Kinderchirurgie*, **41**, 45–47.

Lorber, J. (1971) 'Results of treatment of myelomeningocele: an analysis of 524 unselected cases, with specific reference to possible selection for treatment.' *Developmental Medicine and Child Neurology*, **13**, 279–303.

—— Sillanpaa, M., Greenwood, N. (1978) 'Convulsions in children with hydrocephalus.' *Zeitschrift für Kinderchirurgie*, **25**, 346–351.

—— Salfield, S.A.W. (1981) 'Results of selective treatment of spina bifida cystica.' *Archives of Disease in Childhood*, **56**, 822–830.

Lord, J., Varzos, N., Behrman, B., Wicks, J., Wicks, D. (1990) 'Implications of mainstream classrooms for children with spina bifida.' *Developmental Medicine and Child Neurology*, **32**, 20–29.

Luthy, D.A., Wardinsky, T., Shurtleff, D.B., Hollenbach, K.A., Hicock, D.E., Nyberg, D.A., Benedetti, T.J. (1991) 'Cesarean section before the onset of labour and subseqent motor function in infants with meningomyelocele diagnosed antenally.' *New England Journal of Medicine*, **324**, 662–666.

Macnab, G.H. (1965) 'The development of the knowledge and treatment of hydrocephalus.' *Developmental Medicine and Child Neurology*, **7** (Suppl. 11), 1–9.

Mapstone, T., Rekate, H., Nulsen, F., Dixon, M., Glaser, N., Jaffe, M. (1984) 'Relationship of CSF shunting and IQ in children with myelomeningocele: a retrospective analysis.' *Childs Brain*, **11**, 112–118.

Mazur, J.M., Aylward, G.P., Colliver, J., Stacey, J., Menelaus, M. (1988) 'Impaired mental capabilities and hand function in myelomeningocele patients.' *Zeitschrift für Kinderchirurgie*, **43**, 24–27.

McAndrew, I. (1979) 'Adolescents and young people with spina bifida.' *Developmental Medicine and Child Neurology*, **21**, 619–629.

McClone, D.G., Czyzewski, D., Raimondi, A.J., Sommers, R.C. (1982) 'Central nervous system infections as a limiting factor in the intelligence of children with myelomeningocele.' *Pediatrics*, **70**, 338–342.

Milhorat, T.H., Hammock, M. (1972) '"Arrested" versus normal pressure hydrocephalus in children.' *Clinical Proceedings of the Children's Hospital, Washington*, **28**, 168–173.

Miller, E., Sethi, L. (1971) 'The effect of hydrocephalus on perception.' *Developmental Medicine and Child Neurology*, **13**, 77–81.

Minns, R.A., Sobkowiak, C., Skardatsou, A., Dick, K., Elton, R.A., Brown, J.K., Forfar, J.O. (1977) 'Upper limb function in spina bifida.' *Zeitschrift für Kinderchirurgie*, **22**, 493–506.

Moilanen, I., Meira, L., Serlo, W., Wendt, L. (1985) 'Psychosocial adaptions of shunted hydrocephalic children.' *Zeitschrift für Kinderchirurgie*, **40**, 31–33.

Murch, R.J., Cohen, L. (1989) 'Relationships among life stress, perceived family environment and psychological distress of spina bifida adolescents.' *Journal of Pediatric Psychology*, **14**, 193–214.

O'Hagan, F., Sandys, E.J., Swanson, W.I. (1984) 'Educational provision, parental expectation and physical disability.' *Child: Care, Health and Development*, **10**, 31–38.

O'Hare, A.E., Brown, J.K., Aitken, K. (1991) 'Dyscalculia in children.' *Developmental Medicine and Child Neurology*, **33**, 356–361.

Pappo, I., Meyer, S., Winter, S., Nissan, S. (1988) 'Treatment of faecal incontinence in children with spina bifida by biofeedback and behavioural modification.' *Zeitschrift für Kinderchirurgie*, **43**, 36–37.

Parfitt, V. (1979) *The Development of Number Concepts in Children with Differing Degrees of Spina Bifida and Hydrocephalus.* University of Loughborough: Ph.D. thesis.

Pearson, A.M., Carr, J., Halliwell, M.D. (1985) 'The self concept of adolescents with spina bifida.' *Zeitschrift für Kinderchirurgie*, **40**, 27–30.

—— —— (1988) 'The handwriting of children with spina bifida.' *Zeitschrift für Kinderchirurgie*, **43**, 40–42.

Prigatano, G.P., Zeiner, H.K., Pollay, M., Kaplan, R. (1983) 'Neuropsychological functioning in children with shunted uncomplicated hydrocephalus.' *Childs Brain*, **10**, 112–120.

Rapport, M.D., Bailey, J.S. (1985) 'Behavioral physical therapy and spina bifida: a case study.' *Journal of Pediatric Psychology*, **10**, 87–96.

Raimondi, A.J., Soare, P. (1974) 'Intellectual development in shunted hydrocephalic children.' *American Journal of Diseases of Children*, **127**, 664–680.

Rosenbaum, P., Barnitt, R., Brand, H.L. (1975) 'A developmental intervention programme designed to overcome the effects of impaired movement in spina bifida infants.' *In* Holt, K.S. (Ed.) *Movement and Child Development. Clinics in Developmental Medicine, No. 55.* London: SIMP with Heinemann Medical; Philadelphia: J.B. Lippincott.

Rutter, M. (1977) 'Brain damage syndromes in childhood: concepts and findings.' *Journal of Child Psychology and Psychiatry*, **18**, 1–21.

—— Graham, P., Yule, W. (1970) *A Neuropsychiatric Study in Childhood. Clinics in Developmental Medicine, Nos 35/36.* London: SIMP with Heinemann Medical; Philadelphia: J.B. Lippincott.

Sattler, J.M. (1982) *Assessment of Children's Intelligence.* Philadelphia: W.B. Saunders.

Scherzer, A.L., Gardner, G.G. (1971) 'Studies of the school age child with meningomyelocele: 1. Physical & intellectual development.' *Pediatrics*, **47**, 424–430.

Schwartz, E. (1974) 'Characteristics of speech and language development in the child with myelomeningocele and hydrocephalus.' *Journal of Speech and Hearing Disorders*, **39**, 465–468.

Selker, R.G., Steward, M., Cairns, N., Chalub, E. (1973) 'Effect of "elapsed time" and "insults" on mental development in hydrocephalus.' *Journal of Surgical Research*, **14**, 478–482.

Sella, A., Foltz, E.L., Shurtleff, D.B. (1966) 'A three year developmental study of treated and untreated hydrocephalus in children.' *Journal of Pediatrics*, **69**, 88.

Sklayne, K.D. (1982) *Factors Governing the School Placement of Children with Spina Bifida and Hydrocephalus.* University of Manchester: Ph.D. thesis.

Spain, B. (1974) 'Verbal and performance ability in preschool children with spina bifida.' *Developmental Medicine and Child Neurology*, **16**, 773–780.

Spaulding, B., Morgan, S. (1986) 'Spina bifida children and their parents: a population prone to family disfunction?' *Journal of Pediatric Psychology*, **11**, 359–374.

Stambrook, M., Cardoso, E., Hawryluk, G., Eirikson, P., Piatek, D., Sicz, G. (1988) 'Neuropsychological changes following the neurosurgical treatment of normal pressure hydrocephalus. *Archives of Clinical Neuropsychology*, **3**, 323–330.

Stanworth, A. (1969) *Squint in Hydrocephalus: An Analysis of Cases in Strabismus.* London: Henry Kimpton.

Stark, G.D., Drummond, M. (1970) 'Spina bifida as an obstetric problem.' *Developmental Medicine and Child Neurology*, **12** (Suppl. 22), 157–160.

Stellman, G.R., Bannister, C.M. (1982) 'The first three years: a comparative study of the developmental assessment of premature and full term hydrocephalic children.' *Zeitschrift für Kinderchirurgie*, **37**, 182–183.

—— —— (1985) 'Factors predicting developmental outcome in premature infants with hydrocephalus due to intraventricular haemorrhage.' *Zeitschrift für Kinderchirurgie*, **40**, 24–26.

Stough, C., Nettlebeck, T., Ireland, G. (1988) 'Objectively identifying the cocktail party syndrome among children with spina bifida.' *The Exceptional Child*, **35**, 23–30.

Strauss, A.A., Lehtinen, L.E. (1947) *Psychopathology & Education of the Brain Injured Child, Vol. 1.* New York: Grune & Stratton.

Taylor, E.M. (1961) *The Psychological Appraisal of Children with Cerebral Defects.* Cambridge, Mass.: Harvard University Press.

Tew, B. (1979) 'The "cocktail party syndrome" in children with hydrocephalus and spina bifida.' *British*

Journal of Disorders of Communication, **14**, 89–101.
—— (1984) 'Teacher's ranking of learning difficulties found among spina bifida children.' *Link*, **8**, 17–19.
—— (1986) 'The adolescent with spina bifida: academic achievement and employment prospects.' *British Journal of Special Education*, **13**, 22–26.
—— (1988) 'Spina bifida children in ordinary schools: handicap, attainment and behaviour.' *Zeitschrift für Kinderchirurgie*, **43**, 46–48.
—— (1989a) 'Spina bifida and hydrocephalus.' *In* Jones, N. (Ed.) *Special Educational Needs Review, Vol. 2.* Lewes: Falmer Press. pp. 127–141.
—— (1989b) *The Physical, Psychological and Educational Abilities of a Series of Spina Bifida Children Subjected to a Selective Surgical Treatment Policy. End of Grant Report.* Peterborough: ASBAH.
—— Laurence, K.M. (1972) 'The ability and attainments of spina bifida patients born in South Wales between 1956 and 1962.' *Developmental Medicine and Child Neurology*, **14** (Suppl. 27), 124–131.
—— —— (1973) 'Mothers, brothers and sisters of spina bifida patients.' *Developmental Medicine and Child Neurology*, **15** (Suppl. 29), 69–76.
—— —— Samuel, P. (1974) 'Parental estimates of the intelligence of their physically handicapped child.' *Developmental Medicine and Child Neurology*, **16**, 494–501.
—— —— (1975) 'The effects of hydrocephalus on intelligence, visual perception and school attainments.' *Developmental Medicine and Child Neurology*, **17** (Suppl. 35), 129–135.
—— —— (1978a) 'Ocular defect, intellectual and motor performance in children with spina bifida cystica.' *Zeitschrift für Kinderchirurgie*, **25**, 324–330.
—— —— (1978b) 'Differences in reading achievement between spina bifida children attending normal schools and those attending special schools.' *Child: Care, Health and Development*, **4**, 317–326.
—— —— Richards, A. (1980) 'Inattention among children with hydrocephalus and spina bifida.' *Zeitschrift für Kinderchirurgie*, **31**, 381–386.
—— —— (1983) 'Spina bifida children's intelligence test scores on school entry and at school leaving.' *Child: Care, Health and Development*, **9**, 13–17.
—— Evans, R., Thomas, M., Ford, J. (1985) 'The results of a selective treatment policy on the cognitive abilities of children with spina bifida.' *Developmental Medicine and Child Neurology*, **27**, 606–614.
—— Jenkins, V. (1990) 'Factors affecting employability among young adults with spina bifida and hydrocephalus.' *Zeitschrift für Kinderchirurgie*, **45**, 34–36.
Thomas, A.P., Bax, M.C.O., Smyth, D.P.L. (1989) *The Health and Social Needs of Young Adults with Physical Disabilities. Clinics in Developmental Medicine, No. 106.* London: Mac Keith Press with Blackwell Scientific; Philadelphia: J.B. Lippincott.
Turner, A. (1968) 'Upper limb function of children with myelomeningocele.' *Developmental Medicine and Child Neurology*, **28**, 790–798.
Wallace, S.J. (1973) 'The effect of upper limb function on mobility of children with myelomeningocele.' *Developmental Medicine and Child Neurology*, **15** (Suppl. 29), 84–91.
Wallander, J.L., Varni, J., Babani, L., Banis, H., Wilcox, K. (1988) 'Children with chronic physical disorders: maternal reports of their psychological adjustment.' *Journal of Pediatric Psychology*, **13**, 197–212.
—— Feldman, W., Varni, J. (1989a) 'Physical status and psychosocial adjustment in children with spina bifida.' *Journal of Pediatric Psychology*, **14**, 89–102.
—— Varni, J. W., Babani, L., Banis, H., DeHaan, C., Wilcox, K. (1989b) 'Disability parameters, chronic strain and adaptation of physically handicapped children and their mothers.' *Journal of Pediatric Psychology*, **14**, 23–42.
Wedell, K. (1973) *Learning and Perceptual Motor Disability in Children.* London: Wiley.
Welch, K. (1980) 'The etiology and classification of hydrocephalus in childhood.' *Zeitschrift für Kinderchirurgie*, **31**, 331–335.
Wills, K.E., Holmbeck, G.N., Dillon, K., McClone, D.G. (1990) 'Intelligence and attainments among children with myelomeningocele.' *Journal of Pediatric Psychology*, **15**, 161–176.
Zeiner, H., Prigatano, G., Pollay, M., Biscoe, C., Smith, R. (1985) 'Ocular motility, visual dysfunction of neuropsychological impairment in children with shunted, uncomplicated hydrocephalus.' *Childs Nervous System*, **1**, 115–122.
Ziviani, J., Hayes, A., Chant, D. (1990) 'Handwriting: a perceptual motor disturbance in children with myelomeningocele.' *Occupational Therapy Research*, **10**, 12–26.

179

11

THE EFFECT OF NEURAL TUBE DEFECTS ON THE FAMILY AND ITS SOCIAL FUNCTIONING

Janet Carr

Each child that enters a family alters to some extent the structure and functioning of that family. Other family members make way for and adjust to the newcomer, experience some degree of deprivation from the new competitor for attention, and also some degree of reward from the new companion or playmate. Where the child is disabled the normal balance between positive and negative expectations may be disrupted. The new family member may need a larger share of available resources, of time, energy, attention and caring; and the contribution that s/he can be expected to make is uncertain.

Some writers have felt this effect to be mainly an adverse one (Goldie 1966, Younghusband *et al.* 1970), others that families suffer severe strain (Anderson and Spain 1977) and need considerable support in the task of coping with the disabled child (Walker *et al.* 1971, Tew 1974).

Studies in widely differing areas of childhood disability have concluded that the burden of providing care for a disabled child falls squarely on the mother, and much interest has been shown in the effect this has on her. Almost universally, mothers of disabled children are found to have higher scores overall on measures of stress than mothers of non-disabled children. Table 11.I gives the mean scores from a number of studies on one such measure, Rutter's Malaise scale (Rutter *et al.* 1970).

All the mean scores for mothers of disabled children are higher than those of the non-disabled with the exception of mothers of Down syndrome children in the Surrey survey (whose mean is however higher than that of their own control group). The highest mean score in Table 11.I, nearly double that of most other groups, is that obtained from mothers of very severely disabled children who had applied for help to the Family Fund* (Bradshaw 1980). Evidence of increased stress is shown not only by mean scores but also by the proportions of mothers with very high scores. Thirty-two per cent of Dorner's (1975) group had malaise scores of 7 or more, as did 28 per cent and 26 per cent of mothers in the Greater London Council (GLC) study who completed the malaise scale when their child was aged 11 and again at 12 (Carr *et al.* 1983). In contrast, only 11 per cent of mothers of non-disabled children in two separate studies had scores of 7 or more (Rutter *et al.* 1975,

---

*A special fund established by the British government in the wake of the thalidomide tragedy, and administered by the Joseph Rowntree Memorial Trust, based in York.

TABLE 11.I

Mean scores on Rutter's Malaise scale of mothers of disabled and of non-disabled children

		Mean scores, mothers of:	
		disabled children	non-disabled children
Dorner 1980*		5.13	
Tew and Laurence 1973*		6.08	
Carr *et al.* 1983*:	6 yrs	4.86	
	11 yrs	4.59	
	12 yrs	4.57	
Wallander *et al.* 1989**		5.7	
Ferguson and Watt 1980†		5.1	
Carr 1988†		3.5	
Bradshaw 1980‡		9.02	
Rutter *et al.* 1970			3.2
Rutter *et al.* 1975			4.15
Carr 1988			2.3

*	=	mothers of children with spina bifida
**	=	mothers of children with spina bifida and cerebral palsy
†	=	mothers of children with learning disability
‡	=	mothers of children with mixed, very severe, disability

Carr, in preparation), the difference between Dorner's and Rutter's figures being significant at the 0.001 level.

Some studies have not found mothers of disabled children to score more highly on measures of stress: Spaulding and Morgan (1986) could find no differences between mothers of non-retarded spina bifida children and mothers of non-disabled controls. They referred to studies of families of chronically ill children in support of their thesis that the functioning of these families is little different from that of families in the general population. But they cautioned against extrapolating their results to other groups; in particular they felt that 'It is likely that the combination of mental retardation and spina bifida would result in a different picture of child and family functioning', an expectation supported by findings from the South Wales study (Tew and Laurence 1975) but not by those from the GLC study (Carr *et al.* 1983).

Nevertheless the majority of studies of physically and mentally disabled children (only a minority of the latter have been instanced here) have concluded that such families do show higher levels of stress overall. So what are the factors that produce this stress? McCormick *et al.* (1986), using a scale developed by Stein and Riessman (1980), explored the impact on the family of the child's condition (spina bifida) and related this to the abilities, activities and health problems of the child, socio-demographic characteristics of the family, expenses incurred and parental perception of the child's health. The higher the 'impact' score, the more severe was the effect on family life. Higher scores were related to single parent status, low maternal education and family income, and to extra expenses; and, where the child was concerned, to limitation on activities (such as walking, toileting and play), IQ below 70 and parental perception of the child's health. Level of lesion and presence of a shunt were not significantly associated with higher scores. Overall the mean 'impact' score of 44.6 was similar to that of 48.0 derived from a sample of children with a variety of chronic illnesses. The major predictors of high impact on the family were limitations on the child's activities and the parents' perception of the child's health, followed by resources need (*e.g.* education, insurance and family income), number of visits to the doctor and father's employment status. It is interesting that it was the family's perception of the child's abilities and health, rather than health status as such (*i.e.* level of lesion), that had an effect; while although no normative data are given it seems feasible that many of the factors noted—poor educational, financial, social and employment status and overcrowding in the home—would be likely to have an impact on any family regardless of the child's condition.

Several studies have explored the effect of the different levels of disability. It would seem almost self-evident that mothers of very severely disabled children would be more stressed than those of the more lightly disabled and these expectations have been supported in some studies. Mothers whose children with spina bifida were incontinent, immobile, had IQs of less than 80, and attended special schools had higher Malaise scores than mothers whose children were more lightly disabled (Tew and Laurence 1975). In their group of 20 families of spina bifida children, Nevin *et al.* (1979) found families with a child with severe physical problems to be significantly more likely to be stressed. Kazak and Williams-Clark (1986) found a nonsignificant trend for mothers of the more severely disabled children to report more stress, and both mothers and fathers to report more in areas of the child's distractability and activity if the child were severely rather than more lightly disabled. Other studies, however, have not been able to identify a significant relationship between degree of disability in the child and measures of stress in the mother. Wallander *et al.* (1989) found no relationship between mother's Malaise score and the child's disability, and Dorner (1975) found no relationship between any aspect of the child's condition and maternal depression. Bradshaw (1988), reporting on one of the largest studies of families of very severely affected children, showed that mother's Malaise score was not related to measures of the child's condition, type of impairment, or degree of disability. Similarly in the GLC study there was no association between maternal Malaise score and locomotor disability, incontinence, intelligence (or the combination of all three), measures of the child's dependency, or length or number of hospital admissions (Carr *et al.* 1983). Bradshaw (1980) showed that mothers of children requiring attention at night had higher Malaise scores, but no such effect was seen in the GLC study.

Working mothers had lower Malaise scores in Bradshaw's (1980) but not in the GLC study, although the 'unrestricted paid work' referred to in Bradshaw's study may have differed from the working conditions of the mothers in the GLC study.

Again Bradshaw (1988) indicated that Malaise scores were lower when 'net disposable resources' increased; but help from the Family Fund, including financial help, made no significant difference to Malaise scores. Stress was not influenced by age of the mother or child, family composition, housing conditions or degree of restriction of the mother (Bradshaw 1988). Similarly in the GLC study, although disability (locomotor disability, incontinence and the two combined) was strongly related to the parents' social life, and in particular to the mother's ability to go out on her own during the day, no effect of social restriction was seen on maternal Malaise scores. Paternal involvement had no noticeable effect on Malaise scores, nor did the presence or otherwise of a confidante, nor whether the mother had recently visited the doctor.

In the Scottish families with children with learning disabilities studied by Ferguson and Watt (1980), social class was highly significant: but in the GLC study, the trend to higher Malaise scores in working-class families was not significant.

Factors which have been found significantly related to Malaise scores include the general health and behaviour of the child; the feeling that relations and friends gave enough help (Bradshaw 1988); mothers' ratings of their own health; and especially whether or not mothers felt they were depressed or troubled by their nerves (Carr *et al.* 1983). All these factors are based on subjective data, on feelings and opinions expressed by the mothers, and not on objective findings. Bradshaw commented that 'None of the really independent variables examined either in combination or separately is making a great impact on the level of stress experienced by mothers as measured by the Malaise score . . . There may be other independent factors that have not been uncovered in this study which are important determinants of stress but we are confident that no external factors that could account for much variation in the Malaise score had been overlooked' (Bradshaw 1980).

Marital relationships and divorce

Parents coping with the anxiety, sadness and physical exhaustion caused by the needs of a spina bifida child might be expected to find strains appearing in their marriage, and this possibility has been investigated. In parents of very young spina bifida children (two years or less), two thirds of the parents felt their relationship had not been affected and a further 12 per cent that the family had been drawn closer together. In just under a quarter the relationship had deteriorated and in three (1.5 per cent) it had broken down (Walker *et al.* 1971). Of the 29 parents in Martin's (1975) study, 17 per cent thought the marriage was unchanged and nearly half (45 per cent) that the parents had been brought closer together, while over a third (38 per cent) felt the marriage was stressed. Martin also found that five out of 34 spina bifida children (15 per cent) were not living with their natural parents, compared with two out of 119 (1.7 per cent) of the control group, a difference significant, at the 0.006 level. However, figures from the Family Fund showed that 'the only disabling condition with a significantly lower proportion of families headed by a single parent than would be expected in a normal population is spina bifida (10.3 per cent)' (Bradshaw 1988).

In a longitudinal study, Tew *et al.* (1974) examined marital harmony after the birth of the child and again eight to nine years later. At birth, 70 per cent in both the index and control groups had satisfactory marriages, but in the later study this was the case in only 46 per cent of the index families, while in the controls the figure had improved slightly to 79 per cent, the difference between the two groups now being significant at the 0.001 level. In a follow-up of the same groups at 18 years, marital harmony, as judged by an experienced social worker, did not differ between the groups, with three quarters of the index and four fifths of the controls being judged to have harmonious relationships (Evans *et al.* 1986).

In one study (Kazak and Williams-Clark 1986), marital satisfaction was related to severity of the spina bifida child's condition, but in an unexpected direction: marital satisfaction was highest for both mothers and fathers of the more severely disabled children and lowest for those of the least severely disabled. This study then lends support to the view that having a disabled child can bring a family closer together, and suggests that the more severe the child's disability the stronger is this effect.

Evans *et al.* (1986) found no differences in divorce rates between families with and without a spina bifida child, and similar findings are revealed by other studies (Tew *et al.* 1974, Dorner 1975, Martin 1975). So we must be sceptical about the claim by Romans-Clarkson *et al.* (1986), that 'Most writers have found considerable marital conflict present in families with handicapped children, often resulting in an increased rate of divorce', referencing four studies: two of those cited do not mention divorce (Gath 1972, Dupont 1986) and a third (Sabbeth and Leventhal 1984) describes six controlled studies, including two of spina bifida children, none of which found a higher divorce rate for the families of disabled than of non-disabled children.

Social life
Studies of social networks suggest that families of disabled children are not more isolated than other families (Kazak and Williams-Clark 1986), although network density (the extent to which members of the network know and interact with each other, a factor which has been related to stress) was higher for disabled children's families (Kazak and Williams-Clark 1986, Kazak 1987).

Less severely stressed families were the more likely to be involved in recreational interpersonal and community activities (Nevin *et al.* 1979), although it is not clear whether only the less stressed families were able to put their energies into these activities or whether the activities themselves were a stress protector.

In the GLC spina bifida survey, over half the mothers could rarely or never leave their children in the day, and this was significantly related to locomotor disability and to both locomotor and incontinence problems. Only the combined disability rating was significant for evening outings for the parents together. Eighty per cent of the families took their children on outings 'fairly often', the degree to which they did this being similar to that of families with a non-disabled child. However, mothers of the more severely disabled children found this much more difficult and needed much more help than mothers of the less disabled children, both when the children were very small (Anderson and Spain 1977) and later at 11 (Carr *et al.* 1983). No such effect was seen on holidays: there was no relationship between the number of holidays families had had, either with or without the child, and the child's level of disability.

Where the child is more severely disabled, mothers could be expected to have more severely restricted social lives which could be related to greater stress. Dorner (1975) found a close relationship between impaired mobility of the child and restricted social life for the parent. He did not investigate the effect of social restriction on depression, but depression was not related to the child's mobility. The GLC study found mobility, and mobility and incontinence combined, to be strongly related to restrictions on the parent's social life, but as already discussed these restrictions were not related to measures of stress in the mothers.

Effect on the fathers
In families of non-disabled children, fathers have been shown to be playing an increasingly active role with their children (Newson and Newson 1963, 1976) and this participation was also considered in fathers of children with spina bifida. In the GLC study over half the fathers of those 11- and 12-year-olds who needed help were said to help a great deal. However, this varied with the task concerned: about half helped with childcare, and three quarters looked after the children while the mother was out and played with them (though more would play indoor than outdoor games with them). Contrary to the expectation that fathers would do more for the more severely disabled child, where more help was needed, significantly more fathers of continent than of incontinent children took them out. Relationships with locomotor disability were not significant, though there was a tendency for more fathers of non-disabled children to play with them, both in and out of doors. Fathers generally did not seem to make particular efforts to involve themselves with the more disabled child and incontinence seemed especially difficult for fathers to cope with.

Evans *et al.* (1986) looked at similar factors over a longer period of time. At three years, control fathers were slightly more likely to be involved in dressing, bathing and reading to the child, but the majority of both groups were involved at least sometimes in these activities. At 15 years index fathers were significantly more likely than controls to be involved in the child's personal care but less likely to be involved when all activities (including homework, sport and hobbies) were considered. By 18 years both groups of fathers were less involved than previously but even at this time 30 per cent of the fathers were at least sometimes involved in personal care of the spina bifida child, and this was not affected by the father's age or employment nor by the child's sex.

Looking at personal satisfaction and health, Kazak and Williams-Clark (1986) obtained data from mothers and fathers separately but found no differences between them regarding marital satisfaction or stress. Spaulding and Morgan's (1986) study yielded similar results. In the GLC study, where almost all the data were contributed by the mothers, less than a quarter (21 per cent) of the fathers were said to be in poor or very poor health, and only 7 per cent to have been troubled with their nerves in the past year, compared with 43 per cent and 36 per cent respectively of the mothers. Evans *et al.* (1986) reported that the health of fathers of spina bifida children and controls did not differ until the child was about 14 years old, when significantly fewer of the index fathers were said to have good health (48 per cent *vs* 80 per cent, significant at less than the 0.001 level). By the time the children had reached 18 years this process had gone further and index fathers reported more health problems than mothers and fathers of the controls, and also more than their own wives. Although differences in the incidence of individual problems were not significant, index fathers had a particularly high level of orthopaedic problems, and a higher level than the control fathers of indigestion, bowel problems and nervous troubles, although in the latter they were outstripped by mothers in both groups.

In the South Wales study no differences in social class were seen at any point between the two groups. By 18 years, however, 22 per cent of fathers of spina bifida children were claiming invalidity benefit compared with only 4 per cent of the controls (Evans *et al.* 1986).

Effect on siblings
Parents worry that a disabled child may have an adverse effect on the other children in the family, and views have been put forward in support of this thesis (Walker *et al.* 1971) and against it (Seligman 1983). One much quoted study showed that sibs of children with spina bifida were almost four times as likely to show signs of maladjustment as measured by the Bristol Social Adjustment Guide (BSAG) (Stott 1963) as were sibs of controls (Tew and Laurence 1973). However the spina bifida child's position in the family had no effect on the sibs' BSAG scores, and contrary to expectations sibs of the most lightly disabled children presented as the least well adjusted, having the highest mean BSAG score (19), followed by that of the severely disabled group (17.3). Well below these came that for the group with moderate disabilities (8.27). The significance of these differences is not given but clearly there was no straightforward relationship between degree of disability in the index child and maladjustment in the sibs.

In the GLC spina bifida survey, health and behaviour problems of sibs of 11-year-olds with spina bifida were no greater than those of sibs of children with Down syndrome or of controls (Carr and Hewett 1982). Nearly half the mothers of the spina bifida children (45 per cent) thought the other sibs had suffered from the presence of the disabled child: that holidays and outings were more difficult, that the sibs had been overrelied on, had missed out on attention or had had to put up with the plenitude of hospital visits when the spina bifida child was young. Fourteen per cent felt the other children had benefitted, mainly through gaining extra compassion and awareness of the difficulties faced by disabled people. Nearly a quarter (24 per cent) felt the other children had both benefitted and suffered, and 17 per cent that the disabled child had not affected the other children's lives. No relationship could be found between the child's disability level and benefit, but locomotor disability, and locomotor disability and incontinence combined, were related at the 0.05 and 0.001 level respectively with the judgement that the sibs had been adversely affected. The idea that locomotor disability was the most hampering to the families was borne out by the list of activities—walks, trips out, going out on the spur of the moment—which the families missed. 'You can't ever just get up and go, it's got to be planned all the time' is a common complaint (Carr *et al.* 1983).

Nevertheless the majority of sibs are said to be helpful and understanding, and few show jealousy or resentment (Anderson and Spain 1977). Less than half the mothers in the GLC survey felt there was jealousy between the children, compared with 54 per cent in the Nottingham and 30 per cent in the Surrey surveys of normal children. None of the measures of the relationships between spina bifida children and their sibs showed any effect of the degree of the child's disability, nor could any difference be found on these measures between the non-disabled and the disabled spina bifida children (Carr *et al.* 1983).

Financial factors

Evidence has accumulated to show that families with a disabled child suffer financial disadvantage (Social Policy Research Unit 1981, Baldwin 1985). Paternal earnings have been found not to be significantly affected (Piachaud *et al.* 1981, Evans *et al.* 1986), though Baldwin demonstrated that while this was broadly true for fathers of disabled children in manual occupations, those in non-manual occupations earned substantially less than their counterparts without a disabled child. However, the studies agree about women's employment, especially as the children in the family grow older. Few differences are found when there is a young child in the family (whether or not the child is disabled), but differences emerge when the youngest child is aged six plus and still more after the age of 11. Fewer mothers of 18-year-olds with spina bifida were working (42 per cent compared with 65 per cent of controls), and they earned less (Evans *et al.* 1986). Piachaud *et al.* (1981) showed conflicting effects: in one-child families the mother was less likely to work and worked shorter hours, whereas the reverse was true in three-child families. It may be that in a larger family there are older children who can act as carers for the disabled child; financial pressures may be more insistent and the women themselves may have more need to work as a respite from home life. Baldwin (1985) demonstrated clearly that, with increasing age of the youngest child, women with a disabled child were disadvantaged in their ability to work and in their hours and earnings. Mothers of the more severely disabled—especially of children with fits and severe difficulties in mobility and communication—had more problems in working than the mothers of children without these disabilities.

So work and earnings are markedly reduced in families with a disabled child. Statutory allowances (*e.g.* the attendance allowance) go only some of the way towards closing the gap between the incomes of families with and without a disabled child. These allowances are intended to compensate families for the extra expense of having a disabled child. Baldwin (1985) found that while such families spent less on alcohol, adult clothing and housing (all areas where presumably the adults could forgo their own non-essential outlay), they spent more on food, fuel, transport, household goods and services, and children's clothing. These expenses added up to a total of £5.43 per week (equivalent to £11.83 at 1988 prices). It seems that families are not adequately compensated, but are in fact quite severely penalised financially for having a child with spina bifida.

Ethnic and cultural factors

Most research into the stress on families with a spina bifida child have considered families which were predominantly white, European, American or Australasian. For families who do not fall within these boundaries, the difficulties and stresses may be even more severe. Battle and Gobble (1982) suggested that black American families with a spina bifida child are likely to be especially disadvantaged because of their higher rate of unemployment and poverty, reduced health-care benefits, and reluctance to use medical services that would demand payment in advance. Looking further afield, to Nigeria, the picture changes to the point where it becomes barely recognisable. In a review of one year's intake (Oyewole *et al.* 1985), all but two cases were seen before the child was eight weeks old. Most families had long, difficult journeys to the hospital, 14 per cent travelling 400 to 600 kilometres, and almost 50 per cent of the mothers travelling without an adult companion. Seventy-four of the 76 couples had never heard of the condition, 21 attributed it to witchcraft and 16 fathers blamed it on the mother's hours of work, which necessitated her being out at times when spirits were abroad. Whether the child received surgical treatment was related to the mother's educational level: all four children of mothers who had completed higher education were surgically treated, compared with 45 per cent of those whose mothers had had primary education and 12 per cent of those of mothers who were illiterate. Where treatment had been instituted and had shown that no further surgery would be useful, families (from all ethnic groups and social classes) stopped coming to the clinic. In their home setting mothers had tried to hide the child's condition from neighbours, and families urged the mother to get rid of the child. The traditional source of support in this society—the extended family—was almost totally lacking and the authors concluded that many defaulters (those that did not return to the clinic) must have died early deaths. 'No information exists in Nigeria on the long-term problems of children with spina bifida' (Oyewole *et al.* 1985).

Help for the families

Families have traditionally received help from a range of medical and educational sources. Few have received psychological help, but group therapy has been proposed where intrafamily difficulties exist (Apodaca 1982, Clarke 1986) while behavioural methods may be valuable in enabling the parents to deal with learning and management problems in their children (Carr 1982, Feldman and Varni 1982, Feldman *et al.* 1983). A programme of social work intervention resulted in maternal Malaise scores decreasing from a mean of 8.5 to 6.9, while there was a fall from 7.7 to 6.9 in a comparison group of mothers (Bradshaw 1988). On a more practical level it is clear that families suffer considerable financial disadvantage from the presence of a child with spina bifida, and it seems obvious that they need financial help. One-off financial provision, such as that provided by the Family Fund, has had little effect in alleviating stress (Bradshaw 1988), but this is not to say that an adequate and permanent entitlement would not give more effective relief. Bradshaw (1988) argued eloquently that families have a moral right to this because 'society needs women to have babies to survive', and all members of society run the risk of having a disabled child. Without the care given by parents, society would be landed with a crippling financial burden. The families, in Bradshaw's words, 'have an unanswerable moral claim to adequate support'.

Conclusions

With the myriad problems faced by children with spina bifida—incontinence, locomotor problems, hydrocephalus, infections, intellectual difficulties and repeated hospitalisation—it would not be surprising if families of such children were stressed, depressed, overburdened and complaining. Although families can be found to fit this description the surprise is that they are comparatively few. While studies of families are often effectively studies of the mothers, consideration has also been given to fathers and sibs. Many fathers give a good deal of help with their children but this help continues (understandably perhaps) to be far below that given by the mothers, and to be concerned predominantly with supervision and play rather than with practical tasks, especially where incontinence is concerned. Anderson and Spain (1977) showed how much of a tie it is for mothers who are the only ones who can change or empty a child's incontinence appliance. They wrote: 'This whole area of incontinence is one where it is most essential to involve the father', but this does not seem to have happened to a great extent. The health of fathers of spina bifida children is generally better than that of the mothers, at least while the child is young, and at all ages they suffer less than their wives from nervous troubles. Although fathers are often closely concerned with their disabled children, mothers may be subject to more severe anxiety because of their greater level of day-to-day contact.

Although the South Wales study found that siblings of spina bifida children were more likely to be maladjusted, few objective measures have shown the sibs to be disadvantaged and this is in accordance with reports from studies of the sibs themselves (Hart and Walters 1981). Mothers, on the other hand, felt their children had suffered and were more likely to think this where the child was disabled, especially where there was a locomotor disability. Mothers were only too aware of the limitations that the child's condition imposed on family activities (especially those involving physical exertion), and of how much the other children missed out on this account. Mothers 'seemed to take a slightly more pessimistic view of the restrictions than siblings, according to Hart and Walters (1981). Where there is a disabled child in the family, parents are often worried about the effect on their other children, and parents of the physically disabled child in particular may take some comfort from the comparatively robust view taken by the siblings themselves.

A common finding is that mothers of disabled children show evidence of greater stress than mothers of non-disabled children. There is also much agreement that socio-economic factors, and the mother's subjective view of the conditions of her life, are positively associated with her level of stress. Much more difficult to show, however, is a clear relationship between this stress and factors which an outsider might think would cause it. Objective measures of factors such as the child's disability in all its various forms: dependency, limitations on the parents' social life, health and living conditions are seldom found to be significantly related to maternal stress. The exception is the South Wales study: the children seemed to have reasonably similar levels of disability to the children in the GLC study, but social class patterns were different, with the GLC study containing a much higher proportion of social class I and II families (19 per cent *vs* 7 per cent) and a lower proportion of social class V (2 per cent *vs* 33 per cent). Ferguson and Watt (1980) showed low social class to be associated with increased Malaise scores, but the present data do not show whether the differences between the South Wales and the GLC studies are in any way due to differences in social class. Since a relationship between factors related to the child's condition and stress in the mother would be expected and easy to understand, the absence of such a relationship poses a problem. Bradshaw (1980) suggested that stress is 'determined by internal factors, the physiology and personality of the mother' and that situations and events which would be rated as stressful by a disinterested observer seem to have remarkably little selective effect on the degree of stress that mothers report.

An exception to this statement is the general finding of higher levels of stress in mothers of affected than of unaffected children. Since these children include those with minimal levels of disability it is not easy to account for this finding. Perhaps having a child with any kind of abnormality is enough to raise a mother's anxiety level: she may not know nor want to consider how her child's disability compares with another's—*i.e.* whether her child's disability is 'better' or 'worse' than another's. If her child has a disability, then the world may seem uncertain and ominous. She cannot be sure how serious the threat is, and her peace of mind is gone.

This is merely hypothetical, and does not accord well with personal memories of the many cheerful and relaxed families with spina bifida children. Nevertheless, if there is any truth in it, it suggests that services and support should be freely available not only to families of the severely disabled but to families of *all* disabled children: they all carry an increased burden.

REFERENCES

Anderson, E.M., Spain, B. (1977) *The Child with Spina Bifida.* London: Methuen.
Apodaca, L.R. (1982) 'Group therapy for parents of children with spina bifida: evaluating the model.' *Spina Bifida Therapy*, **4**, 217–226.
Baldwin, S.M. (1985) *The Costs of Caring. Families with a Disabled Child.* London: Routledge and Kegan Paul.
Battle, S.F., Gobble, J.T. (1982) 'The effect of spina bifida on blacks.' *Spina Bifida Therapy*, **4**, 209–216.
Bradshaw, J.R. (1980) *The Family Fund.* London: Routledge and Kegan Paul.
—— (1988) 'The social impact of childhood disablement.' *Zeitschrift für Kinderchirurgie*, **43** (Suppl. 2), 5–11.
Carr, J. (1982) 'A behavioural approach to problems of motivation in the spina bifida child.' *Zeitschrift für Kinderchirurgie*, **37**, 184–186.
—— (1988) 'Six weeks to twenty one years old: a longitudinal study of children with Down's syndrome and their families.' *Journal of Child Psychology and Psychiatry*, **29**, 407–431.
—— Hewett, S. (1982) 'Children with Down's syndrome growing up.' *Association for Child Psychology and Psychiatry News*, **10**, 10–13.
—— Pearson, A., Halliwell, M. (1983) *The GLC Spina Bifida Survey: Follow-up at 11 & 12 Years.* London: Research and Statistics Branch, County Hall.
Clarke, E. (1986) 'The use of single session collectivities with families of spina bifida children.' *Social Work with Groups*, **9**, 103–111.
Dorner, S. (1975) 'The relationship of physical handicap to stress in families with an adolescent with spina bifida.' *Developmental Medicine and Child Neurology*, **17**, 765–776.
—— (1980) 'Personal communication.' *In* Bradshaw, J.R. (Ed.) *The Family Fund.* London: Routledge and Kegan Paul.
Dupont, A. (1986) 'Socio-psychiatric aspects of the young severely mentally retarded and the family.' *British Journal of Psychiatry*, **148**, 227–234.
Evans, O., Tew, B., Laurence, K.M. (1986) 'The fathers of children with spina bifida.' *Zeitschrift für Kinderchirurgie*, **41** (Suppl. 1), 42–44.
Feldman, W.S., Varni, J.W. (1982) 'A parent training program for the child with spina bifida.' *Spina Bifida Therapy*, **4**, 77–89.
—— Manella, K.J., Varni, J.W. (1983) 'A behavioural parent training programme for single mothers of physically handicapped children.' *Child: Care, Health and Development*, **9**, 157–168.
Ferguson, N., Watt, J. (1980) 'The mothers of children with special needs.' *Scottish Educational Review*, **12**, 21–31.
Gath, A. (1972) 'The effects of mental subnormality on the family.' *British Journal of Hospital Medicine*, **8**, 147–150.
Goldie, L. (1966) 'Psychiatry of the handicapped family.' *Developmental Medicine and Child Neurology*, **8**, 456–462.
Hart, D., Walters, J. (1981) *Brothers and Sisters of Physically Handicapped Children.* (Unpublished manuscript.)
Kazak, A.E. (1987) 'Families with disabled children: stress and social networks in three samples.' *Journal of Abnormal Child Psychology*, **15**, 137–146.
—— Williams-Clark, M. (1986) 'Stress in families of children with myelomeningocele.' *Developmental Medicine and Child Neurology*, **28**, 220–228.
Martin, P. (1975) 'Marital breakdown in families of patients with spina bifida cystica.' *Developmental Medicine and Child Neurology*, **17**, 757–764.
McCormick, M.C., Charney, E.B., Stemmler, M.M. (1986) 'Assessing the impact of a child with spina bifida on the family.' *Developmental Medicine and Child Neurology*, **28**, 53–61.

191

Nevin, R.S., Easton, J.K.M., McCubbin, H.I.M., Birkebak, R.R. (1979) 'Parental coping in raising children who have spina bifida cystica.' *Zeitschrift für Kinderchirurgie*, **28**, 417–425.

Newson, J., Newson, E. (1963) *Patterns of Infant Care in an Urban Community*. London: George Allen & Unwin.

—— —— (1976) *Seven Years Old in the Home Environment*. London: George Allen & Unwin.

Oyewole, A., Adeloye, A., Addeyokunnu, A.-A. (1985) 'Psychological and cultural factors associated with the management of spina bifida cystica in Nigeria.' *Developmental Medicine and Child Neurology*, **27**, 498–503.

Piachaud, D., Bradshaw, J., Weale, J. (1981) 'The income effect of a disabled child.' *Journal of Epidemiology and Community Health*, **35**, 123–127.

Romans-Clarkson, S.E., Clarkson, J.E., Dittmer, I.D., Flett, R., Linsell, C., Mullen, P.E., Mullin, B. (1986) 'Impact of a handicapped child on the mental health of parents.' *British Medical Journal*, **293**, 1395–1397.

Rutter, M., Tizard, J., Whitmore, K. (1970) *Education, Health and Behaviour*. London: Longmans.

—— Yule, B., Quinton, D., Towland, O., Yule, W., Berger, M. (1975) 'Attainment and adjustment in two geographical areas: III—some factors accounting for area differences.' *British Journal of Psychiatry*, **126**, 520–533.

Sabbeth, B.F., Leventhal, J.M. (1984) 'Marital adjustment to chronic childhood illness: a critique of the literature.' *Pediatrics*, **73**, 762–768.

Seligman, M. (1983) 'Sources of psychological disturbance among siblings of handicapped children.' *The Personnel and Guidance Journal*, **May**, 529–531.

Social Policy Research Unit (1981) *The Financial Consequences of Disablement in Children. Summary, Conclusions & Policy Implications*. Working Paper, DHSS 77 6/81 SB.

Spaulding, B.R., Morgan, S.B. (1986) 'Spina bifida children and their parents: a population prone to dysfunction?' *Journal of Pediatric Psychology*, **11**, 359–374.

Stein, R.E.K., Reissman, C.K. (1980) 'The development of an impact-on-family scale: preliminary findings.' *Medical Care*, **18**, 456–472.

Stott, D.H. (1963) *The Social Adjustment of Children, 2nd Edn*. London: University of London Press.

Tew, B. (1974) 'Spina bifida: family and social problems.' *Special Education*, **1**, 17–20.

—— Laurence, K.M. (1973) 'Mothers, brothers and sisters of spina bifida patients.' *Developmental Medicine and Child Neurology*, **15** (Suppl. 29), 69–76.

—— Payne, H., Laurence, K.M. (1974) 'Must a family with a handicapped child be a handicapped family?' *Developmental Medicine and Child Neurology*, **16** (Suppl. 32), 95–98.

—— Laurence, K.M. (1975) 'Some sources of stress found in mothers of spina bifida children.' *British Journal of Preventive and Social Medicine*, **29**, 27–30.

Walker, J.H., Thomas, M., Russell, I.T. (1971) 'Spina bifida and the parents.' *Developmental Medicine and Child Neurology*, **13**, 462–476.

Wallander, J.L., Varni, J.W., Babani, L., Banis, H.T., Dehaan, C.B., Wilcox, K.T. (1989) 'Disability parameters, chronic strain and adaptation of physically handicapped children and their mothers.' *Journal of Pediatric Psychology*, **14**, 23–42.

Younghusband, E., Birchall, D., Davie, R., Kellmer Pringle, M.L. (Eds) (1970) *Living with Handicap*. London: National Bureau for Co-operation in Child Care.

12
GROWTH AND PUBERTY IN CHILDREN WITH CONGENITAL HYDROCEPHALUS

R. Brauner, M. Fontoura and R. Rappaport

Precocious or advanced puberty is the most frequent endocrine manifestation in children treated for non-tumoral hydrocephalus. It can result in a reduction in final adult height, for advanced skeletal maturation leads to premature fusion of the epiphyses. Spinal growth is also reduced by myelomeningocele. Adults treated for hydrocephalus show other abnormalities, including growth hormone deficiency (Barber and Garvan 1979), and primary or secondary amenorrhea with gonadotropin secretion levels suggests a central deficiency or abnormal hypothalamic control (Caporal *et al.* 1983).

This chapter reports the precocious and advanced pubertal development and final height of children who have been treated in the neonatal period for congenital hydrocephalus. We define the criteria used to survey growth and puberty and the therapeutic indications for improving the final height of these children.

Normal pubertal and growth development
Puberty is initiated by the activation or deinhibition of pulsatile secretion of gonadotropin releasing hormone (GnRH) from the hypothalamus. This leads to increased circulating pituitary gonadotropins—luteinising hormone (LH) and follicle stimulating hormone (FSH)—and changes of LH pulsatility. The number and amplitude of the LH peaks increase gradually throughout puberty. Gonadotropin secretion induces gonadal development and steroid secretion, testosterone from testes in boys and oestradiol from ovaries in girls. These hormones are responsible for the gonadarche. The adrenals also affect pubic hair development by increasing dehydroepiandrosterone (DHA) secretion. This stage, called adrenarche, occurs at seven or eight years of age, before gonadarche. It is probably controlled by a central factor that is different from gonadotropins or corticotropin.

Puberty includes the appearance of secondary sexual characteristics and the acceleration of growth. Sexual characteristics appear between eight and 13 years in girls, and between nine and 14 years in boys, in 95 per cent of cases. Pubertal stages are rated from stage 1 (prepubertal) to stage 5 (adult development) (Marshall and Tanner 1969, 1970). In girls, the first sign is breast enlargement and/or pubic hair development which occurs at a mean age of 11.5 years. Menarche occurs at a mean interval of two years after the clinical onset of puberty. In boys, the first sign is enlargement of the testes which occurs at a mean age of 11.6 years. Testicular dimensions greater than 30×20mm indicate activation of the hypothalamo-

193

pituitary-gonadal axis. Growth accelerates during puberty in both sexes: annual height gain increases from 5cm before puberty to 8 or 9cm during the pubertal growth spurt. The mean age at this spurt is 12 years in girls and 14 years in boys. The mean total height gain between the clinical onset of puberty and final height is 27.6 ± 3.6cm in boys and 25.3 ± 4.1cm in girls (Tanner *et al.* 1976). The mean total increase in height between first menstruation and final height is 7cm when first menstruation occurs at 13 years. Pubertal growth acceleration is due to the separate or combined effect of three hormones : sex steroids, growth hormone and insulin-like growth factor I (IGFI).

Precocious and advanced puberty in hydrocephalus

Children with hydrocephalus may have various types of advanced pubertal development: (i) central or true precocious puberty due to premature activation of the hypothalamo-pituitary-gonadal axis with onset before eight years in girls and before nine years in boys; (ii) advanced puberty with onset between eight and 10 years in girls and between nine and 11 years in boys; (iii) premature pubarche or adrenarche, which is a variation of normal pubertal development. It is important to diagnose these situations in order to determine the most appropriate therapeutic approach.

General features

Hydrocephalus is responsible for 5 to 8 per cent of cases of central precocious puberty: 24/294 (8 per cent) in our data, 11/205 (5 per cent) in the report by Kaplan and Grumbach (1990) and 5 per cent in a Japanese study (Tomono *et al.* 1983). In our study of 24 cases, hydrocephalus was congenital in 11 cases and acquired in 13. The characteristics of precocious puberty in each group were similar. Among patients with hydrocephalus, the frequency of central precocious puberty (CPP) is 11 per cent (De Luca *et al.* 1985) or 6 per cent in hydrocephalus associated with myelomeningocele (Meyer and Landau 1984). The supposed pathogenesis of precocious puberty in hydrocephalus is the increased pressure on the hypothalamic region inducing a premature activation of the hypothalamo-pituitary-gonadal axis. However, precocious puberty also occurs in children with arrested hydrocephalus or functional derivation with normal ventricular size or minimal enlargement on CT scan. In children with myelomeningocele, precocious puberty occurred only in those with hydrocephalus (Meyer and Landau 1984). A chronic minimally increased intraventricular pressure may be involved in the induction of precocious puberty.

Diagnosis

PRECOCIOUS PUBERTY

Eleven children were seen in our unit for precocious puberty secondary to congenital hydrocephalus (Table 12.I). The great predominance of girls (10 girls to one boy) was at variance with other reports (13 girls to six boys). As the onset of

194

TABLE 12.I

Characteristics of the patients with CPP secondary to hydrocephalus

Case	Sex	Onset CPP (yrs)	CA (yrs)	BA-CA (yrs)	Pubertal stage	Oe2/T	LH peak iu/l	FSH peak iu/l
1	F	5.2	5.8	1.1	P2 B3	40	21	36
2	F	7.0	8.0	0	P2 B2	25	5.3	6.7
3	F	7.5	8.0	0	P2 B2	95	11	9.7
4	F	7.8	8.2	2.8	P3 B3	10	26	9
5	F	7.8	8.4	2.6	P2 B3	25	—	—
6	F	7.8	8.8	0.2	P2 B3	70	7	6.7
7	F	7.9	8.1	-2.1	P2 B2	15	2.1	10
8	F	8.0	8.4	-0.4	P2 B3	56	18	8.4
9	F	8.0	9.0	0.6	P2 B2	45	68	9.8
10	F	8.0	9.0	2.5	P4 B3	55	12.5	4.8
11	M	8.2	9.0	3.5	P3 50 × 25mm		18	8.4

CPP = central precocious puberty; CA = chronological age; BA = bone age; P = pubic hair; B = breast stage; Oe2 = oestradiol (pg/ml); T = testosterone (ng/ml). Age at diagnosis of hydrocephalus was <0.3 mths in 9 cases (case 1 at 2 yrs; case 5 at 8 mths).

TABLE 12.II

Comparison of the characteristics of the patients with CPP secondary to suprasellar arachnoid cyst and congenital hydrocephalus

	Female/male ratio	CA (yrs)	BA-CA	Plasma Oe2 (pg/ml)	Testosterone (ng/ml)	LH/FSH peak ratio	LH peak iu/l	FSH peak iu/l
Arachnoid cyst	5:4	7.8 ± 1.7	1.3 ± 0.4	58 ± 12	2.4 ± 0.8	2.2 ± 0.3	18.5 ± 3.7	8.3 ± 1.5
Hydrocephalus	10:1	7.6 ± 0.3	1.0 ± 0.5	40 ± 6	4.0	1.6 ± 0.6	18.9 ± 5.9	11.0 ± 2.8

CA = chronological age; BA = bone age; Oe2 = oestradiol.

195

precocious puberty is 'late', a precocious increase in testicular volume in boys with hydrocephalus may have been missed in the absence of systematic evaluation. The etiology of hydrocephalus was: myelomeningocele in six cases and ventricular malformation in five cases. The onset of precocious puberty was rather late, between seven and eight years, except in one case. At first evaluation, all the girls presented with breast and pubic hair development, as evidence of true precocious puberty. The boy presented with an increase in testicular volume, indicating hypothalamo-pituitary-gonadal activation. Bone age, evaluated on x-rays of the hand and wrist according to the atlas of Greulich and Pyle (1970), was advanced by more than 1 SD (nine months to one year) in five out of 11 cases. Plasma oestradiol was at a pubertal level (>25pg/ml or 92pmol/l) in eight out of 10 cases. It was in the prepubertal range in the two remaining cases. This situation usually corresponds to the onset of puberty. As cyclical variations of plasma oestradiol may occur, repeated determination of plasma oestradiol and evaluation of oestrogenic activity by vaginal smears was necessary in these cases. In the boy, as is usual in boys with true precocious puberty, plasma testosterone was in the pubertal range (>0.5ng/ml) at the first evaluation. The gonadotropin response to GnRH test (100µg/m2 IV) was of pubertal type with a predominant LH response and an LH/FSH peak ratio higher than in most cases. Such a response is taken into account when treatment is discussed.

Other pituitary functions were also evaluated. None of the patients presented abnormality of growth hormone secretion under pharmacological stimulation, plasma basal or insulin-induced hypoglycaemia cortisol, basal prolactin, thyroxin or urinary concentration capacity. We therefore conclude that precocious puberty is the only endocrine disorder induced by hydrocephalus (Meyer and Landau 1984). This is at variance with the multiple deficiencies reported in five adults with normal pressure hydrocephalus who had their hypophyseal function assessed (Barber and Garvan 1979). We arrived at the opposite conclusion in children with increased intracranial pressure secondary to a congenital suprasellar arachnoid cyst. Of the 11 patients examined, four had isolated CPP and five had CPP associated with growth hormone deficiency. Three of them also had thyrotropin deficiency (Table 12.II). The peak LH/FSH ratio was higher in this group with precocious puberty (2.2 ± 0.3) than in those with hydrocephalus (1.6 ± 0.4 iu/l). The higher hypothalamo-pituitary pressure induced by the arachnoid cyst may be responsible for the pituitary deficiencies. Neurosurgical decompression of the arachnoid cyst led to a regression of precocious pubertal development in three reported cases (Segall *et al.* 1974, Clark *et al.* 1988, Sweasey *et al.* 1989), with the LH peak decreasing. However, we observed no similar regression in our patients; endocrine abnormalities persisted in spite of effective derivation in all cases (Brauner *et al.* 1987, Pierre-Kahn *et al.* 1990).

ADVANCED PUBERTY
Advanced puberty occurs more frequently in children with hydrocephalus than in

the general population. Ten girls were seen in our unit for advanced puberty secondary to congenital hydrocephalus. Their mean age at onset of puberty was 8.7 ± 0.2 years. At first evaluation, their mean bone age advance over chronological age was 1.2 years. Their mean predicted final height was −2 SD below their target height, which was 0.5 SD. At the last evaluation, eight had menstruated, with a mean age at first menstruation of 10.4 years, confirming other findings that the mean menarcheal age in girls with neural tube defects is significantly lower than that of the general population (Dalton and Dalton 1978). Advanced puberty may reduce final height and require therapy.

Treatment

The therapeutic indications are principally associated with the risk of final height reduction: premature secretion of sex steroids may induce premature cartilage fusion. GnRH analogues induce desensitisation of the pituitary gonadotropin receptors. They are the first choice for therapy as they induce full and permanent suppression of the pituitary gonadal axis and then of the gonadal activity. Breast development regresses and menstruation disappears in girls treated with GnRH analogues. Growth rate decreases to a prepubertal range (4 to 6cm/yr). Bone age progression decreases to less than one year by year of chronological advancement (see Fig. 12.1). This leads to an improvement in the predicted final height (Rappaport *et al.* 1987, Manasco *et al.* 1989). At the onset of therapy, GnRH analogues are responsible for menstruation in 20 to 30 per cent of girls. This menstruation results from the initial gonadotropin stimulation by GnRH analogues, before their inhibitory effect begins. The inclusion of cyproterone acetate at the on-set of GnRH analogue therapy usually prevents or reduces the duration and the intensity of the genital bleeding. We use the following protocol: cyproterone acetate (25mg/m2/d orally) 15 days before and one month after the first GnRH analogue injection. We use a long-acting form (Decapeptyl®, D-Trp^{6}GnRH analogue).

GnRH analogue therapy induces regression of secondary sexual characteristics, arrests the decrease in predicted final height, and probably improves it. But it is not certain whether such a therapy is appropriate for all children with precocious and advanced puberty secondary to congenital hydrocephalus. In our experience with idiopathic CPP, the risk of final height reduction is present in all boys and in only about 70 per cent of girls, as there are spontaneously regressive or slowly evolving forms in girls (Fontoura *et al.* 1989). In hydrocephalus, oestrogenisation seems to be progressive in most of the girls. Therefore we suggest that GnRH analogue therapy be initiated in all children with precocious puberty secondary to hydrocephalus, except those with a small breast development and plasma oestradiol below 25pg/ml. In these girls, a longitudinal twice-yearly survey may help to identify cases in which GnRH analogue therapy is necessary; we suggest waiting three to six months before beginning such therapy. We have observed one regressive case and treatment could be postponed by three years in another girl. A test of the gonadotropin response to GnRH may be helpful in arriving at a

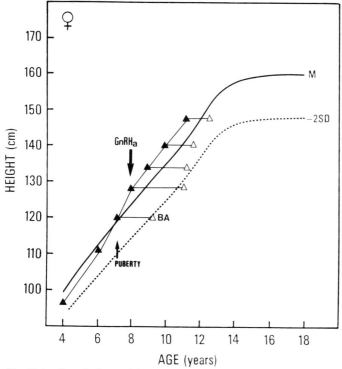

Fig. 12.1. Growth in a girl suffering from central precocious puberty secondary to congenital hydrocephalus. Pubertal development occurred at seven years. GnRH analogue therapy decreased bone age (BA) progression and thus preserved growth capacity.

therapeutic decision, as we have shown that an LH predominant response indicates a more marked hypothalamic activation and is seen predominantly in the evolving forms (Brauner *et al.* 1991). GnRH analogue therapy is also indicated in the developing forms of advanced puberty (onset between eight and 10 years), as these patients frequently have advanced bone ages. The height standard deviation score before puberty is also important, as we believe that the need to stop puberty is greater in children with expected genetic short stature prior to pubertal development.

Final height

There are few data on the final height of children with hydrocephalus. In those treated with cyproterone acetate or medroxyprogesterone for CPP, the predicted final height at the last evaluation was 1 to 1.7 SD below the target parental height (De Luca *et al.* 1985, Brauner *et al.* 1987). Children with myelomeningocele had lower heights than those with hydrocephalus secondary to other causes. In children with myelomeningocele the trunk was short, reflecting abnormal vertebral structure and growth (Greene *et al.* 1985). The growth of the arms was not affected, and the authors suggest that this feature excludes an endocrine factor. Bone age advance over chronological age was found in this group from nine years in girls and from 10 years in boys. This is an additional argument for initiating GnRH therapy early in cases with precocious or advanced puberty.

Our experience indicates that the occurrence of precocious or advanced pubertal development in children who have been treated in the neonatal period for hydrocephalus rarely indicates failure of the derivative process. The diagnosis of precocious or advanced pubertal development is based on clinical survey: increased testicular volume in boys and breast development in girls. This advanced pubertal development induces a risk of reduced final height as the majority of forms are progressive. GnRH analogues are indicated in the majority of cases of hydrocephalus with premature pubertal development, though the other pituitary functions are usually normal during childhood. However growth hormone deficiency has been reported in adults with hydrocephalus and in children having raised intracranial pressure secondary to congenital suprasellar arachnoid cysts. In children with congenital hydrocephalus, decreased growth velocity requires evaluation of the growth hormone response for pharmacological stimulation and plasma IGFI concentration as well as the measurement of plasma thyroxine. This permits diagnosis of the growth hormone deficiency and substitution therapy. An apparently normal growth velocity may persist in patients with the combination of precocious puberty and growth hormone deficiency. However at the same time bone age will advance with a definite risk of final short stature. These patients require a combined treatment with growth hormone and an LHRH analogue.

Follow-up of growth and puberty is needed in all these patients, based on periodic clinical evaluation including growth, bone maturation and testicular volume in boys, and development of the sexual characteristics in both sexes.

Summary
In children treated for congenital hydrocephalus, final height may be reduced by advanced skeletal maturation prior to puberty, reduced spinal growth associated with myelomeningocele, and advanced pubertal development. Central precocious puberty (CPP) is due to premature activation of the hypothalamo-pituitary axis with onset before eight years in girls and before nine years in boys. The reported frequency of CPP in this population is 6 to 11 per cent with great predominance in girls. The diagnosis is based on the clinical survey: increased testicular volume in boys and breast development in girls. The therapeutic indications are principally associated with the risk of final height reduction: the premature secretion of sex steroids may induce premature cartilage fusion. GnRH analogues are the first choice for therapy as they induce a suppression of the pituitary gonadal axis leading to an improvement in the predicted final height. They are indicated in the majority of cases of hydrocephalus with progressive pubertal development. In children the other pituitary functions are usually normal. However growth hormone deficiency and amenorrhoea have been reported in adults with hydrocephalus. The

presentation of these endocrine disorders suggests an impairment of hypothalamic control. Although some evidence was presented in favour of the role of increased intraventricular pressure, most cases develop precocious puberty at a time when there is no evidence of disturbed intracranial pressure.

ACKNOWLEDGEMENTS

We thank M. Lacroix for the preparation of this manuscript and Drs A. Pierre-Kahn, J.F. Hirsch, D. Renier and C. Sainte-Rose (Neurosurgical Unit, Hôpital des Enfants Malades) for sending us their patients.

REFERENCES

Barber, S.G., Garvan, N. (1979) 'Hypopituitarism in normal-pressure hydrocephalus.' *British Medical Journal*, 1, 1039–1041.
Brauner, R., Pierre-Kahn, A., Nemedy-Sandor, E., Rappaport, R., Hirsch, J.F. (1987) 'Pubertés précoces par kyste arachnoidien suprasellaire.' *Archives Françaises de Pédiatrie*, **44**, 489–493.
—— Rappaport, R., Nicod, C., Malandry, F., Thibaud, E., Pierre-Kahn, A., Renier, D., Sainte-Rose, C., Hirsch, J.F. (1987) 'Pubertés précoces vraies au cours de l'hydrocéphalie non tumorale.' *Archives Françaises de Pédiatrie*, **44**, 433–436.
—— Malandry, F., Fontoura, M., Prevot, C., Souberbielle, J-C., Rappaport, R. (1991) 'Idiopathic central precocious puberty in girls as a model of the effect of plasma estradiol level on growth, skeletal maturation and plasma IGFI.' *Hormone Research* (in press).
Caporal, R., Segrestaa, J.M., Dorf, G. (1983) 'Endocrine expressions of hydrocephalus. A case of primary amenorrhea revealing a stenosis of the foramen of Magendie.' *Acta Endocrinologica*, **102**, 161–166.
Clark, S.J., Van Drop, C., Conte, F.A., Grumbach, M.M., Berger, M.S., Edwards, M.S.B. (1988) 'Reversible true precocious puberty secondary to a congenital arachnoid cyst.' *American Journal of Diseases of Children*, **142**, 255–256.
Dalton, M.E., Dalton, K. (1978) 'Menarcheal age in the disabled.' *British Medical Journal*, **2**, 475.
De Luca, F., Muritano, M., Rizzo, G., Pandullo, E., Cardia, E. (1985) 'True precocious puberty: a long term complication in children with shunted non-tumoral hydrocephalus.' *Helvetica Paediatrica Acta*, **40**, 467–472.
Fontoura, M., Brauner, R., Prevot, C., Rappaport, R. (1989) 'Precocious puberty in girls: early diagnosis of a slowly progressing variant.' *Archives of Disease in Childhood*, **64**, 1170–1176.
Greene, S.A., Frank, M., Zachmann, M., Prader, A. (1985) 'Growth and sexual development in children with meningomyelocele.' *European Journal of Pediatrics*, **144**, 146–148.
Greulich, W.W., Pyle, S. (1970) *Radiographic atlas of skeletal development of the hand and wrist, 2nd Edn.* Stanford: Stanford University Press.
Kaplan, S.L., Grumbach, M.M. (1990) 'Pathogenesis of sexual precocity.' *In* Grumbach, M.M., Sizonenko, P.C., Aubert, M.L. (Eds) *Control of the Onset of Puberty.* Baltimore: Williams and Wilkins.
Manasco, P.K., Pescovitz, O.H., Hill, S.C., Jones, J.M., Barnes, K.M., Hench, K.D., Loriaux, D.L., Cutler, G.B. Jr. (1989) 'Six years results of luteinizing hormone releasing hormone (LHRH) agonist treatment in children with LHRH-dependent precocious puberty.' *Journal of Pediatrics*, **115**, 105–108.
Marshall, W.A., Tanner, J.M. (1969) 'Variations in the pattern of pubertal changes in girls.' *Archives of Disease in Childhood*, **44**, 291–303.
—— —— (1970) 'Variations in the pattern of pubertal changes in boys.' *Archives of Disease in Childhood*, **45**, 13–23.
Meyer, S., Landau, H. (1984) 'Precocious puberty in myelomeningocele patients.' *Journal of Pediatric Orthopedics*, **4**, 28–31.

Pierre-Kahn, A., Capelle, L., Brauner, R., Sainte-Rose, C., Renier, D., Rappaport, R., Hirsch, J.F. (1990) 'Presentation and management of suprasellar arachnoid cysts.' *Journal of Neurosurgery*, **73**, 355–359.

Rappaport, R., Fontoura, M., Brauner, R. (1987) 'Treatment of central precocious puberty with an LHRH agonist (buserelin): effect on growth and bone maturation after three years of treatment.' *Hormone Research*, **28**, 149–154.

Segall, H.D., Hassan, G., Ling, S.M., Carton, C. (1974) 'Suprasellar cysts associated with isosexual precocious puberty.' *Radiology*, **111**, 607–616.

Sweasey, T.A., Venes, J.L., Hood, T.W., Randall, J.B. (1989) 'Stereotaxic decompression of a prepontine arachnoid cyst with resolution of precocious puberty.' *Pediatric Neurosciences*, **15**, 44–47.

Tanner, J.M., Whitehouse, R.M., Marubine, E., Resle, L.F. (1976) 'The adolescent growth spurt of boys and girls of the Harpenden growth study.' *Annals of Human Biology*, **3**, 109–126.

Tomono, Y., Maki, Y., Ito, M., Nakada, Y. (1983) 'Precocious puberty due to postmeningitic hydrocephalus.' *Brain Development*, **5**, 414–417.

13
SEXUALITY, SEX AND SPINA BIFIDA

Pat Edser and Gillian Ward

Many people with spina bifida have difficulty achieving a mature sexual relationship as they reach adulthood. To some extent a spinal-cord lesion will make a difference to sexual function, but it should not form a barrier to achieving a satisfying and fulfilling adult relationship. The term 'sexual dysfunction' describes the psychological difficulties which impede achievement of a relationship in which sexual capacity and satisfaction are fully expressed. Sexual dysfunction may occur in the able-bodied, and some of the contributory factors are identical to those experienced by the physically disabled, but the individual with spina bifida has other problems which often lead to dysfunction.

The aim of this chapter, therefore, is (i) to explore the reasons why adolescents and adults with spina bifida may have difficulties achieving mature personal and sexual relationships, (ii) to help the professionals working with them to find acceptable solutions to these problems, and (iii) to explain the effect of a spinal-cord lesion (with or without hydrocephalus) on sexual function.

Psychosexual development
Psychosexual development describes the process of sexual development taking into account psychological as well as physical factors.

A baby finds it comfortable, warm and safe to be cuddled, which encourages the mother to prolong body contact. As they grow, small children begin to explore their own bodies and get satisfaction and pleasure from playing with their genitals. By the time they start school, they have begun role-playing and learning games with other children, *e.g.* mothers and fathers, doctors and nurses.

Identification with the same sex occurs shortly after and a child plays primarily with peers of the same sex, sharing their sexual experiences. Children gradually develop a realistic role definition for themselves as either male or female.

Secondary sexual characteristics develop at puberty, and there begins an uncertain interest in the opposite sex with frequent retreats to the same sex peer group.

Adolescence is a state of rapid growth: physical, psychological, intellectual and emotional. The adolescent experiments sexually to gain satisfaction, starts masturbating, and increases heterosexual contacts. Adulthood is characterised by the ability to establish and maintain social and sexual relationships.

Disabled children are born into a sheltered environment. Often their sexual nature is denied by parents from their earliest years. As they grow up, they become aware of sexuality in many of the ways able-bodied children do: through TV, cinemas, gossip and magazines. But unlike able-bodied children, their social activity is closely supervised. Due to limitations of mobility, access to social functions and opportunity to mix with peers is hindered. Sexual expressions of behaviour are often discouraged, and psychosexual development can become distorted because of the attitudes of other people.

Able-bodied children gradually acquire ownership and respect for their bodies. When they are small, body care is in control of the mother, who hands it over slowly as their children grow up. Various parts are handed over at different times, the genitals being among the last to be the responsibility of the youngster.

Disabled children may never be allowed to 'own' or be responsible for even the non-sexual parts of their bodies—one more area of difficulty in relating to themselves and to their sexuality (Craft and Craft 1978).

These are the first stages in the denial of sexuality by the parents, which usually continues throughout adolescence.

Parent/adolescent relationship

Physically disabled adolescents are so dependent on their parents that it is very difficult for them to express disapproval, and their lack of social experience means that they become more dependent on parents for friendship.

Young people may feel trapped within the family: they know that they have to be 'looked after', and must therefore be ready with a smile of gratitude. They are afraid that if they express disapproval, they may be rejected by parents and others. So they remain nice enough to ensure the continuation of love and care. They know that it would be cruel to be anything but thankful to their parents, though at the same time they may be bursting with pent-up feelings of anger and frustration, which often come to a head during the teenage years.

Another factor within this parent/adolescent relationship is the difficulty experienced by young people in learning how to (or being allowed to) make choices and decisions for themselves. This skill may be no more involved than choosing what to wear, buying clothes, deciding which cinema to go to, or whether to do homework or meet a friend. But these are all fundamental decisions we have to make as we grow up and learn to relate to others and act responsibly. Young disabled people, who have these decisions made for them, or do not have the chance to face the situations that produce them, are doubly handicapped. Young people who rely on parents for all their personal care and decision-making will find it difficult to develop emotionally and sexually.

It is often difficult for parents to accept that their able-bodied adolescents are having a sexual relationship. For some the thought of their disabled child being involved in a sexual relationship is too much to bear. It seems to be the last major hurdle to be faced in the life of their child, for which parents seem ill prepared.

Parents are helped with the physical problems of caring for a disabled child, but rarely are they helped to cope with the emerging sexuality of a child and issues such as menstruation and sex education.

They may find it difficult to think of their disabled child being a sexual partner. They may fear that the adolescent will always be rejected sexually, and may therefore try to protect rather than encourage risk-taking. Subconsciously, parents may feel that their adolescent would be better off without sex education or a sexual relationship.

Most parents want their disabled child to have as normal a life as possible, but often they themselves will have no idea about the effect of disability on sexual function, and may be too embarrassed to talk about the subject, and be unsure of where to go for help or advice. That is why it is so important for professionals involved with the family to raise the subject at some time. Often all that parents need is 'permission' to look upon their disabled child as a sexual being, and a suggestion of where to go for advice.

Friendships and social integration

Most disabled teenagers want to have friends, and often report having close or 'best' friends. However, relationships which a socially active able-bodied teenager would regard as superficial may be inappropriately interpreted by the inexperienced spina bifida adolescent as having much greater importance. Most disabled teenagers do seem to have friends at school. However, lack of contact with friends remains a constant concern for most people with spina bifida. Dorner (1976) found that 40 per cent of spina bifida adolescents had no friends outside school or college.

This effect is possibly greater in Britain than in some countries, because a large proportion of children with spina bifida attend special schools which distance children from neighbourhood peer groups. In addition catchment areas of the special schools are often so large that school friends can live very great distances from each other, limiting contact outside school. Disabled teenagers do not have the finance, independence of movement or social skills to exploit the possibilities open to able-bodied teenagers. Without doubt they miss out on socialising and interacting with their peers.

Anderson and Clarke (1982) found that many adolescents with a disability were worried about the reaction of a boyfriend or girlfriend to their disability. Over one third were worried about explaining the visible aspects of their disability, but the main worry was that this would make them unattractive and that they would never find a boyfriend or girlfriend. This is not an unrealistic worry, as it is well known in the field of social psychology that attraction between individuals is based on perception of similarity of attitudes and physical attributes. Success occurs when people aspire to achieve relationships within a group of others who are likely to share those perceptions (Duck 1977). Thus able-bodied adolescents may find the disabled too dissimilar to choose them initially as potential partners, while physically disabled youngsters often express a preference for able-bodied peers as ideal partners. Efforts have to be made by parents and professionals to encourage young people to make contact with a suitable range of peers, and to pursue some form of social activity outside the home, which should include contact with both disabled and able-bodied peers.

Youngsters rarely have the opportunity to share their anxieties relating to adolescence and sexuality (Dorner 1977), and their distress and dissatisfaction can go unrecognised. Therefore they should be made aware of sources of help and support, and given opportunities for individual and group counselling. It is important that young people have a sound knowledge of their disability and the effect it will have on personal and sexual relationships.

Sex education
The extent of sexual knowledge in neurologically disabled teenagers and adults tends to be limited. In a study of 63 adolescents with spina bifida, only 45 per cent knew how children were conceived (Dorner 1977). Disabled students entering further education colleges were found to have a partial and confused understanding of several subjects including menstruation, intercourse, conception, abortion and sterilisation (Brown 1980). In contrast, knowledge of childbirth was substantially correct. Because of lack of social integration, disabled adolescents are cut off from contemporary sources of education which are so influential for able-bodied teenagers. Disabled teenagers are much more dependent on 'official' sources of information such as teaching (Dorner 1980, Bancroft 1983). The importance of appropriate structured sex education is paramount.

A sex education programme should deal with anatomy, menstruation and reproduction, intercourse, conception, pregnancy and birth, contraception, sexual behaviour (*e.g.* masturbation), the effect of disability on sexual function, genetic counselling, marriage and parenting. When giving sex education to those with spina bifida, it can never be assumed that they understand apparently simple words or phrases (*e.g.* vagina and penis). Often they will say they understand, because they have probably heard the words before, while having little understanding of their meaning. Ignorance about their genitals is common. Often they have never looked or touched, and may be convinced that because they are disabled, their genitals will be abnormal. Whether or not the individual has hydrocephalus, there may be impaired body awareness and proprioception (*i.e.* awareness of the position of the body in space), which will affect understanding. Factual information needs to be repeated frequently, bearing in mind the possibility of short concentration span and short-term memory difficulty. If possible, literature and videos should be made available to every disabled child for home reference.

Sex education should be presented in the context of family life, of loving relationships and respect for others. It should be part of a programme of personal and social development. Emphasis should be on the development of relationships, distinguishing family from friends, friends from strangers, and the awareness of what sort of bodily contact is considered acceptable. This is particularly important with disabled children as they are a vulnerable group, and at risk of being sexually exploited by parents or carers (Evans and McKinlay 1989).

Masturbation

Many people still do not talk about masturbation easily. Some professionals working in residential establishments, schools and day centres may have come across the problem of the disabled person masturbating in public. How this is dealt with depends on personal feelings about masturbation. It should be recognised that masturbation in private is a totally normal adolescent activity. In addition, sexual frustration in the disabled is frequently underestimated; masturbation may be the only way of releasing such frustrations. While some staff may feel very strongly that masturbation is wrong and harmful, and may overreact, others may just turn a blind eye. If possible, staff should be encouraged to discuss it with the person, and teach them that there is a time and place for such activity.

Homosexuality

The sexual preference of a man or woman should be their personal choice. However, the subject of homosexuality is still controversial. As in any other section of the population, there will be disabled people who are homosexual. A disabled person is already in a minority group, and one can see only too clearly the dilemma of being disabled and homosexual.

Menstruation

Some girls with spina bifida can begin menstruation early, at seven or eight years old (De Luca *et al.* 1985). They must be prepared for this event in a sensitive and caring way, and the young girl can be helped to see this as a normal state of development, rather than another difference between herself and her peers. The early onset of puberty in either sex may be related to past or present hydrocephalus, and puberty (including menstruation) can be delayed by hormonal treatment, which is free of harmful side-effects (see Chapter 12).

Genetic counselling

The risk of an individual with spina bifida parenting a baby with spina bifida is approximately one in 25. If both parents have spina bifida, the risk increases to about one in 10.

Genetic counselling involves giving factual information about genetics, particularly the risks involved and the tests available. People have the opportunity to talk over their anxieties connected with having disabled children and about terminating a pregnancy. In the UK there are regional clinical genetics departments throughout the country. Referrals to such centres are often made by a family practitioner.

The role of the professional

As important as sex education for the adolescent is having respect for one's body. This can be lacking in children with spina bifida, who often have little idea of modesty or privacy. This may be maintained by the attitude of their medical attendants and carers. Professionals frequently have difficulty seeing the disabled as real people, and their treatment of individuals too often concentrates exclusively on the body, and does not recognise the importance of developing the mind and personality. Moreover professionals are in some ways also responsible for the development of the sexuality of the disabled person. During a physical examination, this is often not taken into consideration. The lack of respect for an individual's privacy and dignity does nothing to help disabled people develop worthwhile attitudes toward themselves. Instead it encourages them to think of themselves as objects that nobody respects, rather than as people. This is unhealthy and damaging to self-esteem.

A great deal of damage to personality development is done when professionals talk down to disabled young people, who have an equal right to information about themselves as the parents (Ayrault 1981).

Sex and sexuality are difficult to deal with in many contexts, and understand-ably many professionals take the easy way out and ignore the subject. This may reflect their own problems with attitudes towards sex and disability. It prevents them from giving appropriate advice and support to young people, and effectively denies them their sexuality.

Attitudes to sex depend on parental upbringing, sex education and personal sexual experience. Staff training is essential if professionals are to overcome their own biases and to respond positively to the sexual needs of young people. Recently there have been increasing opportunities for this, with conferences and workshops addressing the issue of disability and sexuality. Training should deal with (i) how attitudes are formed and how they can be changed, (ii) ways of helping staff feel more comfortable and confident in discussing sexuality and sex, and (iii) adequate training to ensure that teachers in particular are better equipped to give appropriate sex education.

The effect of disability on sexual function
Spina bifida usually does not limit a female's fertility. Even though there may be a lack of genital sensation, sexual function is not affected. It may be necessary to use an additional lubricant when attempting intercourse, as vaginal lubrication is lessened or absent with lower cord level involvement. Orgasm following clitoral stimulation may not be possible, although it has been known for some females with paralysis from waist level to be aware of a very sensitive spot in or around the vagina. New erogenous zones such as lips, ear-lobes, breasts, nipples and armpits can be discovered and developed. A number of females can experience orgasm which, in terms of physical reactions, strongly resembles the experience of a healthy able-bodied female (Cole 1975).

The male with spina bifida is often unable to attain an erection. This is dependent on the level of the lesion. If the spina bifida is in the thoracic or lumbar cord, psychogenic erections are very unlikely. In turn, this varies according to the severity of the spina bifida male. Ejaculation is possible, but unlikely, for the lower thoracic spina bifida. If it does occur, it will probably be retrograde. Lower thoracic and lumbar spina bifida will usually inhibit both psychogenic and reflexogenic erections. Ejaculation is most often experienced by persons with sacral level spina bifida. There is some evidence to suggest that fertility in these males is unlikely (Sloan 1991).

If impotence is a problem it is necessary to establish whether the cause is physical or psychological. A simple test can be carried out to discover if the male attains erections during sleep. This involves wrapping a strip of paper round the shaft of the penis before sleep, fixing the ends with a postage stamp. An erection during sleep will break the stamp. The erectometer (Bard Ltd, Sunderland, UK) is a commercially produced version of this device. If there are erections during sleep, it can be assumed that the problem is psychological and may be helped by counselling. Psychological causes of impotence are experienced by the able-bodied as well as the disabled, but even if the cause is physical, psychosexual counselling may be of great help to the man in coming to terms with his limitations, so that limited function does not become dysfunction. He may need advice on how to satisfy a partner if intercourse is not possible, and how to obtain stimulation if his genital area is not sensitive. He may well benefit from the advice of an experienced urologist to discuss aids, prostheses, and medical treatment which may enable erection.

Physical methods of treatment

The PIPE technique (Papavarine induced penile erection), which has been widely used for some years, consists of an injection into the penis which produces an erection. This can be self administered. However there are complications, including the possibility of erection lasting several hours, which may necessitate hospital treatment.

Prostheses

INTERNAL

A prosthesis consisting of flexible rods to stiffen the penis can be surgically implanted in the corpora cavernosa. Several different types of rod are available. The simplest consist of plastic which bends at the base so the penis can be pointed downwards for convenience. However, the penis remains at its erect length which can be a disadvantage. A more elaborate inflatable rod is available, with a small pump which is implanted in the scrotum and is pumped up and released at the press of a button. The advantage is that the penis increases in girth as well as becoming erect, but remains more or less at its erect length after deflation.

EXTERNAL

The Correctaid (Genesis Medical) is a custom-fitted penile sheath made from thick rubber; erection is effected by vacuum. ErecAid (Cory Bros) also employs a

208

vacuum, and a silicon rubber ring is placed over the base of the penis after engorgement.

Positions
If sexual intercourse is possible it may be necessary to try several different positions to find one which is comfortable and pain-free. Often it is not possible for the man to lie on top of the woman, but either partner can take a more active role depending on their strength and mobility. Sometimes women with spina bifida have difficulty in separating their thighs sufficiently. By placing a firm cushion or pillow below her hips, and perhaps another between her legs, her body may be held in a position in which this problem is overcome. It must be stressed to the individual that intercourse is not the only way to achieve satisfaction for either partner, and counselling in other techniques should be available.

Incontinence and sex
Indwelling catheters do not have to be removed before intercourse. The man simply bends his catheter over the erect penis, or keeps it in place with tape or a sheath. However, a more satisfactory solution is to teach the man to remove and reinsert his catheter.

A woman's catheter does not interfere with intercourse, but again she can be taught to remove and reinsert her catheter.

If intermittent catheterisation is used, the bladder can be emptied before sex. A penile appliance can simply be removed before sexual intercourse. People may worry, however, that urine may escape during intercourse, and this issue needs to be discussed. Ostomy bags should ideally fit well with no leaks, but it is important to ensure that there is no odour. Bags should be emptied before intercourse, and can be covered with suitable material if desired.

It is advisable to ensure that the bowel is as empty as possible before intercourse, using an enema, suppository or manual evacuation if necessary.

Some people with spina bifida may not be able to achieve full intercourse. They must be counselled that satisfaction is not reliant on orgasm, but can be the result of good communication and shared intimacy in whatever way is pleasing to both partners.

Marriage
Most parents look forward to a time when their children will be married and possibly have children of their own. The situation may be very different for the parents of a disabled child. In this context, 'child' is the operative word: many parents still talk about a 30- or 40-year-old son or daughter as a child, and continue to treat them as such. While the child is still very young, parents need to be encouraged to believe that separation will be possible, and that they need not be afraid of permanent and never-ending care (Greengross 1980).

More and more young people with spina bifida are living independently or in sheltered accommodation; many are married and have had children. The ultimate goal for most couples in love is marriage, and this is equally true for the disabled.

Being a parent
If one or both parents are disabled, baby care will present them with many practical problems. Most problems can be overcome, however, sometimes with varying degrees of support from the social services and other agencies.

Counselling
It is necessary for doctors and other professionals seeing parents and child to enquire whether there are any problems or anxieties about sexual matters. Few parents or children will ask for help initially, but may be able to in the future.

Many professionals seem afraid of raising the subject of sexuality as they deem themselves unable to give expert advice. They should be aware of suitable agencies which can offer such counselling, and of the referral procedure.

A programme of counselling should be established by people who have:
(1) experience of sex education and counselling of able-bodied teenagers
(2) detailed knowledge of the nature of spina bifida
(3) specific genetic counselling skills
(4) awareness of the psychological aspects of physical disability during adolescence, and
(5) information about, or can provide, group and/or individual counselling (Dorner 1977).

In England and Wales the Association for Spina Bifida and Hydrocephalus (ASBAH), like similar organisations in other countries, has for many years been aware of the emotional difficulties facing adolescents and their parents, particularly in the area of sexuality. Counselling services from such organisations are available to the person with spina bifida and their families. An integral part of this service should be the provision of training courses for professionals, parents and young people on disability and sexuality.

Summary and recommendations
Sexual dysfunction among the disabled is common, and may be related to psychological and emotional factors as well as physical limitations. Such factors may include poor sex education, difficulties in relationships with parents and peers, lack of opportunity for appropriate peer-group interaction, and inadequate advice and counselling from professionals.

Greater research is required to establish the physical and emotional needs of the disabled and to devise sex-education programmes for them and their carers. It has to be recognised that the disabled, like all humans, are sexual beings and have a right to enjoy the same social, emotional, and sexual contact as the able-bodied. This can be achieved with appropriate education, support and counselling.

Parents and professionals need to examine their attitudes to sex and disability.

If a professional feels unable to deal with the subject, a referral should be made to a person with the relevant expertise.

Professionals should discuss with parents the importance of emotional and physical independence and should encourage parents to share their feelings about their child's emerging sexuality. Counselling should be made available to parents, and appropriate sex education and counselling should be routinely available to children and adolescents.

Teachers, care staff and all professionals working with disabled people need specific training in sexuality, sex and disability.

The most important thing is to listen to what the disabled tell us about their sexual needs and feelings. Having listened, it is our responsibility to respond in a sensitive and constructive way. To ignore what we hear is to deny young disabled people a fundamental human need: the right to enjoy love and be loved, and to experience sexual fulfilment.

REFERENCES

Anderson, E.M., Clarke, L. (1982) *Disability in Adolescence*. London: Methuen.
Ayrault, E.W. (1981) *Sex, Love and the Physically Handicapped*. New York: Continuum.
Bancroft, J. (1983) *Human Sexuality and its Problems*. London: Churchill Livingstone.
Brown, H. (1980) 'Sexual knowledge and education of ESN students in centres of further education.' *Sexuality and Disability*, **3**, 215–220.
Cole, T.M. (1975) 'Sexuality and physical disabilities.' *Archives of Sexual Behaviour*, **4**, 389–403.
Craft, M., Craft, A. (1978) 'Psycho-sexual development.' *In Sex and the Mentally Handicapped—A Guide for Parents and Carers*. London, Boston: Routledge and Kegan Paul.
De Luca, F., Muritano, M., Rizzo, G., Pandullo, E., Cardia, E. (1985) 'True precocious puberty: a long-term complication in children with shunted non-tumoral hydrocephalus.' *Helvetica Paediatrica Acta*, **40**, 467–472.
Dorner, S. (1976) 'Adolescents with spina bifida.' *Archives of Disease in Childhood*, **51**, 439–444.
—— (1977) 'Sexual interest and activity in adolescents with spina bifida.' *Journal of Child Psychology and Psychiatry*, **18**, 229.
—— (1980) 'Sexuality and sex education for the handicapped teenager.' *Journal of Maternal and Child Health*, **5**, 356–360.
Duck, S. (Ed.) (1977) *Theory and Practice in Interpersonal Attraction*. London: Academic Press.
Evans, A.L., McKinlay, I.A. (1989) 'Sex education and the severely mentally retarded child.' *Developmental Medicine and Child Neurology*, **31**, 98–103.
Greengross, W. (1980) *Sex and the Handicapped Child*. Rugby: National Marriage Guidance Council (Relate).
Sloan, S.L. (1991) 'Sexual issues in spina bifida.' *Spotlight*, **June**.

INDEX